Atlas of Human Chromosome Heteromorphisms

Atlas of Human Chromosome Heteromorphisms

Edited by

Herman E. Wyandt, PhD, FACMG
Associate Professor of Pathology
Director of Cytogenetics
Center for Human Genetics
Boston University School of Medicine
Boston, Massachusetts, USA

Vijay S. Tonk, PhD, FACMB
Professor of Pediatrics
(with joint appointments in Pathology
and in Obstetrics and Gynecology)
Director of Cytogenetics and Medical
Genetics
Texas Tech University
Health Sciences Center
Lubbock, Texas, USA

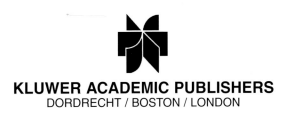

KLUWER ACADEMIC PUBLISHERS
DORDRECHT / BOSTON / LONDON

Library of Congress Cataloging-in-Publication Data

Atlas of human chromosome heteromorphisms / editors, Herman E. Wyandt and Vijay S. Tonk.
   p.; cm.
  Includes index.
  ISBN 1-4020-1303-5 (alk. paper)
   1. Human chromosomes – Atlases. 2. Chromosome polymorphism – Atlases. I. Wyandt,
Herman Edwin, 1939– II. Tonk, Vijay S.
  [DNLM: 1. Chromosomes, Human – Atlases.]

2003051681

ISBN 1-4020-1303-5

Published by Kluwer Academic Publishers,
P.O. Box 17, 3300 AA Dordrecht, The Netherlands

Sold and distributed in North, Central and South America
by Kluwer Academic Publishers,
101 Philip Drive, Norwell, MA 02061, USA

In all other countries, sold and distributed
by Kluwer Academic Publishers, Distribution Center,
P.O. Box 322, 3300 AH Dordrecht, The Netherlands

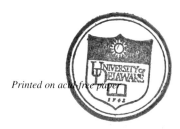
Printed and bound by Emirates Printing Press, Dubai.

DEDICATION

We dedicate this work to our families, to Linda, to Sunita and Sahil, and to Sachi who will not be forgotten.

Contents

CONTENTS

Authors

Mauricio Arcos-Burgos, PhD
Medical Genetics Branch
National Institute of Health NIH
Bethesda, MD, USA

Syed M. Jalal, PhD
Cytogenetics Laboratory
Division of Laboratory Genetics
Department of Laboratory
Medicine and Pathology
Mayo Clinic and Mayo Foundation
Rochester, MN, USA

Rhett P. Ketterling, MD
Division of Laboratory Genetics
Department of Laboratory
Medicine and Pathology
Mayo Clinic and Mayo
Foundation
Rochester, MN, USA

Roger V. Lebo, PhD
Department of Pathology
Children's Hospital Medical Center
of Akron, OH, USA

Brynn Levy, MSc (Med), PhD
Departments of Human Genetics
and Pediatrics
Mount Sinai School of Medicine
New York, NY, USA

R. Ellen Magenis, MD
Department of Molecular and
Medical Genetics and Child
Development and Rehabilitation
Center
Oregon Health Sciences University
Portland, OR, USA

Susan Bennett Olson, PhD
Department of Molecular and
Medical Genetics
Oregon Health Sciences University
Portland, OR, USA

Shivanand R. Patil, PhD
Department of Pediatrics
University of Iowa College of
Medicine
Iowa City, IA, USA

Willmar Patino, PhD
Wilson Genetics Laboratory
Department of Obstetrics and
Gynecology
George Washington University
Medical Center
Washington, DC, USA

Vijay S. Tonk, PhD
Departments of Pediatrics and
Pathology
Texas Tech University Health
Sciences Center
Lubbock, TX, USA

Gopalrao V.N. Velagaleti, PhD
Departments of Pediatrics and
Pathology

University of Texas Medical Branch
Galveston, TX, USA

Peter E. Warburton, PhD
Department of Human Genetics
Mount Sinai School of Medicine
New York, NY, USA

Herman E. Wyandt, PhD
Center for Human Genetics
Boston University School of
Medicine
Boston, MA, USA

Foreword

Critical to the accurate diagnosis of human illness is the need to distinguish clinical features that fall within the normal range from those that do not. That distinction is often challenging and not infrequently requires considerable experience at the bedside. It is not surprising that accurate cytogenetic diagnosis is also often a challenge, especially when chromosome study reveals morphologic findings that raise the question of normality.

Given the realization that modern human cytogenetics is just over five decades old, it is noteworthy that thorough documentation of normal chromosome variation has not yet been accomplished. One key diagnostic consequence of the inability to distinguish a "normal" variation in chromosome structure from a pathologic change is a missed or inaccurate diagnosis.

Clinical cytogeneticists have not, however, been idle. Rather, progressive biotechnological advances coupled with virtual completion of the human genome project have yielded increasingly better microscopic resolution of chromosome structure. Witness the progress from the early short condensed chromosomes to the later visualization of chromosomes through banding techniques, high-resolution analysis in prophase, and more recently to analysis by fluorescent in situ hybridization (FISH).

Pari passu with these advances has been the recognition of normal variation in chromosome morphology with each progressive step in microscopic resolution. Most recently, the advent of analysis by FISH aimed at determination of specific subtelomeric deletions revealed that about 5% of individuals with "idiopathic" mental retardation are accounted for by these submicroscopic telomeric rearrangements. An emerging salutary lesson is that some of the sub-telomeric deletions have been observed in entirely normal subjects, and a number of benign familial variants have been documented. Moreover, we now know that demonstration of a subtelomeric deletion in an individual with unexplained mental retardation should nevertheless be followed by the same studies in both parents, before any diagnostic conclusion or phenotypic association is reached. Whether or not observed microdeletions in normal subjects reflect population variation or are not associated with a particular phenotype simply because of gene dosage effects (e.g., trisomy or monosomy) remain unknown. While telomeric imbalances that are not pathogenic have been described (including from 10q and 17p), a full appreciation, size assessment and categorization, is yet to be accomplished. Careful adherence to strict epidemiologic principles applied to case ascertainment and selection will be necessary to determine definitive associations and delineation of normal variants.

Dr Wyandt and Dr Tonk, in recognizing the need to organize the established data on chromosomal variants, have gathered the important information for this valuable text. Every clinical cytogeneticist engaged in diagnostic or research studies will want to have this reference work in constant reach to assist in the critical distinction between a benign variant and a pathologic chromosomal rearrangement.

AUBREY MILUNSKY, MBBCh, DSc, FRCP, FACMG, DCH

Preface

Standards of care are rapidly changing in clinical cytogenetics. Today's research almost immediately becomes tomorrow's clinical test. What was once unsolvable becomes approachable with new technologies, almost before the overworked clinician or laboratory director may be aware they are available. This book does not provide a panacea for such problems, nor does it try to distinguish between chromosome variants that are clinically significant and those that are not. It does, however, provide the first comprehensive view of perhaps the most neglected regions of the human karyotype – namely, those regions that are the most variable and at the same time can be the most problematic. In almost every case, where striking variants are observed, parental studies are the first order of business, following which new technologies, if available, may be required. There are numerous examples in this volume where this approach has been and should be followed. This volume is intended for those who do cytogenetics daily, as well as for physicians and counselors who must attempt to understand and present sometimes ambiguous results to their patients. A predictable response of the physician, when confronted with a rare or unusual variant that has not been experienced by the cytogeneticist before, is "Well, what do I tell my patient now?"

In fact, this is a work in progress. Often there is not an easy answer to the question. Ultimately, if the specific question cannot be answered, the query becomes "Where is it reasonable to stop?" In prenatal cases, time and the resources at hand may be the constraints. In other cases it is the goal to answer the question as completely as possible to satisfy the need of the individual or family to know or plan what to expect. In such cases there may not be an immediate endpoint. However, there is always the obligation to present the facts and their limitations to the extent these are known. This is the normal process in genetics. The purpose of this volume is to summarize the known facts about regions of the human karyotype, which have not been summarized in one place before.

HERMAN E. WYANDT, PhD
VIJAY S. TONK, PhD,
Editors

Acknowledgements

This is a review of the work of many investigators spanning more than five decades of cytogenetic research. It is not possible to adequately represent the early efforts of investigators such as A. Craig-Holms, J.P Geraedts, P. Jacobs, H Lubs, W. H. MacKenzie, R.E. Magenis, A.V.N. Mikelsaar, H.J. Muller, S. Patil, P. Pearson, M. Shaw, and many others who perceived the need to study heteromorphisms in populations and who attempted to make order of a complicated topic. We have tried to be thorough in our review but, because of the great volume of literature that has accumulated over time, worldwide, we have inevitably made significant omissions. We regret these oversights and anticipate that our colleagues will inform us of the most serious ones. We also acknowledge the contributions to the literature on the topic by the late Ram S. Verma.

For specific examples of common and rare heteromorphisms, we are grateful for the individual contributions from colleagues around the world. These are acknowledged throughout the book and hopefully will encourage additional contributions of a similar nature in future editions. In this regard, we owe special thanks to Lauren Jenkins at Kaiser Permanente Medical Group (San Jose), who provided us with a significant number of examples of chromosome heteromorphisms without which we may never have started. We must also acknowledge the use of archived material from our laboratories. The cytogenetic technologists and technicians who helped in providing additional examples from these sources include: Xin Li Huang (supervisor), Alex Dow, Agen Pan, Zhen Kang, Xiao Wu, Xiuqi Li, Xiaoli Hou, Hong Shao and Yan Li in the Center for Human Genetics at Boston University, and Manju G. Jayawickrama, Caro E. Gibson, Ken L. Futrell, Eun Jung Lee and Amantia S. Kennedy in the Cytogenetics Laboratory at Texas Tech University. Sun Han Shim (cytogenetics fellow, CHG) also provided key examples of FISH variants. For the remainder, we would be remiss if we did not acknowledge the large amount of published material for which we obtained permission to reproduce in this volume.

This project would not have been completed without the support of our respective departments. In this regard, we are grateful to the following individuals in the Department of Pediatrics, Texas Tech University Health Sciences Center in Lubbock, TX: Richard M. Lampe, M.D., Chairman; Surendra K. Varma, M.D., Vice Chairman; John A. Berry, Administrator; Rebecca L. Timmons and Stephanie S. Stephens, Medical Secretaries; and Leandra Gomez, Coordinator. We are similarly grateful to the following individuals in the Center for Human Genetics, Boston University School of Medicine, Boston, MA: Marilyn McPhail,

ACKNOWLEDGEMENTS

Medical Secretary; Judy Heck, Administrator; Aubrey Milunsky, MB.B.Ch., D.Sc., Professor of Human Genetics, Pediatrics, Pathology and Obstetrics & Gynecology and Director of the Center for Human Genetics and Jeff Milunsky, M.D., Associate Professor of Pediatrics, Genetics and Genomics and Associate & Clinical Director of the Center for Human Genetics.

We also owe specials thanks for critical review of the manuscript to: David Morgan, M.D., Associate Professor of Pathology and Pediatrics, Texas Tech University; Shafiq A Khan, Ph.D., Associate Professor, Clinton C. MacDonald, Ph.D., Associate Professor and Simon C. Williams, Ph.D., Associate Professor, Department of Cell Biology and Biochemistry, Texas Tech University; and Golder Wilson, M.D, Professor of Pediatric Genetics, Texas Tech University.

We must also thank Peter Butler and staff at Kluwer Academic Publishers for taking a personal interest in this project and Phil Johnstone and staff at Lancaster Publishing Services Ltd. for remarkable compliance with our suggestions in nearly all aspects of the organization and printing of this volume. Any deficiencies or failings, therefore, are our own.

List of Atlas Contributors

Numbers in parentheses with a "c" prefix represent specific atlas contributions. Some variants that were submitted were not able to be included because of redundancy. Nevertheless, those individuals or institutions are listed, but are not followed by "c" number(s). In other instances, submissions were of published material so that appropriate citations have been made accordingly in the text, figure or plate where used, but have not been given "c" number(s). We encourage continued submission of variants, or useful data, which have not already been included in this volume, for possible inclusion in future editions.

Zamecnikova Adriana (c5, c6)
Department of Genetics
National Cancer Institute
Klenova, Slovakia

Arturo Anguiano, PhD (c17, c29)
Quest Diagnostics Incorporated
San Juan Capistrano, California, USA

Petr Baliček, MD (c16)
Division of Medical Genetics
University Hospital
Kráklové, Czech Republic

Peter A. Benn, PhD (c11)
Division of Human Genetics
University of Connecticut Health Center
Farmington, Connecticut, USA

J.J.M. Engelen, PhD (c40)
Department of Molecular Cell Biology and Genetics
Universiteit Maastricht
The Netherlands

James M. Fink, MD, PhD (c37, c38)
Hennepin County Medical Center
Minneapolis, Minnesota, USA

Center for Human Genetics (c1)
Boston University School of Medicine
Boston, Massachusetts, USA

Cheong Kum Foong (c31, c32)
Cytogenetic Laboratory
Kandang Kerbau Women's and Children's Hospital
Singapore

Cytogenetics Laboratory
Texas Tech Health Sciences Center
Lubbock, Texas, USA

Steven L. Gerson, PhD (c18)
Dianon Systems
Stratford, Connecticut, USA

Patricia N. Howard-Peebles, PhD
Genetics and IVF Institute
Fairfax, Virginia, USA

Lauren Jenkins, PhD (c2)
Kaiser Permanente Medical Group
San Jose, California, USA

James Lespinasse, MD (c10)
Laboratoire de Cytogénétique
Centre Hospitalier
Chambéry cedex, France

Thomas Lynch, MD
Anzac House
Rockhampton Old, Australia

Jim Malone (c39)
Akron Children's Hospital
Akron, Ohio, USA

Patricia M. Miron, PhD
(c7, c8, c9, c33, c34, c35, c36)
Brigham and Women's Hospital
Boston, Massachusetts, USA

Emelie H. Ongcapin, MD (c12)
Department of Pathology
Saint Barnabas Medical Center
Livingston, New Jersey, USA

Sayee Rajangam
Department of Anatomy
St Johns Medical College
Bangalore, India

Birgitte Roland, MD (c30)
Department of Histopathology
Foothill Hospital
University of Calgary, Canada

Jacqueline Schoumans
(c19, c20, c21, c22, c23, c24, c25,
c26, c27, c28)
Department of Medical Genetics
University Hospital Haukeland
Bergen, Norway

Cathy M. Tuck-Miller (c15)
Department of Medical Genetics and
Genetics-Birth Defects Center
University of South Alabama
Mobile, Alabama USA

Sharon L. Wenger, PhD (c3, c4)
Department of Pathology
West Virginia University
Morgantown, West Virginia, USA

K. Yelavarthi, PhD (c13, c14)
Northwest Center for Medical
Education
Gary, Indiana, USA

J. Zunich, PhD (c13, c14)
Northwest Center for Medical
Education
Gary, Indiana, USA

Part I
Review

1
Introduction

HERMAN E. WYANDT

The cornerstone of genetics is variation. No two individuals are alike, nor are their chromosomes. Heteromorphisms represent microscopically visible regions on chromosomes that are variable in size, morphology and staining properties in different individuals. Literally meaning "other or different forms", the term "heteromorphism" is often used interchangeably with the terms "variant" or "polymorphism". Polymorphism, however, is more correctly used in other contexts, implying multiple identifiable forms of a gene or molecule rather than of chromosome morphology. The term "normal variant" is often used, but is less precise. The main distinction is that heteromorphism can be seen under the microscope, whereas a polymorphism or normal variant might not. Because of widespread usage, both "normal variant" and "heteromorphism" are used interchangeably in this book. Heteromorphisms are typically stable, inherited and, by definition, every individual carries at least one form, if not two, for every heteromorphic region on their chromosomes.

Variations in morphology in certain regions of the human genome were noted even before the advent of chromosome banding techniques. In the first Conference on Standardization in Human Cytogenetics in Denver in 1960 [1], chromosomes were divided into Groups A–G based on their relative sizes and positions of the centromeres. The X chromosome fell somewhere in the C group. The Y was distinguished from the G group by its lack of satellites and somewhat distinctive morphology. It was already evident, however, that there was considerable variation in the size of the Y chromosome. By 1963, at the London Conference [2], it was apparent that chromosome 1 in the A group had a secondary

---

*The genetic definition of "polymorphism" is "an identifiable variant form of a molecule or gene that occurs in at least 1% of the population". Variant forms occurring with a lesser frequency are more correctly referred to as mutations. Since heteromorphisms typically represent a continuum, it is often difficult to determine whether or not a particular form in one individual is the same as a similar-appearing form in an unrelated individual. Therefore, frequencies are not precise. For that reason we will avoid the use of the term "polymorphism" in referring to the morphological variants of chromosomes observed under the microscope.

constriction near the centromere as did one pair of chromosomes in the C group (chromosome 9) and one pair (no. 16) in the E group. At the Chicago Conference in 1966 [3], it was generally recognized that there were morphological variations in the short arms of the D- and G-group chromosomes, in the long arm of chromosome 16 and in the long arm of the Y. Although heteromorphisms had been reported in chromosomes 1 and 9 [4–6], it was unclear whether or not clinical abnormalities might be associated [8,9]. It was not until large consecutive newborn studies [10–17] that it became evident that most such variations were probably normal.

In 1968 Donahue et al. [18] mapped the first gene (the Duffy blood group) to an autosome using a large secondary constriction on chromosome 1 as a marker, soon to be followed by mapping of Rh, phosphoglucomutase and amylase to chromosome 1 by linkage. Individual pedigrees in which heteromorphisms have been traced usually do not extend back in time more than a few generations. One of the oldest traceable heteromorphisms, however, is a satellited Y chromosome in a French-Canadian family that by inference could be traced back to its origin, 11 generations or 315 years [19–21].

Despite the fact they are heritable and everyone carries them, the frequency of any specific heteromorphism is often unknown. The largest population studies [10–15] were done on unbanded chromosomes in which only certain types of heteromorphisms were detectable. In 1970–71, chromosome banding techniques became widely used. Q- and C-banding techniques, especially, revealed a much greater variety of heteromorphisms on chromosomes 1, 3, 4, 9, 13–16, 21, 22 and the Y than had previously been suspected [22–24]. Most studies assumed that these heteromorphisms behaved like Mendelian traits, although some suggested there was non-inherited variation between parents and children in a few isolated cases [8,25–28]. Family studies carried out collaboratively in Indiana and Oregon by Magenis et al. [29] revealed Mendelian segregation of a variety of variants of chromosome 1 in 42 two- to four-generation families, with no evidence of discrepancies in the size and nature of variants between parents and children.

Several good-size studies attempted to assess the frequencies of Q- and C-band variants in normal populations [30–34]. Biases in selection as well as technical factors and different methods of scoring have made direct comparisons between these studies difficult. Perhaps the best-designed studies were those of Lubs and colleagues [35,36] that classified C- and G-band variants by size and intensity. C-band size was divided into five levels compared to the size of the non-variant 16p. Q-band variants were divided into five levels of intensity, compared to intensities of selected non-variant regions (see Chapter 3).

Population studies, using different banding techniques, have revealed significant differences in frequencies of some heteromorphisms in different ethnic groups (Chapter 3). Numerous smaller studies of selected populations have associated certain striking heteromorphisms with mental retardation, infertility, increased abortion rate or susceptibility to cancer. Because of the difficulties in study design, however, the outcomes of these studies are often controversial and contradictory. Chapter 4 in this volume deals with the studies in some of these areas.

Chromosomal heteromorphisms also reflect the evolution of the eukaryotic genome. Brightly fluorescent variants, detectable by Q-banding, seem to be of relatively recent origin evolutionarily, showing up only in chimpanzee, gorilla and humans, with only the last two having a brightly fluorescent Yqh [37]. Early molecular studies showed C-band heteromorphism to be composed of different fractions of satellite DNA based on their differing GC content and buoyant densities in CsCl or Cs_2SO_4 gradients [38–43]. Until their study by more refined molecular techniques in the last decade [44–47], however, it was not possible to truly characterize and trace the molecular origins of most heteromorphisms. Such studies are still ongoing. Chapter 8 reveals the results of molecular dissection of at least some classes of repeated sequences, especially the alpha satellite DNAs, in heteromorphic regions, and Chapter 9 gives a detailed description of how information concerning the rates of mutation and evolution of alpha satellite sequences can be extracted from the human genome database [48,49].

The heritability of heteromorphisms has been applied in a variety of ways, ranging from making a simple determination of parental origin of a particular chromosome to detecting maternal contamination in prenatal samples [50] or determining paternity and non-paternity [51–54]. Numerous studies have used heteromorphisms to determine, with surprising accuracy, the mechanisms and parental origins of various aneuploidies [55–57], triploidies [58] and certain structural chromosome imbalances. Chapter 5 includes sections on the use of heteromorphisms in the determination of paternity, maternity or identity of twins and of the meiotic and parental origin of trisomies and other chromosome abnormalities. Because these techniques have now been largely outdated by molecular technologies [59–62], they may seem more of historical than practical interest. However, for the laboratory or researcher who does not always have immediate access to such advanced technologies, application of simple inexpensive chromosome banding techniques can still provide immediate answers.

Chapter 6 in this volume discusses a class of variants that does not fit in with the usual perception of heteromorphism. These involve so-called "euchromatic" regions that are not generally perceived to be variable in size or staining because they presumably contain genetic material. Examples of such variants are rare and some are detectable only by newer molecular technologies. In some cases they may not be variants at all, but may have hidden phenotypic consequences that are not immediately evident until more observations of an identical kind are reported.

The variety of classical techniques for studying human chromosomes has gradually added to the number of potentially detectable heteromorphisms. These techniques are discussed in detail in Chapter 2 and include Q-, G-, R-, C- and G-11 banding, a variety of fluorochromes or combinations of fluorochromes which mimic or reproduce results from the banding techniques mentioned above, and silver staining for nucleolar organizing regions (NOR staining). However, in the late 1980s and early 1990s, molecular and "fluorescence in situ hybridization" (FISH) techniques allowed virtually any DNA sequence to be physically localized to one or more specific chromosomal sites. Chapter 7 outlines some of the current and more widely used FISH techniques for detecting and diagnosing subtle chromosome abnormalities and their origins. The FISH technologies have the potential of characterizing heteromorphisms detected by classical techniques with greater accuracy and precision. This has not been done on any large scale. In fact, only a handful of what might be termed "FISH variants" have been reported [63,64]. Therefore, although we have included a section especially for

FISH, this inclusion is mainly with the anticipation that new variants will be added as time goes on. Some variants that are reported in Chapter 6 and in the FISH section are not definitively determined to be normal variants. There may, in fact, be other genetic factors such as imprinting or uniparental disomy that influence whether these rare or newly found variants are normal or not.

With each new technique come the crucial questions. What, if any, is the clinical relevance of the variable regions detected? Do certain regions that demonstrate particularly striking heteromorphism have any function or do they simply represent "junk" DNA? Are they associated with increased infertility, rates of pregnancy loss, congenital abnormalities or risks for cancer? For many of the variants in this book these questions are still relevant. Large satellites, double satellites, double or triple NORs or observations of increased rates of satellite association have not been convincingly demonstrated to result in increased risk for non-disjunction leading to Down syndrome or other acrocentric trisomies (see Chapter 5A). Pericentric inversions of heterochromatin regions have not been associated with large increased risks for miscarriages or chromosomal imbalances in live-born children due to meiotic recombination. Homologs with large discrepancies in size of their heterochromatic regions do not routinely undergo unequal crossing-over in meiosis to yield deletions/duplications that likewise could result in congenital anomalies and/or mental retardation. In fact, it was shown early that such regions appear to suppress crossing over so that there is a lower rate of recombination leading to imbalance than would normally be expected [65]. Nevertheless, as in all complex topics, there are regions or sites very close to the centromeres of some chromosomes that appear to be preferentially involved in chromosome rearrangement, duplication and deletion. Recent molecular studies reveal some of these regions consist of low-copy, intermediate-size repeated sequences of 100–400 kb in length that typically flank the regions showing high rates of duplications and/or deletions [66–69].

Our purpose with the present volume is to present a pictorial record and summary of the known literature and data on the range of variation representing normal human chromosomal heteromorphism, both common and rare, including, and to the extent possible, an assessment of the relative frequencies or identity of populations where specific heteromorphisms may be especially prevalent. We also have attempted to identify those heteromorphisms which for one reason or another may not be totally innocuous but, in fact, either carry some clinical risk or may be confused with a chromosome rearrangement that does carry a significant risk. There are the rare cases of "jumping satellites" [70–72] that appear to contradict the more frequent observation of the stability of most chromosome heteromorphisms. Inversions in chromosome 9 that have breakpoints just outside the heterochromatic secondary constriction may occasionally be difficult to distinguish from the more typically harmless 9qh inversion seen in as many as 5% of the population [73–76]. Large bright short arms on a chromosome 15, 22 or other autosome might occasionally be a translocation with a Y chromosome. Such translocations can carry genes that place female carriers at risk for gonadoblastoma or male carriers at risk for infertility or prostate cancer [77,78], but the majority appear to have no demonstrable phenotypic effect. The increased degree of accuracy offered by molecular characterization and in situ hybridization can help to answer some of these questions more definitively, at least in individual cases.

INTRODUCTION

The study of heteromorphisms is an ongoing and dynamic process involving changing technologies by which new heteromorphisms are continually being defined as molecular characterization of the human genome progresses. We hope that this volume will provide a vehicle in which new heteromorphisms can be systematically added, and that it will eventually become an indispensable resource for professionals who must daily make determinations of the clinical significance of chromosomal variants in the patients they serve. We hope this also becomes a resource for the researcher who is involved in the study of the structure and function of the human genome as well, because we firmly believe that, as with all biological diversity, even the most apparently unobtrusive structural variation, whether observed in the whole animal or at the chromosome or DNA level, becomes fixed in a population because of some evolutionary advantage. Newer variations that have not become fixed or are more transient may have more unpredictable consequences.

References

1. Denver Conference (1960). A proposed standard system of nomenclature of human mitotic chromosomes. Lancet. i:1063–1065 (1960); reprinted in Chicago Conference (1966), pp. 12–15.
2. London Conference on the Normal Human Karyotype (1963). Cytogenetics. 2:264–268 (1963); reprinted in Chicago Conference (1966), pp. 18–19.
3. Chicago Conference (1966). Standardization in human cytogenetics. Birth Defects: Original Article Series, Vol. 2, No. 2. New York: National Foundation, 1966.
4. Cooper HL, Hernits R (1963). A familial chromosome variant in a subject with anomalous sex differentiation. Am J Hum Genet. 15:465–75.
5. Yunis JJ, Gorlin RJ (1963). Chromosomal study of patients with cysts of the jaw, multiple nevoid basal cell carcinomata and bifid rib syndrome. Chromosoma. 14:146–53.
6. Hakansson L (1966). A case of Werdnig–Hoffman muscular dystrophy with an unusual chromosome complement. Hereditas Genetiskt Archiv. 55:358–61.
7. Moores EC, Anders JM, Emanuel R (1966). Inheritance of marker chromosomes from cytogenetic survey of congenital heart disease. Ann Human Genet. 30:77–84
8. Palmer CG, Schroder J (1971). A familial variant of chromosome 9. J Med Genet. 8:202–8.
9. Lobitz JR, McCaw BK, Hecht F (1972). Giemsa banding pattern of a heritable 1qh+ variant chromosome: a possible partial duplication. J Med Genet. 9: 276–9.
10. Jacobs PA, Melville M, Ratcliffe S, Keay AJ, Syme JA (1974). Cytogenetic survey of 11,680 newborn infants. Ann Hum Genet. 37:359–76.
11. Friedrich U, Nielsen J (1973). Chromosome studies in 5,049 consecutive newborn children. Clin Genet. 4:333.
12. Nielsen J, Sillisen I (1975). Incidence of chromosome aberrations among 11148 newborn children. Humangenetik. 30:1–12.
13. Sergovich F, Valentine GH, Chen ATL, Kinch RAH, Snout MD (1969). Chromosome aberrations in 2159 consecutive newborn babies. N Engl J Med. 280:851–5.
14. Hammerton JL, Canning N, Ray M, and Smith S (1975). A cytogenetic survey of 14,069 newborn infants. I. Incidence of chromosome abnormalities. Clin Genet. 8: 223–43.
15. Walzer S, Gerald PS (1977). A chromosome survey of 13,751 male newborns. In: Hook EB, Porter IH, editors. Population Cytogenetics. New York: Academic Press, pp. 45–61.
16. Lubs HA, Ruddle F (1970). Chromosomal abnormalities in the human population: estimation of rates based on New Haven newborn study. Science. 169:495–7.
17. Hook EB, Porter IH (1977). Population Cytogenetics Studies in Humans. New York: Academic Press.
18. Donahue RP, Bias WB, Renwick JH, McKusick VA (1968). Probable assignment of the Duffy blood group locus to chromosome 1 in man. Proc Natl Acad Sci USA. 61:949–55.
19. Genest P (1972). An eleven-generation satellited Y chromosome. Lancet. i:1073.
20. Genest P (1973). Transmission hereditaire, depuis 300 ans, d'un chromosome Y a satellites dans une lignee familiale. Ann Genet (Paris). 21:237–8 [French].

21. Genest P, Genest FB, Gagnon-Blais D (1983). Un remaniement chromosomique inhabituel. Une translocation telomerique autosomique sur un Y a satellites (Yqs) multicentenaire. Ann Genet (Paris). 26:86–90 [French].
22. Paris Conference (1971). Standardization in human cytogenetics. Birth Defects Original Article Series, Vol. 8, No. 7. New York: National Foundation, 1972; also in Cytogenetics. 11:313–62 (1972).
23. Geraedts JPM, Pearson PL (1974). Fluorescent chromosome polymorphisms; frequencies and segregation in a Dutch population. Clin Genet. 6:247–57.
24. Arrighi FE, Hsu TC (1971). Localization of heterochromatin in human chromosomes. Cytogenetics. 10:81–6.
25. Craig-Holmes AP, Shaw MW (1973). Polymorphism of human C-band heterochromatin. Science. 174:702–4.
26. Fitzgerald PH (1973). The nature and inheritance of an elongated secondary constriction on chromosome 9 of man. Cytogenet Cell Genet. 12:404–13.
27. Craig-Holmes AP, Moore FP, Shaw MW (1975). Polymorphism of human C-band heterochromatin II. Family studies with suggestive evidence for somatic crossing over. Am J Hum Genet. 27:178–89.
28. Sekhon GS, Sly WS (1975). Inheritance of Q and C Polymorphisms. Am J Hum Genet 27:79a.
29. Magenis RE, Palmer CG, Wang L et al. (1977). Heritability of chromosome banding variants. In: Hook EB, Porter IH, editors. Population Cytogenetics. Studies in Humans. New York: Academic Press, pp 179–188.
30. Geraedts JPM, Pearson PL (1974). Fluorescent chromosome polymorphisms; frequencies and segregation in a Dutch population. Clin Genet. 6:247–57.
31. Mikelsaar AV, Kaosaar ME, Tuur SJ, Viikmaa MH, Talvik TA, Laats J (1975). Human karyotype polymorphisms. III. Routine and fluorescence microscope investigation of chromosomes in normal adults and mentally retarded children. Humangenetik. 26:1–23.
32. Muller HJ, Klinger HP, Glasser M (1975). Chromosome polymorphism in a human newborn population. II. Potentials of polymorphic chromosome variants for characterizing the ideogram of an individual. Cytogenet Cell Genet. 15:239–55.
33. Muller HJ, Klinger HP (1975). Chromosome polymorphism in a human newborn population. In: Pearson PL, Lewis KR, editors. Chromosomes Today, Vol. 5. Jerusalem: John Wiley.
34. Lin CC, Gideon MM, Griffith P et al. (1976). Chromosome analysis on 930 consecutive newborn children using quinacrine fluorescent banding technique. Hum Genet. 31:315–28.
35. McKenzie WH, Lubs HA (1975). Human Q and C chromosomal variations: distribution and incidence. Cytogenet Cell Genet. 14:97–115.
36. Lubs HA, Patil SR, Kimberling WJ et al. (1977). Q and C-banding polymorphisms in 7 and 8 year old children: Racial differences and clinical significance: In: Hook E, Porter H, editors. Population Cytogenetic Studies in Humans. New York: Academic Press, pp. 133–59.
37. Pearson P (1973). The uniqueness of the human karyotype. In: Caspersson T, Zech L, editors. Chromosome Identification – Technique and Application in Biology and Medicine. Nobel Symposium. Medicine and Natural Sciences. New York: Academic Press, pp. 145–51.
38. Jones KW, Corneo G (1971). Location of satellite and homogeneous DNA sequences on human chromosomes. Nature (Lond.) New Biol. 233:268–71.
39. Jones KW, Prosser J, Corneo G, Ginelli E (1973). The chromosomal localisation of human satellite DNA III. Chromosoma. 42:445–51.
40. Jones KW, Purdom IF, Prosser J, Corneo G (1974). The chromosomal localisation of human satellite DNA I. Chromosoma. 49:161–71.
41. Gosden JR, Mitchell AR, Buckland RA, Clayton RP, Evans HJ (1975). The location of four human satellite DNAs on human chromosomes. Exp Cell Res. 92:148–58.
42. Ginelli E, Corneo G (1976). The organization of repeated DNA sequences in the human genome. Chromosoma. 56:55–68.
43. Miklos GLG, John B (1979). Heterochromatin and satellite DNA in man: properties and prospects. Am J Hum Genet. 31:264–80.
44. Marcais B et al. (1991). On the mode of evolution of alpha satellite DNA in human populations. J Mol Evol. 33:42–8.
45. Warburton PE, Haaf T, Gosden J, Lawson D, Willard HF (1996). Characterization of a chromosome-specific chimpanzee alpha satellite subset: evolutionary relationship to subsets on human chromosomes. Genomics. 33(2):220–8.
46. Willard HF (1991). Evolution of alpha satellite. Curr Opin Genet Dev. 1:509–14.

47. Meyer E, Wiegand P, Rand SP, Kuhlmann D, Brack M, Brinkmann B (1995). Microsatellite polymorphisms reveal phylogenetic relationships in primates. J Mol Evol. 41:10–14.
48. Pennisi E (2000). Human genome. Finally, the book of life and instructions for navigating it. Science. 288:2304–7.
49. Macilwain C (2000). World leaders heap praise on human genome landmark. Nature. 405:983–4.
50. Olson S, Buckmaster J, Bissonnette J, Magenis E (1987). Comparison of maternal and fetal chromosome heteromorphisms to monitor maternal cell contamination in chorionic villus samples. Prenat Diagn. 7:413–17.
51. Hauge M, Poulsen H, Halberg A, Mikkelsen M (1975). The value of fluorescence markers in the distinction between maternal and fetal chromosomes. Humangenetik. 26:187–91.
52. Olson SB, Magenis RE, Rowe SI, Lovrien EW (1983). Chromosome heteromorphism analysis in cases of disputed paternity. Am J Med Genet. 15:47–55.
53. Olson SB, Magenis RE, and Lovrien EW (1986). Human chromosome variation: the discriminatory power of Q-band heteromorphism (variant) analysis in distinguishing between individuals, with specific application to cases of questionable paternity. Am J Hum Genet. 38:235–52.
54. Gürtler H, Niebuhr E (1981). The use of chromosome variants in paternity cases. In: 9. Internatianale Tagung der Gesellschaft fur forensisch Blutgruppenkund, Bern: Wurzburg, Schmitt & Meyer, pp. 597–601.
55. Magenis RE, Overton KM, Chamberlin J, Brady T, Lovrien E (1977). Prenatal origin of the extra chromosome in Down's syndrome. Hum Genet. 37:7–16.
56. Juberg RC, Mowrey PN (1983). Origin of nondisjunction in trisomy 21 syndrome: all studies compiled, parental age analysis, and internal comparisons. Am J Med Genet. 16:111–16.
57. Mikkelsen M, Poulsen H, Grinsted J, Lange A (1980). Non-disjunction in trisomy 21: study of chromosomal heteromorphisms in 110 families. Ann Hum Genet. 44:17–28.
58. Jacobs PA, Szulman AE, Funkhouser J, Matsuura JS, Wilson CC (1982). Human triploidy: relationship between parental origin of the additional haploid complement and development of partial hydatidiform mole. Ann Hum Genet. 46:223–31.
59. Lorber BJ, Grantham M, Peters J, Willard HF, Hassold TJ (1992). Nondisjunction of chromosome 21: comparisons of cytogenetic and molecular studies of meiotic stage and parent of origin. Am J Hum Genet. 51:1265–76.
60. Redline RW, Hassold T, Zaragoza MV (1998). Prevalences of partial molar phenotype in triploidy of maternal and paternal origin. Hum Pathol. 29:505–11.
61. Zaragoza MV, Surti U, Redline RW, Millie E, Chakravarti A, Hassold TJ (2000). Parental origin and phenotype of triploidy in spontaneous abortions: predominance of diandry and association with the partial hydatidiform mole. Am J Hum Genet. 66:1807–20.
62. Hopman AHN, Raap AK, Landegent JE, Wiegant J, Boerman RH, Van der Ploeg M (1988). Non-radioactive in situ hybridization. In: Molecular Neuroanatomy. Amsterdam: Elvesier, editor. pp. 43–68.
63. Stergianou K, Gould CP, Walters JJ, Hulten MA (1993). A DA/DAPI positive human 14p heteromorphism defined by in situ hybridization using chromosome 15-specific probes D15Z1 (satellite III) and p-TRA-25 (alphoid). Hereditas. 119: 105–10.
64. Ballif BC, Kashork CD, Shaffer LG (2000). The promise and pitfalls of telomere region-specific probes. Am J Hum Genet. 67:1356–9.
65. Jacobs PA (1977). Human chromosome heteromorphisms (variants). Progr Med Genet. 2:251–74.
66. Mazzarella R, Schlessinger D (1998). Pathological consequences of duplications in the human genome. Genome Res. 8:1007–21.
67. Lupski JR (1998). Genomic disorders: structural features of the genome can lead to DNA rearrangements and human disease traits. Trends Genet. 14:417–22.
68. Ji Y, Eichler EE, Schwartz S, Nicholls RD (2000). Structure of chromosome duplicons and their role in mediating human genomic disorders. Genome Res. 10:597–610.
69. Emanuel BS, Shaikh TH (2001). Segmental duplications: an expanding role in genomic instability and disease. Nature Rev. 2:791–800.
70. Farrel SA, Winsor EJT, Markovik VD (1993). Moving satellites and unstable chromosome translocations. Am J Med Genet. 46:715–20.
71. Gimelli G, Porro E, Santi F, Scappaticci S, Zuffardi O (1976). "Jumping" satellites in three generations: a warning for paternity tests and prenatal diagnosis. Hum Genet. 34:315–18.
72. Livingston GK, Lockey JE, Witt KS, Rogers SW (1985). An unstable giant satellite associated with chromosomes 21 and 22 in the same individual. Am J Hum Genet. 37:553–60.

73. Howard-Peebles PN, Stoddard GR (1979). Pericentric inversions of chromosome number 9: Benign or harmful? Hum Hered. 29:111–17.
74. Luke S, Verma RS (1993). Genetic consequences of euchromatic band within 9qh region. Am J Med Genet. 45:107.
75. Samonte RV, Conte RA, Ramesh KH, Verma RS (1996). Molecular cytogenetic characterization of breakpoints involving pericentric inversions of human chromosome 9. Hum Genet. 98:576–80.
76. Ramesh KH, Verma RS (1996). Breakpoints in alpha, beta and satellite III DNA sequences of chromosome 9 result in a variety of pericentric inversions. J Med Genet. 33:395–8.
77. Lau, YF (1999). Gonadoblastoma, testicular and prostrate cancers and the TSPY gene. Am J Hum Genet. 64:921–27.
78. Lau Y, Chou P, Iezzoni J, Alonzo J, Komuves L (2000). Expression of a candidate gene for the gonadoblastoma locus in gonadoblastoma and testicular seminoma. Cytogenet Cell Genet. 91:160–4.

2
Methods of Studying Human Chromosomes and Nomenclature. The Normal Human Karyotype

GOPALRAO V.N. VELAGALETI AND VIJAY S. TONK

Ever since the elucidation of the correct human chromosome number (2n = 46) by Tijo and Levan [1], clinical cytogenetics has become an important branch of medical genetics. It was natural that this epoch-making discovery was soon followed by discovery of various numerical chromosomal abnormalities such as trisomy 21 [2], trisomy 13 [3], trisomy 18 [4] and sex chromosome abnormalities that included monosomy X [5], XXY [6] and XXX [7]. Several of these important observations were followed by breakthroughs in the technological aspects of cell cultures, which had been a stumbling block in routinely studying human chromosomes. Two independent investigators, Nowell [8] and Moorehead *et al.* [9], described a simple method of cell culture to study human chromosomes, thus paving the way for the clinical cytogenetics revolution.

2.1 BASIC MORPHOLOGY

Each human chromosome consists of two arms joined by a "centromere". The two arms are termed p for the usually shorter arm and q for the longer arm. Centromeres are essential structures where the mitotic spindles attach during cell division. The centromere is a complex structure with mostly repetitive DNA that is associated with a trilaminar plate structure called the "kinetochore". Microtubules attach to the kinetochore and help in directing the chromosome movements along the spindle [10]. While the kinetochore structure and many centromere proteins that are essential for the spindle fiber attachment are conserved during evolution, the centromeric DNA sequences are not conserved among the eukarotyic organisms. In humans the centromeric DNA consists of large blocks of middle-repetitive DNA known as alpha satellite DNA that is AT (adenine, thymidine)-rich. These repeats consist of a basic monomeric sequence of 170 bp arranged in a head to tail manner. The total length of centromeric DNA varies from chromosome to chromosome, as does the sequence of the 170 bp monomer between and within the chromosomes [11–13]. Several studies with in situ hybridization, and the discovery of the centromeric protein B (CENP-B), suggested that alpha satellite DNA constituted the centromere [12]. However, later studies have shown that associated DNA sequences do not always function as centromeres and are not conserved during centromere evolution [14–16]. Recent studies of marker chromosomes that are mitotically stable with no apparent alpha satellite DNA, in humans and *Drosophila*, further strengthen the proposal that alpha satellite DNA may not be necessary for centromeric function [17–21]. The structure of the centromere and the role of centromeric DNA remain not fully understood.

Depending on the location of the centromere, human chromosomes can be classified into three groups. When the centromere is located in the middle with both arms being more or less equal in length, the chromosome is called "*metacentric*". In the human karyotype, chromosomes 1, 3, 16, 19 and 20 are metacentric or near-metacentric. When the centromere is located off-center with one arm longer than the other, the chromosome is called "*submetacentric*". Chromosomes 2, 4, 5, 6–12, X, 17 and 18 are submetacentric. When the centromere is almost at the end of the chromosome with one arm markedly smaller than the other, the chromosome is called "*acrocentric*". Chromosomes 13, 14, 15, 21 and 22 are acrocentric and are distinguished by the presence of satellites or secondary constrictions. *Secondary constrictions* are unstained regions or gaps in the short arms that contain nucleolar organizing genes (NORs) [12,22]. Such secondary constrictions commonly separate a small segment of chromosome called a "*satellite*" from the short arm. In such cases the secondary constriction is referred to as a "*satellite stalk*" since it connects the satellite to the chromosome short arm. Secondary constrictions are also a distinctive feature of the pericentromeric regions of chromosome 1, 9 and 16. These constrictions do not contain NOR's but consist of repetitive DNA sequences that contribute to "*constitutive heterochromatin*" surrounding each human centromere [23]. They stain dark with C-banding and show considerable variation in length. Sometimes they are shorter than the average (e.g. 1qh−, 9qh− and 16qh−; the h refers to heterochromatin) and sometimes many times longer than the average (e.g. 1qh+, 9qh+ and 16qh+). Since repetitive DNA sequences in these regions are not normally transcribed, variation in the content of this DNA is considered to be a clinically insignificant, normal heteromorphism [24,25].

The chromosome ends contain special structures called "telomeres". Telomeres provide stability to the chromosomes by stabilizing the linear ends of DNA molecules and are essential structures for maintaining the integrity of chromosomes. They contain the simple DNA sequence, TTAGGG [26], repeated many times up to 10 kb at the end of each chromosome arm. Unlike centromere sequences, this simple telomere repeat is conserved throughout evolution. An RNA-containing enzyme, "telomerase", adds new repeat units to the ends of chromosomes to maintain telomere length. Over time, decreased telomerase function is thought to result in progressive shortening of telomeres leading to senescence and cell death [27].

2.2 NOMENCLATURE

From the beginning it was recognized that standardization was needed in describing human chromosomes. To this end, several prominent investigators met in

Denver in 1960 [28] at the invitation of Dr T. T. Puck. The group, led by Dr C. E. Ford, reached a consensus in the formulation of a common system. The autosomes were serially numbered, 1 to 22, in the order of descending length. The sex chromosomes continued to be referred to as the X and Y. Also, the autosomes were classified into seven distinct groups, with chromosomes within a group arranged in descending order of length (Table 2.1). In order to arrange the chromosomes in a karyotype, three primary measurements were used: the total length of the chromosome relative to the total length of the haploid set with the X chromosome; the arm ratio, the length of the long arm relative to the length of short arm; and centromeric index, expressed as the ratio of length of short arm to the length of the entire chromosome. In 1963, at the London Conference, the previously identified seven groups of chromosomes were designated by the letters A to G, and the secondary constrictions were recognized.

Significant changes in nomenclature were again made after the discovery of Q-banding by Caspersson *et al.* [29]. With the ability to identify each individual chromosome based on banding patterns, it became essential to incorporate the latest developments into the existing nomenclature resulting in the "Paris Conference (1971)" [30] and its supplement [31]. The major highlights of these documents are: (1) introduction of mosaicism and chimerism, (2) designation of chromosome bands, (3) codes for describing the various banding methods and (4) designation of heteromorphic variants. After Caspersson *et al.* showed the presence of alternating dark and bright fluorescence patterns called bands on chromosomes, the Paris Conference document published a diagrammatic representation of the banding patterns of each chromosome called an "ideogram" (Fig. 2.1). In order to identify individual bands a distinct system of nomenclature was used.

Table 2.1 Architecture of human chromosomes (adapted from Paris Conference, 1971) [30]

Group 1–3	Large chromosomes in terms of length with centromeres located at approximate center. Based on the length, it is easier to distinguish* these three chromosomes.
Group 4–5	Large sub-metacentric chromosomes with very short short arms. It is difficult to distinguish between chromosome 4 and 5 without banding,* but chromosome 4 is slightly longer than chromosome 5.
Group 6–12	The most difficult group to distinguish.* All are sub-metacentric chromosomes of medium length. The X-chromosome is included in this group because of its length and architecture.
Group 13–15	Medium-sized chromosomes with centromeres at one end (acrocentric). They are easy to distinguish from other groups but difficult to distinguish within the group.* All of them may show satellites with considerable variation in length and size of satellites.
Group 16–18	Short chromosomes with either metacentric (chromosome 16) or sub-metacentric chromosomes (chromosomes 17 and 18).
Group 19–20	Short metacentric chromosomes. Often can be confused with chromosome 16.*
Group 21–22	Very short, acrocentric chromosomes, easy to recognize by their size, but difficult to distinguish from each other.* Chromosome 22 is actually longer than chromosome 21. The Y chromosome is often included in this group because of its morphological similarity.

*These comments refer to unbanded chromosome preparations. In banded preparations of adequate quality, all pairs can be easily distinguished, one pair from another.

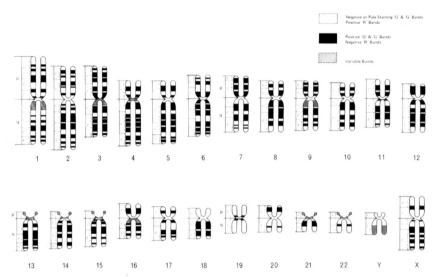

Fig. 2.1 Ideograms of human chromosomes (Reproduced with permission from Paris Conference (1971). Standardization in human cytogenetics. Birth Defects Original Article Ser VII, 7. New York: National Foundation, 1972)

The chromosome arms were subdivided into regions that included distinct landmarks helpful in the identification of each chromosome. The regions were numbered in sequential order starting at the centromere and progressing towards the telomere, for each arm. With development of higher resolution banding techniques the regions have been divided into bands and sub-bands based on the light and dark staining patterns (see Part II for the most current ideograms from ISCN 1995). Sequential numbering of regions, bands and sub-bands facilitates the identification of a specific area of the chromosome that is involved in a rearrangement.

Subsequent improvements to the human chromosome nomenclature became systematic with the election of a standing committee to amend the nomenclature and with renaming the nomenclature document as "An International System for Human Cytogenetic Nomenclature" (ISCN 1978) [32]. All subsequent documents pertaining to nomenclature are referred to as ISCN followed by the year in which the document is published. The most recent such document, ISCN 1995 [33], was the result of several significant changes and technological developments both in clinical and cancer cytogenetics. Until ISCN 1995, cancer cytogenetics had a separate nomenclature document, ISCN 1991 [34]. ISCN 1995 is the most comprehensive document describing human cytogenetic nomenclature to date, because it incorporates both constitutional and cancer cytogenetics into one uniform system of nomenclature. It also provides uniform guidelines for describing emerging molecular cytogenetic techniques and results. The ISCN 1995 document provides detailed descriptions of human chromosomes, heteromorphisms, and basic guidelines for reporting normal as well as abnormal chromosomes using various cytogenetic techniques. The reader is referred to ISCN 1995 for a comprehensive review of human cytogenetic nomenclature in its most current form.

2.3 CHROMOSOME BANDING TECHNIQUES

The ability to identify individual chromosomes and their structure based on alternating light and dark-staining patterns revolutionized the study of human chromosomes. The ability to distinguish each human chromosome by its banding pattern heralded the banding era and the ability to identify the majority of structural chromosome abnormalities and their consequences. Once it was shown that it was possible to obtain this banding on human chromosomes using fluorescence, there quickly followed further technological improvements using Giemsa staining after various treatments to obtain the same banding pattern – called "G-banding" (Fig. 2.2a). Because of the ease with which the G-banded chromosomes can be analyzed under light microscopes, it has become the banding method of choice in the majority of laboratories around the world.

In order to differentiate the various banding methods the Paris Conference devised a three-letter coding system. In this system the first letter describes the type of banding, the second letter the technique or the agent used to obtain the banding pattern, and the third letter to describe the stain used. For example, G-banding obtained by using trypsin and Giemsa stain is described by the three-letter code GTG (Table 2.2). The following are brief descriptions of some of the more commonly used banding methods.

2.3.1 Q banding (QFQ)

With the introduction of quinacrine banding by Caspersson *et al.* [35], it was possible to identify all of the human chromosomes with certainty, and thus this discovery is one of the most important in the era of clinical cytogenetics. Figure 2.2b shows an example of Q bands. While Q-banding was a remarkable discovery, the banding method has drawbacks. Prolonged exposure of fluorescence to UV light results in fading of the bands, making the technique unsuitable for extended microscopic analysis. Also, the expense of fluorescence microscopes is cost-limiting for many laboratories.

Mechanisms: Caspersson and colleagues at the Karolinska Institute with an American team of biochemists at Harvard Medical School headed by S. Farber and G. Foley set out to test or design fluorescent molecules that would preferentially bind to specific nucleotide pairs in DNA, which they hoped to be able to detect spectrophotometrically [36]. The first molecule tested was quinacrine mustard dihydrochloride (QM), a nitrogen mustard analog of the antimalarial drug, quinacrine. The dye, first applied to Vicia faba *and* Trillium erectum, *revealed brightly fluorescent bands that distinguished the individual plant chromosomes. The findings led Caspersson and Zech [37] to apply QM staining to human chromosomes, with the discovery that the end of the long arm of the Y chromosome was brightly fluorescent – bright enough that the human Y chromosome could be easily detected in interphase as well as in metaphase cells. With refinements, QM-banding produced banding patterns that were specific for each human chromosome. Caspersson* et al. *[37] suggested that the pattern of fluorescent bands in terms of their intensity was dependent on the amount of DNA and its ability to bind quinacrine mustard. However, their suggestion that GC- (guanine and cytosine)-rich regions of DNA accounted for bright fluorescence was found not to be the case.*

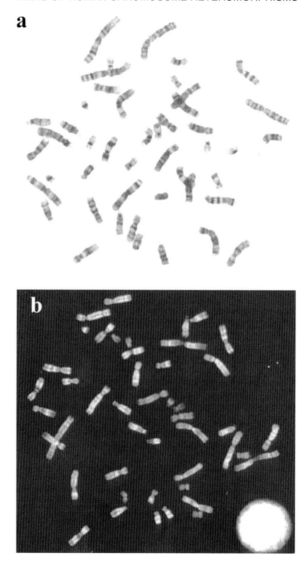

Fig. 2.2   (a) Metaphase showing typical G-banding. (b) Metaphase showing typical Q-banding

Several investigators showed that the AT-rich regions of DNA corresponded to the bright fluorescent bands obtained with quinacrine mustard [38–41]. Weisblum and DeHaseth [38] showed that, rather than preferential binding, this difference in intensity of fluorescence reflected a difference in quenching of the QM molecule. AT-richness alone, however, is not the sole determinant of the intensity of Q-banding. The actual differences in relative percentages of AT vs. GC in different regions are not as great as might be implied. The periodicity of

Table 2.2 Banding nomenclature (adapted from Paris Conference Supplement, 1975) [32]

G-Banding	
GTG	G bands by trypsin and Giemsa stain
GTL	G bands by trypsin and Leishman stain
GTW	G bands by trypsin and Wright's stain
GPG	G bands by pancreatin and Giemsa stain
GAG & GSG	G bands by acetic saline and Giemsa stain
GUG	G bands by urea and Giemsa stain
Q-Banding	
QFQ	Q bands by fluorescence and quinacrine stain
QFH	Q bands by fluorescence and Hoechst 33258 stain
C-Banding	
CBG	C bands by barium hydroxide and Giemsa stain
R-Banding	
RFA	R bands by fluorescence and acridine orange stain
RHG	R bands by heating and Giemsa stain
RBA	R bands by BudR and acridine orange stain

interspersion of GC within short highly repetitive AT-rich sequences appears to play a significant role [41].

2.3.2   G-banding (GTG)

G-banding, introduced in 1971 by Sumner *et al.* [42], overcame the two most significant problems of Q-banding and thus became the more widely used banding technique in the majority of clinical cytogenetics laboratories. Figure 2.2a shows a metaphase with typical G-banding. G-banding as it is practiced today has undergone several changes. The various acronyms of GTG, GTW, GTL and GAG all represent the variations used to obtain the same banding pattern that can be seen and analyzed using standard light microscopy. While the original G-banding method used acid fixation with saline treatment followed by Giemsa staining (GAG) [42,43], application of proteolytic enzymes such as trypsin [44,45] and or pancreatin [46,47] are simpler and have improved the banding pattern. Also, the blood stains, Wright's or Leishman's, are often used instead of Giemsa, depending on the laboratory's experience and preference. The G bands, obtained either by enzymatic or chemical pretreatment, irrespective of the blood stain used, resemble Q bands and are known to represent AT-rich regions of the chromosomal DNA (Table 2.3b) [48].

Mechanisms: Mixtures of thiazin dyes present in Giemsa, Leischman, Wright or Romanowski blood stains, all can produce banding patterns under the right conditions. It is obvious from the variety of treatments that produce G-banding that more than one mechanism is involved. The most reliable and widely used treatment is mild proteolytic digestion with trypsin [44,45]. However, the precise role of nucleoproteins in G-banding has not been determined [48–53]. Extraction of histones also seems to have little effect [54–56]; in fact, very little protein is lost from chromosomes in various G-banding treatments [50]. Furthermore, it is evident that there is an underlying structural integrity of the chromosome that is revealed in the "chromomere pattern" of very long chromosomes in meiosis

17

Table 2.3 (a) Different classes of chromosome bands and techniques for their recognition. Modified from Sumner (1994) [72]. (b) Properties of euchromatic bands.

	Class	
Heterochromatin	*Euchromatin*	*Special*
C-banding	G-banding	Ag-NOR staining
G-11 banding	Q-banding	Cd-banding
Q-banding	R-banding	Immunofluorescent
Distamycin/DAPI	T-banding	staining with CREST
	Replication banding	serum
Positive G-/Q-bands, negative R-bands, pachytene chromomeres	*Negative G-/Q-bands, positive R-bands, interchromomere regions*	
Early condensation	Late condensation	
Late-replicating DNA	Early-replicating DNA	
AT-rich DNA	GC-rich DNA	
Tissue-specific genes	Housekeeping genes	
Long intermediate repetitive DNA sequences (LINEs)	Short intermediate repetitive DNA sequences (SINEs)	

[57,58]. This pattern in non-banded meiotic chromosomes is identical to the pattern of G-banded metaphase chromosomes (see ISCN 1995).

The relationship between DNA structure and the binding of components making up Giemsa dye mixtures is not totally understood. Treatments that loosen the integrity of underlying DNA structure appear to be most effective, suggesting that certain Giemsa components bind to condensed DNA in monomeric form and to looser DNA structure in polymeric form [59,60]. The more the individual dyes components become stacked, the greater the shift to the lower absorption spectra (purple or pink). In monomer form the shift is to the blue end of the spectrum. Such a shift in color, based on a dye's ability to become stacked in polymer form, is referred to as metachromacy. Some Giemsa components are more metachromatic than others. Methylene blue, azure A, azure B, and thiazin show varying degrees of metachromacy determined by the number of methyl groups present on the dye molecule [59–61]. Eosin, which is also a component of Giemsa dyes, shows no metachromacy but appears to have a differential staining effect when combined with the other components.

Although the correlation is not yet completely understood, regions of condensed chromatin tend to be AT-rich and replicate their DNA late, whereas GC-rich regions tend to be less condensed and replicate their DNA earlier (Table 2.3) [48]. DNA-binding proteins thought to be involved in maintaining chromosomal structural integrity form the nuclear matrix and include topoisomerases that appear to have a basic role in the control of gene activity [62–64]. It may be that the nuclear matrix proteins hold AT-rich regions together, making them less easily available for DNA replication and at the same time allowing dye to bind only in monomer form so that they stain more intensely. Conversely, GC-rich regions that are gene-rich and transcriptionally active may be more loosely bound and consequently bind dye in polymer form and so that they stain less intensely.

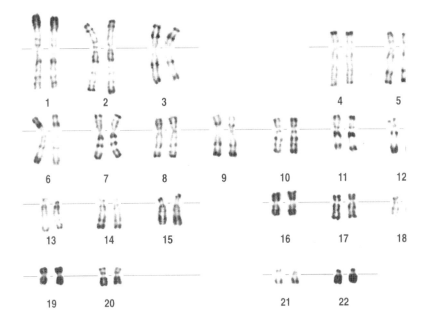

Fig. 2.3 The R-banded human karyotype (Courtesy of B. Dutrillaux) (Reproduced with permission from ISCN (1995). An International System for Human Cytogenetic Nomenclature (1995), Mittelman F, editor. Basel: S. Karger.)

2.3.3 R-banding (RHG)

Dutrillaux and Lejeune [65] introduced a banding technique involving treatment of chromosomes in saline at high temperature (87°C), followed by Giemsa staining that resulted in a reverse pattern of G or Q bands. They called this "*reverse banding*" and, since the method involved heating with Giemsa stain, it has been described as a "RHG" banding. R bands are most useful in identifying abnormalities involving the terminal regions of chromosomes, which are lighter staining by G- and or Q-banding. Figure 2.3 shows an R-banded human metaphase. Inconsistencies in reproducibility of this RHG method led to the development of alternate methods to produce R-banding. Various fluorescent chemicals such as acridine orange and chromomycin A3/methyl green [66–68] can also be used to obtain R-banding (Table 2.4). However, because of the technical difficulties or fluorescence requirements, R-banding is still not used in many laboratories.

2.4 SPECIALIZED BANDING TECHNIQUES

Other banding techniques such as C-banding, G-11 staining, silver staining for nucleolar organizer regions, distamycin/DAPI, etc. were introduced subsequently. Most of these techniques have limited application and none is used for the purpose of primary chromosome identification. While each of these banding methods lacks the universal application of G-, Q-, or R-banding methods, they are

19

Table 2.4 Fluorescent DNA ligands used in human chromosome staining, base affinity and type of banding when used with counter stain. Modified from Verma and Babu [68]

Primary dye	Affinity	Counterstain	Banding	Ref(s)
DAPI	AT	Distamycin A*	DAPI/DA	
DIPI	AT	Netropsin	DAPI/DA	
		Pentamidine	DAPI/DA	
Hoechst 33258	AT	Distamycin A*	DAPI/DA	
		Netropsin	DAPI/DA	
		Actinomycin D‡	QFH bands	
		Chromomycin A$_3$	QFH bands	
7-Aminoactino-mycin D	GC	Methyl green*	R bands (enhanced)	
Chromomycin A$_3$	GC	Distamycin A*	R bands (enhanced)	
Mithramycin	GC	Malachite green*	R bands (enhanced)	
Olivomycin	GC	Distamycin A	R bands (enhanced)	
		Netropsin	R bands (enhanced)	
		Methyl green*	R bands (enhanced)	
Coriphosphin		Methyl green	R bands (modified)	
Quinacrine/quinacrine mustard	GC (low)		Q bands	

*Non-fluorescent with AT affinity.
‡Non-fluorescent with GC affinity.

useful for demonstrating or characterizing many of the heteromorphisms described in this book. These are specialized banding methods.

2.4.1 C-banding (CBG)

C-banding is a method to stain the constitutive heterochromatin at the centromeres and secondary constrictions of human chromosomes. During their experiments with in situ hybridization of tritium-labeled satellite DNA to mouse chromosomes, Pardue and Gall [69] noted that constitutive heterochromatin at the centromeres of mouse chromosomes stained darker than other chromosomal regions. In 1971, Arrighi and Hsu [70,71] developed a modified technique of sodium hydroxide treatment followed by DNA renaturation and Giemsa staining that eliminated the need for the radiolabeling. However, treatment with sodium hydroxide can be harsh on the morphology of chromosomes. In yet another modification, Sumner [72] substituted barium hydroxide for sodium hydroxide, producing the same C-banding pattern but with less distortion of the chromosome morphology. Hence, many laboratories use CBG banding. Figure 2.4a shows a metaphase with typical C-banding. Since the method selectively stains repetitive or constitutive heterochromatin, it has become one of the important special banding methods for investigating heteromorphic variations at the centromeres, in marker chromosomes and in pericentric inversions.

Mechanisms: The C-banding technique had its basis in the autoradiographic in situ hybridization method developed by Pardue and Gall in 1968 [69]. Isolated highly repetitive DNA that was tritium-labeled hybridized to heterochromatic regions in interphase nuclei. It was subsequently shown to correspond to regions around the centromeres of mouse, human and other mammalian chromosomes. In a modification of the in situ hybridization technique, Arrighi and Hsu [70,71]

20

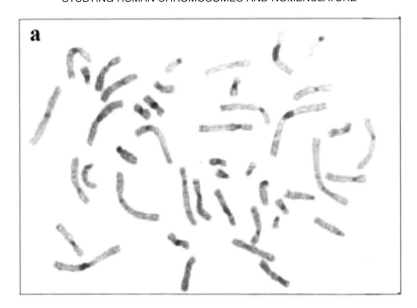

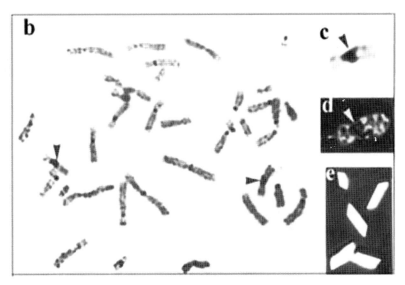

Fig. 2.4 (a) Metaphase showing typical C-banding. (**b–e**) Metaphase showing G-11 banding (Reproduced with modification from Wyandt *et al* (1970). Exp Cell Res. 102: 85–94)

applied Giemsa staining to preparations that were first denatured with 0.07 M NaOH and then incubated in 2 × SSC for several hours. This procedure resulted in intense staining of the heterochromatin around the centromeres, whereas the rest of the chromosome stained pale blue. They postulated this was due to faster reannealing of repetitive DNA in heterochromatin than in the less repetitive DNA sequences elsewhere. Subsequent studies of isolated satellite DNAs [73–78] confirmed that satellite fractions hybridized specifically to regions stained by C-banding.

McKenzie and Lubs [79] were able to produce C-banding by simply treating chromosomes with HCl and prolonged incubation in 2 × SSC. Studies by Comings et al. [50] demonstrated considerable extraction of nucleoprotein and DNA from non-heterochromatic regions by various C-banding treatments, while heterochromatic regions were resistant to such extraction. Furthermore, they demonstrated that hybridization of repetitive sequences in solution was not required for enhancement of staining, but in fact those regions reassociated instantaneously as soon as they were removed from the denaturing NaOH solution. Subsequent incubation in 2 × SSC extracted additional non-heterochromatic DNA. Since incubation that produces C-banding is done for times ranging from a couple of hours to overnight, it is unlikely that much single-stranded DNA remains to bind Giemsa components. Differential staining is more likely due to the greater amount of double-stranded DNA remaining in the heterochromatic regions.

2.4.2 G-11-banding

G-11 staining is used to selectively stain some heterochromatic regions on human chromosomes a deep magenta color in contrast to the pale blue color of the remainder of the chromosome. These include chromosomes 1, 3, 5, 7, 9, 10, 19 and Y. However, there is variability in the intensity of staining at the pericentromeric and satellite regions of acrocentric chromosomes. Such variability is dependent on the individual characteristics of these chromosomes. The G-11 technique utilizes modified Giemsa staining at an alkaline pH [80] and is useful in the study of human heteromorphic variants and pericentromeric inversions, especially on chromosome 9. Figure 2.4b shows a metaphase with typical G-11-banding.

Mechanisms: G-11-banding receives its name from attempts to obtain differential banding of specific chromosome regions by staining in Giemsa at different pH values. The standard pH of the staining solution in G-banding procedures is 6.8–7.0. It was found by Patil et al. [80] that if the alkalinity of some Giemsa mixtures was raised to 9.0, G-banding could be achieved without any other special treatment. Bobrow et al. [81] showed that if alkalinity was raised to pH 11, subcomponents of C bands, especially the secondary constriction (qh region) of chromosome 9, stained a deep magenta color in contrast to the pale blue color of the euchromatic regions. Jones et al. [75] first showed that satellite III DNA, isolated on a silver cesium sulfate gradient, hybridized to the heterochromatic regions of chromosome 9 and to the acrocentric chromosomes. Buhler et al. [77] showed that this magenta-staining DNA, which appears to be especially specific for 9qh, 15p and Yq, corresponded to sites of hybridization of a specific class of highly repetitive satellite III DNA. Other classes of satellite DNAs I–VII were found to be distributed in chromosome 9 and in other chromosomes [78], but satellite III was found mainly in these three chromosomes. The mechanism of G-11-banding is still uncertain. Wyandt et al. [82] tested various components of Giemsa and showed that G-11-banding could be achieved when the right proportions of azure

22

B and eosin Y were mixed at pH 11. When mixed in equimolar amounts, most of the azure B and eosin Y precipitated as large highly reflective trapezoidal crystals of azure-eosinate. Finer crystals appear to be precipitated at magenta-colored sites on chromosomes (Fig. 2.4b and c) [82].

2.4.3   Silver staining (Ag-NOR)

Silver staining is a method to stain the nucleolar organizer regions (NORs) on the human acrocentric chromosomes. NORs, which contain the genes for ribosomal RNA or proteins, were known early to stain with silver [83]. Using this information, Howell *et al.* [84] showed that NORs on chromosomes could be stained with silver nitrate, and called their technique "Ag-SAT". Howell and Black [85] subsequently developed a simplified technique using a colloidal developer for better results. Many laboratories use this method with various modifications. Figure 2.5a shows a metaphase with typical AgNOR staining.

Mechanisms: There is still controversy as to the nature or exact location of this silver staining. While Miller et al. [86] showed that it is not the activity of NOR regions that is responsible for the staining, the actual location of the staining was shown to be the satellite stalks of acrocentric chromosomes and not the satellites themselves [87]. Subsequent experiments by Verma et al. [88] showed that AgNOR-positive chromosomes are those that are found frequently in satellite associations while the Ag-NOR-negative chromosomes are not seen in such associations. Silver staining is an important banding method to study heteromorphic variations in the size and number of NORs, and to characterize marker chromosomes or other structural rearrangements involving the acrocentric chromosomes.

2.4.4   Cd-banding

Cd-banding, used for identification of centromeres, is believed to stain DNA-protein complexes representing the kinetochores or organelles associated with sites of spindle fiber attachment to chromosomes. The technique, first described by Eiberg [89], reveals pairs of dots at presumed centromere locations; hence, the term "centromere dots" (Cd). The technique involves the usual hypotonic treatment of chromosomes followed by a series of fixations starting with a 9:1 ratio of methanol:acetic acid followed by a 5:1 ratio and then the standard 3:1 ratio. One-week-old slides are then incubated in Earle's balanced salt solution (pH 8.5–9.0) at 85°C for 45 min, followed by staining in a dilute solution of phosphate-buffered Giemsa (0.0033 M, pH 6.5). The technique appears to specifically stain only active centromeric regions and not inactive centromeres, secondary constrictions or other variable heteromorphic regions. Hence, it has been useful in identifying the active centromere(s) in dicentric, pseudodicentric and Robertsonian translocations. Figure 2.5 shows a metaphase with typical Cd-banding.

Mechanisms: The mechanism of this technique suggested by Eiberg was that it represented a specific DNA-protein complex. Evans and Ross (1974) [90] suggested the Cd-positive regions represent kinetochores. Nakagome et al. [91,92] and Maraschio et al. [93] studied dicentric and pseudodicentric chromosomes and showed that the Cd-positive regions do appear to correspond only to active centromeres. The presence or absence of specific centromeric proteins associated with centromeric activity have been recently studied with specific fluorescent

23

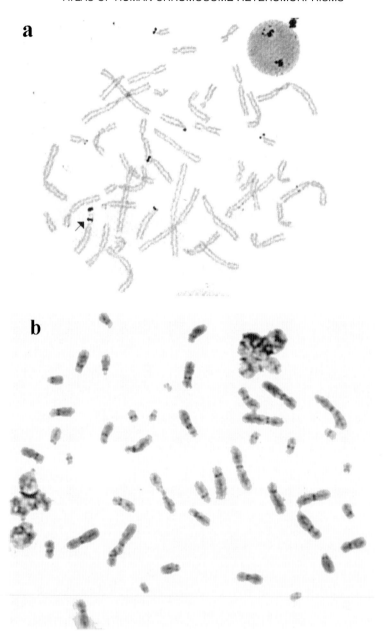

Fig. 2.5 (**a**) Metaphase showing typical Ag-NOR staining. (**b**) Metaphase showing Cd-banding (Reproduced with slight modification and enhancement from Eiben H (1974), New selective Giemsa technique for human chromosomes, Cd staining. Nature 248: 55)

antibodies that distinguish particular proteins associated with active or inactive centromeres [94].

2.5 SISTER CHROMATID EXCHANGE STAINING (SCE)

Sister chromatid exchanges (SCEs) are the result of interchange of DNA between replication products at homologous loci [95]. SCEs at low levels are normally seen in humans and can be demonstrated in somatic cells by incorporating a thymidine analog, 5-bromodeoxyuridine (BrdU) into replicating DNA for two successive cell cycles and subsequent photodegradation of the resulting chromosomes. Staining of metaphases with Hoechst 33258 [96] or with Giemsa following this procedure results in faint staining of one chromatid and strong staining of the other chromatid. A reversal of staining intensity of the two chromatids occurs where there has been an exchange (Fig. 2.6). The technique has been extensively used for testing the mutagenic potential of various chemicals [97], to study cell cycle kinetics [98,99] and to diagnose Bloom's syndrome [100].

Mechanisms: Because of the semi-conservative nature of DNA replication, after two complete pulses of BrdU substitution, one chromatid has both halves of the DNA helix BrdU-substituted (bifilarly labeled) while the other chromatid has only one half of the DNA helix BrdU-substituted (monofilarly labeled). The latter is the basis of differences in staining of sister chromatids that allow detection of SCEs, mainly in non-heterochromatic regions.

2.6 REPLICATION BANDING

Replication banding is most useful in identifying the early- and late-replicating X chromosomes in females or in patients with sex chromosome abnormalities. It is

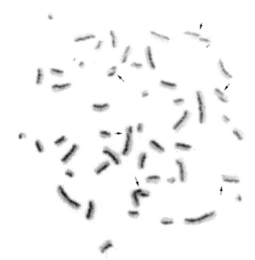

Fig. 2.6   Metaphase showing typical sister chromatid exchanges (SCEs)

well known that one of the X chromosomes in females is inactive, resulting in dosage compensation [101]. It is also known that X chromosome inactivation is random and that the inactive X chromosome initiates and completes DNA synthesis later than the active X and other chromosomes [102–106]. Replication banding, obtained by incorporation of BrdU and subsequent staining with Giemsa or other stains [96], allows distinction of the active and inactive X chromosomes. Variations in replication banding can also be achieved. In the "T pulse" procedure, BrdU is made available at the beginning of the cell cycle and then replaced with thymidine for the last 5–6 hours before the harvest. With the RBG technique (R bands by BrdU and Giemsa), the active or early-replicating chromosome regions that have incorporated BrdU stain pale, whereas late-replicating regions that have incorporated thymidine, such as most of the inactive X chromosome, stain dark. The "B pulse" is the opposite. Thymidine, made available at the beginning of the cell cycle, is replaced with BrdU the last 5–6 hours before harvest. Subsequent Giemsa staining will result in early-replicating chromosome regions appearing dark because they have incorporated thymidine, while the inactive or late-replicating chromosome regions appear pale due to the BrdU incorporation. Figure 2.7 shows a typical metaphase with replication banding.

Banding patterns

The equivalent of Q- and G- or R-banding patterns is achieved depending on whether a B or T pulse is used. If a B pulse is used, a Q- or G-banding pattern is achieved and if a T pulse is used, an R-banding pattern is achieved. Subtle changes in pattern toward the earliest R bands or latest G bands can be achieved by shortening the length of the BrdU pulse. A short T pulse at the very end of the S period can produce what are referred to as T bands (bright or dark bands at the terminal ends of some chromosome arms). These bright bands with a T pulse also correspond to early-replicating GC-rich regions, whereas dull bands correspond

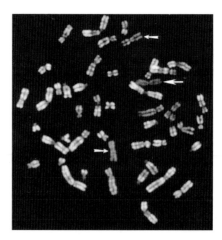

Fig. 2.7 Metaphase with 47, XX, i(Xq) showing replication banding with late-replicating normal X (upper arrow), late replicating i(Xq) (middle, large arrow) and early replicating normal X (lower arrow).

to late-replicating AT-rich regions. The exception to this is the late-replicating X chromosome whose bright bands do not differ in AT:GC content from the less intensely stained bands at the same locations on the early-replicating X.

Lateral asymmetry

An interesting variation of the BrdU labeling technique is the method of detecting lateral asymmetry. The latter is due to an interstrand compositional bias in which one half of the DNA helix is predominantly T-rich and the complementary half is correspondingly A-rich [109]. Since BrdU substitutes for thymidine and not adenine, after one complete pulse of BrdU, the BrdUA-rich strand stains less intensely than the AT-rich strand, resulting in a block of heterochromatin that is more intensely stained on one chromatid than on the other. A more even distribution of thymidine in the two strands results in both chromatids staining similarly in euchromatin or in heterochromatin that does not have interstrand compositional bias. Variation in the size and location of such blocks forms the basis of a subclass of variants in chromosomes 1, 9, 15, 16 and Y [110–112].

2.7   OTHER DNA-BINDING FLUOROCHROMES

A variety of different DNA-binding fluorochromes will produce chromosome banding patterns or enhancement of AT- or GC-rich regions depending on absorption and emission spectra and how they are used in combination (Table 2.3). For instance, the combination of distamycin A (DA) and DAPI produces bright qh regions on chromosome 1, 9 and 16 that correspond to G-11 bands and probably to satellite III DNA. The use of various fluorochromes and their mechanisms of action have been adequately described by others [68] and will not be described in detail here.

2.8   HIGH-RESOLUTION BANDING AND OTHER SPECIAL TREATMENTS

Other treatments and methods that have particular bearing on characterizing heteromorphisms include treatments such as methotrexate added to cultures to synchronize cells in G2 and used for high-resolution chromosome banding. Ethidium bromide intercalates into GC-rich regions during cell culture, a property that is also used to produce elongated chromosomes for high-resolution banding analysis [113]. 5-Azacytidine, and a number of DNA analogs such as FudR, produce very long secondary constrictions such as shown by Balicek and Zizka [114] or can enhance so-called "fragile sites" on chromosomes. Most of these are common fragile sites that can be induced *in vitro* in cells from anyone. Others are "rare" fragile sites that are induced only in cells from certain individuals and are heritable. A few such sites involve oncogenes that are implicated in cancer.

Acknowledgements

The authors wish to thank Ms Linda Merryman and Ms Neli Panova for their excellent technical assistance and for the figures.

References

1. Tijo JH, Levan A (1956). The chromosome number in man. Hereditas. 42:1–6.
2. Lejeune J, Gautier M, Turpin MR (1959). Etude des chromosomes somatiques de neuf enfants mongoliens. CR Acad Sci. (III) 248:1721–2.
3. Patau K, Smith DW, Therman E, Inhorn SL (1960). Multiple congenital anomaly caused by an extra chromosome. Lancet. 1:790–3.
4. Edwards JH, Harnden DG, Cameron AH, Cross VM, Wolff OH (1960). A new trisomic syndrome. Lancet. 1:711–13.
5. Ford CE, Jones KW, Polani PE, de Almeida JC, Briggs JH (1959). A sex chromosome anomaly in a case of gonadal dysgenesis (Turner Syndrome). Lancet. 1:711–11.
6. Jacobs PA, Strong JA (1959). A case of human intersexuality having a possible XXY sex determining mechanism. Nature. 183:302–3.
7. Jacobs PA, Baikie AG, MacGregor TN, Harnden DG (1959). Evidence for the existence of the human superfemale. Lancet. 2:423–5.
8. Nowell PC (1960). Phytohemagglutinin: an initiator of mitoses in cultures of normal human leukocytes. Cancer Res. 20:462–6.
9. Moorhead PS, Nowell PC, Mellman WS, Battips DM, Hungerford DA (1960). Chromosome preparations of leukocytes cultured from human peripheral blood. Exp Cell Res. 20:613–16.
10. Pluta AF, Mackay AM, Ainsztein AM, Goldberg IG, Earnshaw WC (1995). The centromere: hub of chromosomal activities. Science. 270:1591–4.
11. Wevrick R, Willard VP, Willard HF (1992). Structure of DNA near long tandem arrays of alpha satellite DNA at the centromere of human chromosome 7. Genomics. 14:912–23.
12. Therman E, Susman M (1993). Human Chromosomes. New York: Springer-Verlag.
13. Le M-H, Duricka D, Karpen GH (1995). Islands of complex DNA are widespread in *Drosophila* centric heterochromatin. Genetics. 141:283–303.
14. Page SL, Earnshaw WC, Choo KHA, Shaffer LG (1995). Further evidence that CENP-C is a necessary component of active centromeres: studies of a dic(X;15) with simultaneous immunofluorescence and FISH. Hum Mol Genet. 4:289–94.
15. Steiner NC, Clarke L (1994). A novel epigenetic effect can alter centromere function in fission yeast. Cell. 79:865–74.
16. Sullivan BA, Schwartz S (1995). Identification of centromeric antigens in dicentric Robertsonian translocations: CENP-C and CENP-E are necessary components of functional centromeres. Hum Mol Genet. 4:2189–97.
17. Voullaire LE, Slater HR, Petrovic V, Choo KHA (1993). A functional marker centromere with no detectable alpha-satellite III or CENP-B protein:activation of a latent centromere? Am J Hum Genet. 52:1153–63.
18. Brown W, Tyler-Smith C (1995). Centromere activation. Trends Genet. 11:337–9.
19. Depinet TW, Zackowski JL, Earnshaw WC *et al.* (1997). Characterization of neo-centromeres in marker chromosomes lacking detectable alpha-satellite DNA. Hum Mol Genet. 6:1195–204.
20. du Sart D, Cancilla MR, Earle E *et al.* (1997). A functional neo-centromere formed through activation of a latent human centromere and consisting of non-alpha-satellite DNA. Nature Genet. 16:144–53.
21. Williams BC, Murphy TD, Goldberg ML, Karpen GH (1998). Neocentromere activity of structurally acentric mini-chromosomes in *Drosophila*. Nature Genet. 18:30–7.
22. Henderson AS, Warburton D, Atwood KC (1972). Location of ribosomal DNA in the human chromosome complement. Proc Natl Acad Sci USA. 69:3394–8.
23. Brown SW (1996). Heterochromatin. Science. 151:417–25.
24. John B (1998). The biology of heterochromatin. In: Verma RS, editor. Heterochromatin: Molecular and Structural Aspects. Cambridge: Cambridge University Press, pp. 1–147.
25. Verma RS (1998). Heteromorphisms of heterochromatin. In: Verma RS, editor. Heterochromatin: Molecular and Structural Aspects. Cambridge: Cambridge University Press, pp. 276–92.
26. Moyzis RK, Buckingham JM, Cram LS *et al.* (1988). A highly conserved repetitive DNA sequence, $TTAGGG_n$, present at the telomeres of human chromosomes. Proc Natl Acad Sci USA. 85:6622–6.
27. Kipling D, Cooke HJ (1992). Beginning or end? Telomere structure, genetics and biology. Hum Mol Genet. 1:3–6.
28. Denver Conference (1960). A proposed standard system of nomenclature of human mitotic chromosomes. Lancet. i:1063–5.
29. Casperson T, Zech L, Johansson C, Modest EJ (1970). Identification of human chromosomes by DNA-binding fluorescent agents. Chromosoma. 30:215–27.

30. Paris Conference (1971). Standardization in human cytogenetics. Birth Defects Orig Article Ser VII, 7. New York: National Foundation, 1972.
31. Paris Conference (1971), Supplement (1975). Standardization in human cytogenetics. Birth Defects Orig Article Ser XI. New York: National Foundation, 1975.
32. ISCN (1978). An international system for human cytogenetic nomenclature. Birth Defects Orig Article Ser XIV. New York: National Foundation.
33. ISCN (1995). Mitelman F, editor. An International System for Human Cytogenetic Nomenclature. Basel: Karger.
34. ISCN (1991). Mitelman F, editor. Guidelines for Cancer Cytogenetics, Supplement to An International System for Human Cytogenetic Nomenclature. Basel: Karger.
35. Casperson T, Lomakka G, Zech L (1971). The 24 fluorescence patterns of human metaphase chromosomes – distinguishing characters and variability. Hereditas. 67:89–102.
36. Caspersson T, Farber S, Foley GE *et al*. (1968). Chemical differentiation along metaphase chromosomes. Exp Cell Res. 49:219–22.
37. Caspersson T, Zech L, Johansson C (1970). Analysis of human metaphase chromosome set by aid of DNA-binding fluorescent agents. Exp Cell Res. 62:490–2.
38. Weisblum B, DeHaseth PL (1972). Quinacrine, a chromosome stain specific for deoxyadenylate-deoxythymidylate rich regions in DNA. Proc Natl Acad Sci USA. 63:629–32.
39. Ellison JR, Barr HJ (1972). Quinacrine fluorescence of specific chromosome regions. Late replication and high A:T content in *Samoia leonensis*. Chromosoma. 36:375–90.
40. Comings DE, Kovacs BW, Avelino E, Harris DC (1975). Mechanism of chromosome banding. V. Quinacrine banding. Chromosoma. 50:111–45.
41. Michelson AM, Monny C, Kovoor A (1972). Action of quinacrine mustard on polynucleotide. Biochimie. 54:1129–36.
42. Sumner AT, Evans HJ, Buckland RA (1971). New technique for distinguishing between human chromosomes. Nature New Biol. 232:31–2.
43. Drets ME, Shaw MW (1971). Specific banding patterns of human chromosomes. Proc Natl Acad Sci USA. 68:2073–77.
44. Seabright M (1971). A rapid banding technique for human chromosomes. Lancet. 2:971–2.
45. Wang HC, Fedoroff (1972). Banding in human chromosomes treated with trypsin. Nature New Biol. 235:52–4.
46. Muller W, Rozenkranz (1972). Rapid banding technique for human and mammalian chromosomes. Lancet. 1:898.
47. Pearson P (1972). The use of new staining techniques for human chromosome identification. J Med Genet. 9:264–75.
48. Sumner AT (1994). Chromosome banding and identification absorption staining. In: Gosden GR, editor. Methods in Molecular Biology. Chromosome Analysis Protocols. Totowa, NJ: Humana Press, pp. 59–81.
49. Comings DE, Avelino A (1974). Mechanisms of chromosome banding. II. Evidence that histones are not involved. Exp Cell Res. 86:202–6.
50. Comings DE, Avelino E, Okada TA, Wyandt HE (1973). The mechanisms of C- and G-banding of chromosomes. Exp Cell Res. 77:469–93.
51. Sumner AT (1973). Involvement of protein disulphides and sulphydryls in chromosome banding. Exp Cell Res. 83:438–42.
52. Korf BR, Schuh BE, Salwen MJ, Warburton D, Miller OJ (1976). The role of trypsin in the pretreatment of chromosomes for Giemsa banding. Hum Genet. 31:27–33.
53. Holmquist GP (1992). Chromosome bands, their chromatin flavors and their functional features. Am J Hum Genet. 51:17–37.
54. Brown RL, Pathak S, Hsu TC (1975). The possible role of histones in the mechanism of G-banding. Science. 189:1090–1.
55. Holmquist GP, Comings DE (1976). Histones and G-banding of chromosomes. Science. 193:599–602.
56. Retief AE, Ruchel R (1977). Histones removed by fixation. Their role in the mechanism of chromosome banding. Exp Cell Res. 106:233–7.
57. Okada TA, Comings DE (1974). Mechanisms of chromosome banding. III. Similarity between G-bands of mitotic chromosomes and chromomeres of meiotic chromosomes. Chromosoma. 48:65–71.
58. Jhanwar SC, Burns JP, Alonso ML, Hew W, Chaganti RS (1982). Mid-pachytene chromomere maps of human autosomes. Cytogenet Cell Genet. 33:240–8.

59. Comings DE (1975). Mechanisms of chromosome banding. IV. Optical properties of the Giemsa dyes. Chromosoma 50:89–110.
60. Comings DE, Avelino E (1975). Mechanisms of chromosome banding. VII. Interaction of methylene blue with DNA and chromatin. Chromosoma. 51:365–79.
61. Wyandt HE, Anderson RS, Patil SR, Hecht F (1980). Mechanisms of Giemsa banding. II. Giemsa components and other variables in G-banding. Hum Genet. 53:211–15.
62. Saitoh Y, Laemmli (1994). Metaphase chromosome structure: bands arise from a differential folding path of highly AT-rich scaffold. Cell. 75:609–21.
63. Hancock R (2000). A new look at the nuclear matrix. Chromosoma. 109:219–25.
64. Nickerson J (2001). Experimental observations of the nuclear matrix. J Cell Sci. 114:463–74.
65. Dutrillaux B, Lejeune J (1971). Cytogenetique humaine. Sur une nouvelle technique d'analyse du caryotype humain. CR Acad Sci. 272:2638–40.
66. Bobrow M, Collacott HEAC, Madan K (1972). Chromosome banding with acridine orange. Lancet. 2:1311.
67. Wyandt HE, Vlietinck RF, Magenis RE, Hecht F (1974). Colored reverse-banding of human chromosomes with acridine orange following alkaline–formalin treatment:densitometric validation and applications. Humangenetik. 23:119–30.
68. Verma RS, Babu (1995). Human Chromosomes. Principles and Techniques, 2nd edn. Inc, New York: McGraw-Hill.
69. Pardue ML, Gall JG (1970). Chromosomal localization of mouse satellite DNA. Science. 168:1356–8.
70. Arrighi FE, Hsu TC (1971). Localization of heterochromatin in human chromosomes. Cytogenetics. 10:81–6.
71. Hsu TC, Arrighi FE (1971). Distribution of constitutive heterochromatin in mammalian chromosomes. Chromosoma. 34:243–53.
72. Sumner AT (1972). A simple technique for demonstrating centromeric heterochromatin. Exp Cell Res. 75:304–6.
73. Saunders GF, Hsu TC, Getz MJ, Simes EL, Arrighi F (1972). Locations of human satellite DNA in human chromosomes. Nature New Biol. 236:244–6.
74. Jones KW, Corneo G (1971). Location of satellite and homogeneous DNA sequences on human chromosomes. Nature New Biol. 233(43):268–71.
75. Jones KW, Prosser J, Corneo G, Ginelli E (1973). The chromosomal location of human satellite DNA III. Chromosoma 42:445–51.
76. Jones KW, Purdom IF, Prosser J, Corneo G (1974). The chromosomal localization of human satellite DNA I. Chromosoma. 49:161–71.
77. Buhler EM, Tsuchimoto T, Jurik LP, Stalder GR (1975). Satellite DNA III and alkaline Giemsa staining. Humangenetik. 26:329–33.
78. Ginelli E, Corneo G (1976). The organization of repeated DNA sequences in the human genome. Chromosoma 56:55–69.
79. McKenzie WH, Lubs HA (1973). An analysis of the technical variables in the production of C bands. Chromosoma. 41:175–82.
80. Patil SR, Merrick S, Lubs, HA (1971). Identification of each human chromosome with a modified Giemsa stain. Science. 173:821–2.
81. Bobrow M, Madan K, Pearson PL (1972). Staining of some specific regions of human chromosomes, particularly the secondary constriction of No. 9. Nature New Biol. 238:122–4.
82. Wyandt HE, Wysham DG, Minden SK, Anderson RS, Hecht F (1976). Mechanism of Giemsa banding of chromosomes. I. Giemsa-11 banding with azure and eosin. Exp Cell Res. 102:85–94.
83. Ruzicka V (1891). Zur geschichte und kenntnis der feineren structur der nucleolen centraler nervzellen. Anat Anz. 16:557–63.
84. Howell WM, Denton TE, Diamond JR (1975). Differential staining of the satellite regions of human acrocentric chromosomes. Experentia. 31:260–2.
85. Howell WM, Black DA (1980). Controlled silver-staining of nucleolus organizer regions with a protective colloidal developer: A 1-step method. Experientia. 36:1014–15.
86. Miller OJ, Miller DA, Dev VG, Tantravahi R, Croce CM (1976). Expression of human and suppression of mouse nucleolus organizer activity in mouse–human somatic cell hybrids. Proc Natl Acad Sci USA. 73:4531–5.
87. Goodpasture C, Bloom SE, Hsu TC, Arrighi FE (1976). Human nucleolus organizers: the satellites or the stalks? Am J Hum Genet. 28:559–66.

88. Verma RS, Rodriguez J, Shah JV, Dosik H (1983). Preferential association of nucleolar organizing human chromosomes as revealed by silver staining technique at mitosis. Mol Gen Genet. 190:352–4.

89. Eiberg H (1974). New selective Giemsa technique for human chromosomes, Cd staining. Nature. 248:55.

90. Evans HJ, Ross A (1974). Letter: Spotted centromeres in human chromosomes. Nature. 249:861–2.

91. Nakagome Y, Abe T, Misawa S, Takeshita T, Iinuma K (1984). The "loss" of centromeres from chromosomes of aged women. Am J Hum Genet. 36:398–404.

92. Nakagome Y, Nakahori Y, Mitani K, Matsumoto M (1986). The loss of centromeric heterochromatin from an inactivated centromere of a dicentric chromosome. Jinrui Idengaku Zasshi. 31:21–6.

93. Maraschio P, Zuffardi O, Lo CF (1980). Cd bands and centromeric function in dicentric chromosomes. Hum Genet. 54:265–7.

94. Willard HF (1990). Centromeres of mammalian chromosomes. Trends Genet. 6:410–16.

95. Perry P, Wolff S (1974). New Giemsa method for differential staining of sister chromatids. Nature. 261:156–8.

96. Latt SA (1973). Microfluorometric detection of deoxyribonucleic acid replication in human metaphase chromosomes. Proc Natl Acad Sci USA. 70:3395–9.

97. Gebhart E (1981). Sister chromatid exchange (SCE) and structural chromosome aberration in mutagenicity testing. Hum Genet. 58:235–54.

98. Craig-Holmes AP, Shaw MW (1976). Cell cycle analysis of asynchronous cultures using the BudR-Hoechst technique. Exp Cell Res. 99:79–87.

99. Crossen PE, Morgan WF (1977). Analysis of human lymphocyte cell cycle time in culture measured by sister chromatid differential staining. Exp Cell Res. 104:453–7.

100. German J, Crippa LP, Bloom D (1974). Bloom's syndrome. III. Analysis of the chromosome aberrations characteristic of this disorder. Chromosoma. 48:361–6.

101. Lyon MF (1961). Gene action in the X-chromosome of the mouse (*Mus musculus* L.). Nature. 190:372–3.

102. German JL III (1962). DNA synthesis in human chromosomes. Trans NY Acad Sci. 24:395–407.

103. Peterson AJ (1964). DNA synthesis and chromosomal asynchrony. J Cell Biol. 23:651–4.

104. Priest JH, Heady JE, Priest RE (1967). Delayed onset of replication of human X chromosomes. J Cell Biol. 35:483–6.

105. Lyon MF (1972). X-chromosome inactivation and developmental patterns in mammals. Biol Rev. 47:1–35.

106. Latt SA (1975). Fluorescence analysis of late DNA replication in human metaphase chromosomes. Somat Cell Genet. 1:293–321.

107. Sahar E, Latt SA (1978). Enhancement of banding patterns in human metaphase chromosomes by energy transfer. Proc Natl Acad Sci USA. 75:5650–4.

108. Sahar E, Latt SA (1980). Energy transfer and binding competition between dyes used to enhance staining differentiation in metaphase chromosomes. Chromosoma. 79:1–28.

109. Angell RR, Jacobs PA (1975). Lateral asymmetry in human constitutive heterochromatin. Chromosoma. 51:301–10.

110. Lin MS, Alfi OS (1978). Detection of lateral asymmetry in the C band of human chromosomes by BrdU-DAPI fluorescence. Somatic Cell Genet. 4:603–8.

111. Angell RR, Jacobs PA (1978). Lateral asymmetry in human constitutive heterochromatin:frequency and inheritance. Am J Hum Genet. 30:144–52.

112. Gosh PK, Rani R, Nand R (1979). Lateral asymmetry of constitutive heterochromatin in human chromosomes. Hum Genet. 52:79–84.

113. Ikeuchi T (1984). Inhibitory effect of ethidium bromide on mitotic chromosome condensation and its application to high-resolution chromosome banding. Cytogenet Cell Genet. 38:56–61.

114. Balicek P, Zizka J (1980). Intercalar satellites of human acrocentric chromosomes as a cytological manifestation of polymorphisms in GC-rich material. Hum Genet. 54:343–7.

3
Normal Population Studies

HERMAN E. WYANDT AND VIJAY S. TONK

3.1 VARIANTS IN NON-BANDED CHROMOSOMES

The first major population studies of human chromosomes were an eventual
collaborative effort with data collected from 56 952 newborns from six different
countries [1–7]. These, for the larger part, were initiated on unbanded chromosome material and in most centers were based on examination of two to five
metaphases from each subject. The frequency of major chromosome abnormalities from these studies forms the basis of much of the statistical knowledge relating to frequencies of the major chromosome abnormalities, both numerical and
structural. In tabulations of the results of these studies [8], however, there was a
conscious effort to exclude normal morphological variants. The rationale for this
was that, even though variants of certain chromosomes were well known, chromosome banding techniques were discovered before most of these studies were
completed, so that it was quickly realized that accurate determination of variants
in the majority of chromosomes was not possible in non-banded material.
Nevertheless, a specific attempt to assess variants in unbanded chromosomes
from 4482 consecutive newborns was made by Lubs and Ruddle [9] in New
Haven, Connecticut. Their study included 3476 infants of White mothers and
807 infants of Black mothers. All of the children were phenotypically normal
except for one White child with low birth weight. Criteria for the most common
variants were established for chromosomes A1, C9, E16, the short arms and satellites of D and G group chromosomes, and Y long arm. A total of 2131 variants
were scored. A subpopulation was subsequently studied by Q- and C-banding
[10]. The overall frequency of variants (Table 3.1) was found to be nearly twice
as high in Black as in White children. In particular, a metacentric C9 variant (subsequently recognized as a 9qh inversion) was 20 times more frequent in the Black
children (1.24% : 0.06%); a large short arm on a D-group chromosome was four
times more frequent. Consistent with earlier small studies of adult males [11,12],
variants of Y chromosome were not different for Black and White children.
However, a large Y (>E18) was present in one of nine Chinese infants included
in the study and a second large Y was present in the only Turkish infant. Earlier

Table 3.1 Frequencies (%) of variants in Caucasian and Black infants in unbanded chromosomes (adapted from Lubs and Ruddle, 1971 [8])

Description of variant	Caucasian (n = 3476)	Black (n = 807)
1qh+	0.23	0.37
metacentric (C9)	0.06	1.24
Dp+ (= E18p)	13.80	21.18
Dp+ (> E18p)	0.25	0.87
Ds+ (> Dp)	2.24	4.21
Dss (tandem s)	0.09	0.25
Dp−	0.06	0
E16+ (> C6p)	2.04	3.96
E16 < E18	0.55	0.37
Gp+ (= E18p)	2.33	5.58
Gp+ (> E18p)	0.06	0
Gs+ (> Gp)	2.65	4.46
Gss (tandem s)	0.09	0
Totals	24.45	42.49
Y (> F19)	14.53	14.59
Y (> E18)	0.34	0.24
Y (< G22)	0.40	0.48
Y metacentric	0.11	0

studies had shown a high frequency of large Y in Japanese adult males [12]. The basis for the racial differences in variants in these early studies was not known. Lubs and Ruddle speculated that the frequency was lower in White children for one of two reasons: (1) the rate of elimination of unusual variants was more rapid in one race than the other because of a higher risk of associated phenotypic abnormalities; (2) the variants simply represented basic differences in heterochromatin in the two races. Later studies would confirm the second interpretation.

3.2 VARIANTS BY Q- AND C-BANDING

With the development of chromosome banding techniques in the early 1970s, several studies were done to determine the frequencies of variants in the general population by banding [10,13–20]. Criteria used in these and other studies were not standardized and populations selected often-introduced biases, making it difficult to directly compare frequencies in different populations. Nevertheless, there emerged recognition of the chromosome regions that are the most variable. The Standing Committee on Human Cytogenetic Nomenclature [21,22] attempted to devise a system whereby Q- and C-band variants could be numerically classified by size and/or intensity of staining (Table 3.2, Fig. 3.1).

Craig-Holms *et al.* [13–15] did C-banding studies in a series of 20 normal individuals selected at random from blood-bank donors. They classified C-banded heterochromatic regions into four types: (1) centromeres of all chromosomes; (2) acrocentric short arms and satellites; (3) secondary constrictions of

Table 3.2 Examples of how size and intensity descriptions can be expressed numerically (adapted from Paris Conference, 1971 [21])

Size*	Intensity
Q-banding	
1 Very small	1 Negative (no or almost no fluorescence)
2 Small	2 Pale (as on distal 1p)
3 Intermediate	3 Medium (as the two broad bands on 9q)
4 Large	4 Intense (as the distal half of 13q)
5 Very large	5 Brilliant (as on distal Yq)
C-banding	
1 Very small	0 No quantitation of intensity
2 Small	
3 Intermediate	
4 Large	
5 Very large	

*The definitions of "small", "large", etc., should be clearly presented in specific publications where the terminology is employed. A zero (0) may be used in any instance where quantitation is not used.

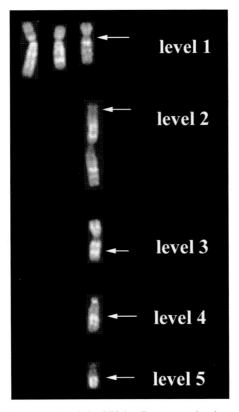

Fig. 3.1 Examples of chromosome bands by QFQ-banding representing the various intensity levels as designated by the Paris Conference in 1971 (see Table 3.2). Level 1 represented by the primary constriction (centromeric region) of most chromosomes (6, 8 and 10 are shown as examples) is the least intense. Level 5 represented by the distal end of the Y chromosome is the most intense (see text for details)

chromosomes 1, 9 and 16; (4) the distal long arm of the Y chromosome. Heteromorphisms involving the last three categories were particularly noted to occur in relatively high frequency. In their study, pairs of chromosomes from each individual were arranged in a line with pairs of the same chromosome or group from the other individuals. Chromosomes 1, 2, 3, 9 and 16 could be separated based on their morphology. The other chromosomes were classified by group. Chromosomes which showed a larger (+) or smaller heteromorphism (−) than others in the group were scored. For example, since chromosomes 17 and 18 could not be distinguished, any chromosome that consistently had a centromere that was larger or smaller than the other three in the group, was scored as having a 1 : 3 pattern and was scored as +; a variant that was larger or smaller in two chromosomes than in the other two had a 2 : 2 pattern and was not scored, etc. The percent of cells showing variation in size between cells was also scored for each chromosome or group. This system detected 20 variants in chromosomes 1, 3, 9 and 16 (Fig. 3.2a) and 11 variants in the remaining groups of chromosomes; eight were in the satellite and centromere regions of the D and G groups and three were in centromeric regions of the E and F groups (Fig. 3.2b). Of the 20 subjects, most had one to four C-band variants. Three had no detectable variants.

Early reports had already recognized variability in the length of the Y long arm [23–26]. The size of the Y varied from smaller than a G-group chromosome to as large as a D-group chromosome in apparently normal and fertile men. By Q-banding it was determined that the length of the brightly fluorescent distal end of the Y accounted for most of these size differences [27–31] and that the distal

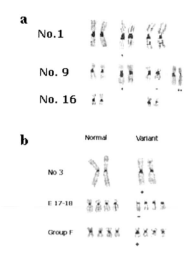

Fig. 3.2 (a) Normal C-band patterns of chromosomes 1, 9 and 16 are shown on the left. The other pairs demonstrate examples of each type of variant for nos. 1, 9 and 16. Additional heterochromatin (+); decreased heterochromatin (−); pericentric inversion (inv) which transposes a portion of heterochromatin to the short arm (Fig. 2, reprinted with permission from Craig-Holmes *et al.* [13]). (b) The normal C-band pattern and variants seen in chromosome no. 3, E 17–18 and group F (Fig. 3, reprinted with permission from Craig-Holmes *et al.* [13])

Q-bright end of the Y was dark by G- and C-banding. In small Y's the Q-bright region is greatly diminished in size or even absent [32,33]. A number of studies revealed racial differences, particularly in the frequency of large Y's. Based on the length of the Y chromosome, it was hypothesized that the large Y could have originated in a population of Mediterranean origin [34]. Other variant forms of the Y in normal males included pericentric inversions and satellited Y's. More detailed discussion of these differences is covered in Part II.

One of the first population assessments of Q-band variants in human autosomes was by Geraedts and Peason [16] in 221 Dutch individuals: 109 were females and 113 were males; 132 of the individuals were from 16 families; 75 individuals were from an additional three families. The Q-banding technique had the advantage that every chromosome could be identified. Furthermore, the variants allowed distinction between many pairs of homologs. Variants were first scored in the oldest generation of the 19 pedigrees with variants passed on from the mother coded as 1 and those from the father as 2. New polymorphisms, introduced in the family by marrriage, were also coded. The frequency of Q-band variants by this system was approximately four per individual with no significant difference between males and females. Excluding chromosomes 1, 9, 16, and the Y, the highest numbers of heteromorphisms were in chromosomes 3 and 13. The numbers of heterozygotes vs. homozygotes were also scored for each chromosome. Hardy-Weinberg expectations were calculated and expectations were met for chromosomes 3, 4, 14, 21 and 22. However, for chromosomes 13 and 15 there was an excess of heterozygotes and a lack of homozygotes. The excess of heterozygotes for heteromorphism of chromosome 13 appeared to come from the maternal side in the case of sons and from the paternal side in the case of daughters. Of interest in this regard, Fogle and McKenzie [35] studied 81 members of a Black kindred studied by sequential Q- and C-banding. Evidence for preferential segregation of Q heteromorphisms was found and was especially distorted for chromosome 13.

Muller and Klinger [17] studied polymorphisms, by C-, Q- and G-banding, in 376 neonates in a New York hospital. Classification of variants was according to the 1971 Paris Conference (Table 3.2). C-band variants of 1, 9 and 16 were compared to the length of the long arm of chromosome 21. Karyotypes were first examined by G-banding. Infants with a chromosome abnormality were excluded from the study. For those included, metaphases were examined by Q-banding alone, by C-banding alone and by Q- and C-banding of the same metaphases. The final classification of variants was made from the latter category. For chromosomes 1, 9 and 16, variations were seen in size or in the position of the centromere. The remaining chromosomes were scored for size of heterochromatin by C-banding and for intensity by Q-banding. C-banding revealed apparent partial inversions of heterochromatin into the short arms in 1.6% of no. 1's, 10.7% of no. 9's and 1.4% of no. 16's. Complete inversion of heterochromatin into the short arm occurred in about 0.6% of no. 9's. Chromosomes 6, 8, 10, 12, and the X had larger than average C bands in <1% of subjects. Chromosomes 7 and 11 had larger bands in 10% and 13% of subjects, respectively. Chromosomes 17–20 occasionally had C bands that were about twice the average size (0.0–2.0%). The D and G groups showed heteromorphisms in the short arm and satellite regions in every chromosome.

Mackenzie and Lubs [19] studied variants in 77 normal newborns from Grand Junction, CO. C-banding was preceded by Q- or G-banding, in some cases on the same cells so that variants on homologs by C-banding could be distinguished. Of 391 variants described, 225 (57.6%) were Q-band variants and 166 (42.4%) were C-band variants. Q-band variants, excluding the Y, were restricted to autosomes 3, 4, 13–15, 21 and 22. C-band variants, while fewer in number, were found to give at least one variant in every chromosome. Except for giant satellites on the acrocentric chromosomes, Q-band and C-band variants often represented different chromosome regions. Overall, an average of approximately five heteromorphisms was found per individual.

Lin *et al.* [20] studied Q-band variants in 930 consecutive newborns in a Canadian population that was 87% White and 13% Black and Oriental. Variants were classified by intensity level as outlined in the Paris Conference (1971), using methods similar to those of McKenzie and Lubs. A bright variable band in chromosome 3 was present in the long arm in 77% of cases. In about 33% this variant was present in both homologs. In <1% of cases the bright variant appeared to be inverted and was in the short arm. All cases were normal, whereas Soudek and Sroka [36] reported a higher incidence of this inverted bright variant in children with mental retardation (see Chapter 4).

Mikelsaar *et al.* [37–39] did several detailed studies of variants by G-banding and by Q-banding in an Estonian population of normal adults and of children with mental retardation. Variants more frequent in men than women included 16q+ in adults; 17ph+, 15p+ and short arm variants of 21 in mental retardation of unknown etiology (MRU); and 15pss in Down syndrome. Variants that were more frequent in children with Down syndrome than in normal adults were 9q+ and 15pss. Variants more frequent in Down syndrome than in MRU were 13ps, 14p+, 15ps+, 15pss and 22p+. Yq++ was also more frequent in MRU, but not significantly different from normal males. One variant in a patient with Downs was 14ps+ (unusually large bright satellites). Combinations of variants (multiple bright regions) in one patient and multiple G-band variants (9q+, 13p−, 17ph− and Yq−) in a second patient were unusual. Overall, Q-banding revealed no significant differences in the autosomes between sexes. Girls with MRU had a higher frequency of bright 3p11q11 than normal females or females with Downs, due to a greater number of homozygotes. Males with Down syndrome showed more frequent heterozygotes of 3p11q11 than normal men or boys with MRU. Girls with mental retardation showed a different distribution of homozygotes vs. heterozygotes for bright 4p11q11 and bright satellites on 15p than normal population. The frequencies of homozygotes for 4p11q11, 13p11q11, 13p13, 15p13 and 17p12 fit Hardy-Weinberg expectations in all populations. However, normal populations showed an excess of homozygotes for 14p13, 21p13, 22p13, 22p11 and 9q12: 14p12 was in excess in males; 21p13 and 22p13 were in excess in females; in MRU 21p13 and 22p13 were in excess in females. There were also differences between males and females for 11q11 and 16q11 in normal populations and for 15p12 in children with mental retardation. Overall, differences between males and females for all classes did not differ and an excess of variants for 13p such as reported by Geraedts and Person [16] was not found. The significance of the specific differences in distributions of variants, if any, has not been clarified in any more up-to-date studies.

38

3.3 THE NEW HAVEN STUDY

A significant attempt to study normal variants in a standardized way was made by Lubs *et al.* [10] in a New Haven study of 7- and 8-year-old children who had been followed from birth. Because the study of 4366 White newborns and 806 Black newborns had been initiated 8 years earlier [9], before banding techniques were available, a subsample of 400 children were selected by a randomization process that included equal numbers of White and Black children with IQs >85 and <85. G-banding was done on all of the children and assessment of variants was done by the new Q- and C-banding techniques. Although the study is not especially large, it was carefully designed. Guidelines for classification of the common chromosome variants by Q- and C-banding were similar to those adopted by the Paris Conference in 1971 [20], and a Supplement to the Paris Conference, published in 1975 [21]. Frequencies and criteria for classifying chromosome variants, described in this study, are referred to throughout much of this book, especially in the summaries of chromosome variants in Part II.

As in the Grand Junction study [19], Q and C band variants studied by Lubs *et al.* were classified as to intensity and/or size. Q-band intensity was divided into five levels, according to Paris Conference criteria (Table 3.2). Because Q- and C-banding were done on the same chromosomes, each chromosome could be ranked in order of its average C-band size (Fig. 3.3). Average C-band size for chromosomes 1, 9, Y and 16 were compared to the short arm of chromosome 16 (Fig. 3.4). Level 1 was ≤ one-half the length of 16p and level 5 was > twice the length of 16p. C-bands of the other chromosomes were classified as small (−) or large (+). Comparisons between Black and White children were made of the frequencies of heteromorphisms at the extreme levels for each chromosome (Table 3.3). Differences were found for chromosomes 4, 12, 18, 19 and 22, with the greatest difference being for chromosome 19. Ten percent of Black children had a large 19cen compared to 0% of White children, although, because of the low numbers of cases, none of these differences was statistically significant. C-band variants for chromosomes 1, 9 and 16 were more frequent, but level 1 variants were still not significantly different in the two races. However, level 5 C-band variants were significantly higher (nearly twice as frequent) in the Black children. Inversions in chromosomes 1 and 9 were classified into three types: 1h partial inversion, 9h partial inversion and 9h complete inversion. Only one 1qh partial inversion was found in Black children; 14 were found in White children. Partial inversions in 9h were more frequent in White than in Black children, but the difference was not significant. However, a significantly higher frequency of complete inversion of 9qh was found in Black children. No inversions in chromosome 16 were found in either race.

For Q-banding, significant differences in frequencies were seen for bright or brilliant heteromorphisms (levels 4 and 5) of the centromeres for chromosomes 3, 4 and for the satellites and short arms of acrocentric chromosomes. A particularly high frequency with a large short arm on chromosome 13 was seen in the Black population. Chromosomes other than 3, 4, the acrocentrics and the Y did not show polymorphisms by Q-banding. Overall, differences in frequencies of Q- and C-band polymorphisms related to IQ were not statistically significant, although large brilliant satellites on 21 were half as frequent in Black children with low IQ

C REGIONS RANKED BY SIZE

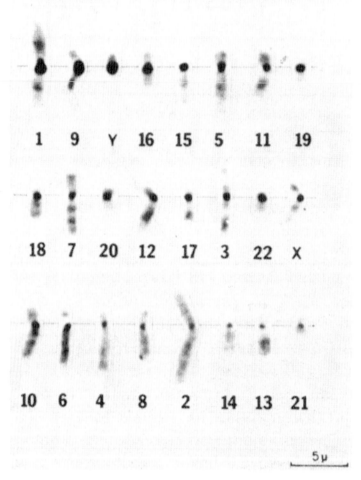

Fig 3.3 C karyotype. In this karyotype chromosomes, previously identified by Q or C banding, are arranged in the order shown. This sequence reflects the estimated average size of the C region for each chromosome from large to small (Fig. 1, reprinted from Lubs *et al.* (1977). In: Hook E, Porter IH, editors. Population Cytogenetic Studies in Humans. New York: Academic Press, pp. 133–59)

and large brilliant satellites on 22 were twice as frequent in White children with low IQ. Again, small numbers of children were represented in each group, and no attempt was made to extend these correlations to other family members. The issues of frequencies of heteromorphisms in selected populations with mental retardation, fetal wastage, aneuploidy or other detrimental effects are more appropriately discussed in the chapter that follows.

The major studies of frequencies of normal variants by Q- and C-banding are summarized in Tables 3.4 and 3.5. Although comparisons of the relative frequencies

CLASSIFICATION OF h REGIONS IN HUMAN CHROMOSOMES 1, 9 AND 16

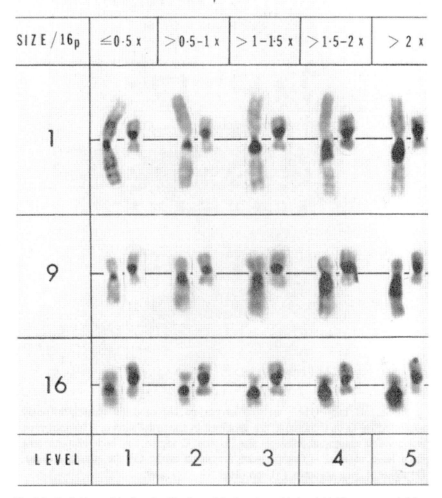

Fig. 3.4 Definitions of the five classifications of the h regions of 1, 9 and 16. These were coded from small to large (1–5). The short arm of 16 was used as a reference standard within the same cell. A code 1, for example, was assigned to an h region of 1, 9 or 16 if its size was judged to be less than half the size of 16p. A code 5 was assigned if it was judged to be more than twice as large as 16 p (Fig. 2, reprinted with permission from Lubs *et al.* (1977). In: Hook E, Porter IH, editors. Population Cytogenetic Studies in Humans. New York: Academic Press, pp. 133–59)

of variants involving different chromosome regions are tabulated, such comparisons do not necessarily identify the same variants or reveal any identifiable origin. As already seen, they mainly represent criteria used in different studies to classify variants into groups that seem most similar in size or intensity of staining. Technical variations in staining, in treatment, in degree of chromosome elongation

41

Table 3.3 Centromere polymorphism frequencies by race (C-banding) [Table 10, reproduced with permission from Lubs et al. (1977). In: Hook E, Porter IH, editors. Population Cytogenetic Studies in Humans. New York: Academic Press, pp. 133–59]

Chromosome region	White (n = 95)			Black (n = 97)		
	Small	Large	Total	Small	Large	Total
2c	1	–	1	–	3	3
3c	3	4	7	3	3	6
4c	3	–	3	3	7	10
5c	–	3	3	6	3	9
6c	2	3	5	1	–	1
7c	–	4	4	1	3	4
8c	–	1	1	–	–	–
10c	1	3	4	1	3	4
11c	6	–	6	3	1	4
12c	–	1	1	–	5	5
13c	2	3	5	5	4	9
14c	1	2	3	3	–	3
15p	–	4	4	–	5	5
15c	6	4	10	9	1	10
17c	4	2	6	2	4	6
18p	1	–	1	–	1	1
18c	9	–	9	7	8	15
19c	2	–	2	4	9	13
20c	6	1	7	1	5	6
21c	–	–	–	–	4	4
22c	1	2	3	4	8	12
Xc	–	5	5	–	1	1
Total	48	42*	90	53	78*	131

*$\chi^2 = 11.21$; $p < 0.005$.

Table 3.4 Frequencies of bright to brilliant Q autosomal variants from five early studies

Chromosome	Geraedts and Pearson, 1974 (n = 221)[a]	Muller et al., 1975 (n = 376)[b]	Lubs et al., 1976 (n = 400)[c]	Lin et al., 1976 (n = 930)[d]	Mikelsaar et al., 1976 (n = 349)[e]
3c	48.4	54.7	46.7	55.5	55.1
4c	2.7	2.8	8.1	14.1	28.4
13p	50.0	44.2	42.9	31.3	72.9
13s		7.5	3.5	1.9	9.3
14p	14.3	2.4	0.0	0.8	0.0
14s		12.3	6.0	0.2	10.2
15p	21.5	2.6	<0.1	0.2	0.0
15s		9.9	5.3	0.9	5.9
21p	24.4	2.6	<0.1	0.1	6.8
21s		16.5	5.1	1.1	0.0
22p	21.9	34.3	1.6	0.3	31.6
22s		26.5	4.9	0.3	5.1

[a]Normal Dutch population; 14 referred for diagnostic work-up had normal phenotype.
[b]Newborn population of 188 males and 188 females from Albert Einstein Hospital in New York.
[c]Randomly selected 7- and 8-year-olds from sequential newborn population, consisting of equal numbers of Blacks and Caucasians; half with IQ < 85; half with IQ ≥ 85.
[d]Consecutive newborns, 493 males and 437 females from St Joseph's Hospital, Ontario; parents consisting of 87% Caucasian and 23% Black or Oriental.
[e]Results from 208 normal adults and 141 mentally retarded children of Estonian nationality.

Table 3.5 C-band heteromorphism frequencies (%) for chromosomes 1, 9, 16 and Y

Chromosome	Holmes, 1971, unspecified C-band (n = 20)	Muller et al., 1975, mixed newborn C-band (n = 367)	McKenzie and Lubs, 1975, White C-band (n = 77)	Lubs et al., 1977 White C-band (n = 194)	Black C-band (n = 190)
1qh−	10	0.6	5	2	5
1gh+	2.50	8.10	12	11	12
1qh part inv		1.60	6	0.45	0.06
1qh total inv		0	0	0	0
9qh−	7.50	0.40	3	5.00	3.00
9qh+	5	8.00	10	7.00	10.00
9qh part inv		11.30	0.45	0.55	0.45
9qh total inv	2.50		1.07	0.13	1.07
16qh−		23.60	39	35	39
16qh+		6.50	4	2	4
16qh part inv		1.40	0	0	0
16qh total inv	5	0	0	0	0

or contraction, and even mutational events can change the appearance of a particular variant within an individual. There are also discrepancies in frequencies because of differences in ethnic origin, age distribution and ascertainment. Nevertheless, the relative frequencies of the most common variants are revealed. Relatively consistent from one study to another is the number of heteromorphisms per individual. By Q- and C-banding this number ranges from 4 to 6 with both techniques.

3.4 ADDITIONAL STUDIES OF RACIAL OR ETHNIC DIFFERENCES

Kuleshov and Kulieva [40] studied the overall frequencies of striking variants by G-banding in 6000 Russian newborns. Variants scored as 1qh+, 9qh+, and 16qh+, were identified as greater than one-quarter of the long arm; Gp+ or Dp+, larger than short arm of 18; Ds+ or Gs+, equal to or greater than the thickness of a long arm chromatid; Dss or Gss (double satellites); Yq+ (Y larger than G-group) and Yq− (Y less than the size of G group); Es+ (satellites on the short arms of chromosomes 17 or 18). The total frequency of these variants combined was 12.8 per 1000 births. They also determined frequencies in married couples with recurrent abortions and in couples with a history of congenital malformation in offspring (see Chapter 4).

Belloni et al. [41] studied a random sample of newborns in Central Italy by C-banding. The frequency of acrocentric variants was higher than reported in other populations.

Potluri et al. [42,43] did qualitative analysis of C-band inversion of 1, 9 and 16 studied in 200 infants in New Delhi (100 males and 100 females). Partial (minor) and half inversions of 1 and 9 were observed at modal levels in both sexes. Homozygous size combinations showed higher incidences than heterozygous size combinations for all three chromosomes. However, higher percentages of 1 and 9 inversions were seen in males than females. The percent of size differences between sexes were not significant. Heterozygous inversion combinations of 1 and 9 were more frequent than homozygous combinations in both sexes. No inversion of chromosome 16 was seen. They also observed a significant correlation between C-band size and inversion. The larger the size of the C band the higher is the incidence of inversion.

3.5 SPECIALIZED BANDING STUDIES

Verma, Dosik and Lubs [45] studied variants by QFQ and RFA techniques in 100 Whites. Six color classes distinguished by RFA and five intensity classes distinguished by QFQ. No consistent relationship was seen between color variants by RFA and intensity variants by QFQ. RFA variant frequencies for 13, 14, 15, 21 and 22 were 33.0, 38.0, 28.0, 50 and 24.5%. QFQ variant frequencies for 13, 14, 15, 21 and 22 were 56.5, 10.0, 10.0, 15.5 and QFQ. RFA revealed more differences between races than QFQ, 10.0%. In a comparable study of 100 American Blacks [46] studied by sequential QFQ and RFA banding, frequencies of QFQ and RFA heteromorphisms were higher in Blacks than in Whites. No racial difference was noted for chromosome 21 by RFA banding.

3.6 SUMMARY

Several groups have studied chromosome variants in different populations. While it is obvious that some common variants such as a large Y are more frequent in some populations than others, variations in the quality of preparations, in staining procedures, in degree of chromatin contraction and biases in selection of subjects make it difficult to directly compare frequencies for most of the other common variants. While controls for technical and methodological variations have been done in a few studies, most of these have involved small samples so that reliable data are not readily available. In this chapter we have tried to present an overview of the most significant studies. The common variants individually occurring in 1% or more of the population are represented in most of these studies. From these studies it is apparent that the different banding techniques, collectively, gave a potentially unique pattern of variants in each individual. Irrespective of population, the number of variants per individual is surprisingly consistent, and seems to be in the range of four to six per individual in an average chromosome preparation. This number becomes higher if extraordinary methods to distinguish subtle differences are used, as in the paternity studies of Olson *et al.* [48].

This chapter has dealt mainly with the findings in normal populations. Whether or not some striking variants, even some that are common, are totally innocuous may still need to be resolved. Distortions in variant frequency either in Hardy-Weinberg distribution or in distribution between sexes tend to be anecdotal or remain unexplained. It should be kept in mind, however, that distinction between normal and subclinical populations is not always easy to make. Review of heteromorphisms in clinical populations is covered in the chapter that follows.

References

1. Lubs HA, Ruddle FH (1970). Chromosome abnormalities in the human population: estimation of rates based on New Haven newborn study. Science. 169:495–7.
2. Jacobs PA, Melville M, Ratcliffe S, Keay AJ, Syme JA (1974). Cytogenetic survey of 11,680 newborn infants. Ann Hum Genet. 37:359–76.
3. Friedrich U, Nielsen J (1973). Chromosome studies in 5,049 consecutive newborn children. Clin Genet. 4:333.
4. Nielsen J, Sillesen I (1975). Incidence of chromosome aberrations among 11148 newborn children. Humangenetik. 30:1–12.
5. Sergovich F, Valentine GH, Chen AT, Kinch RA, Smout MS (1969). Chromosome aberrations in 2159 consecutive newborn babies. N Engl J Med. 280:851–5.
6. Hammerton JL, Canning N, Ray M, Smith S (1975). A cytogenetic survey of 14,069 newborn infants. I. Incidence of chromosome abnormalities. Clin Genet. 8:223–43.
7. Walzer S, Gerald PS (1977). A chromosome survey of 13,751 male newborns. In: Hook EB, Porter IH, editors. Population Cytogenetics. New York: Academic Press, pp. 45–61.
8. Hook EB, Porter IH (1977). Population Cytogenetics Studies in Humans. New York: Academic Press.
9. Lubs HA, Ruddle FH (1971). Chromosome polymorphism in American negro and white populations. Nature. 233:134–6.
10. Lubs HA, Patil SR, Kimberling WJ *et al.* (1977). Q and C-banding polymorphisms in 7 and 8 year old children: racial differences and clinical significance: In: Hook EB, Porter IH, editors. Population Cytogenetic Studies in Humans. New York: Academic Press, pp. 133–59.
11. Starkman MN, Shaw MW (1967). Atypical acrocentric chromosomes in Negro and Caucasian Mongols. Am J Hum Genet. 19:162–73.
12. Cohen MM, Shaw MW, MacCluer JW (1966). Racial differences in the length of the human Y chromosome. Cytogenetics. 5:34–52.
13. Craig-Holmes AP, Shaw MW (1973). Polymorphism of human C-band heterochromatin. Science. 174:702–4.
14. Craig-Holmes AP, Moore FB, Shaw MW (1973). Polymorphism of human C-band heterochromatin. I. Frequency of variants. Am J Hum Genet. 25:181–92.
15. Craig-Holmes AP (1977). C-band polymorphisms in human populations. In: Hook EB, Porter IH, editors. Population Cytogenetics. Studies in Humans. New York: Academic Press, pp. 161–77.
16. Geraedts JPM, Pearson PL (1974). Fluorescent chromosome polymorphisms; frequencies and segregation in a Dutch population. Clin Genet. 6:247–57.
17. Muller HJ, Klinger HP (1975). Chromosome polymorphism in a human newborn population. In: Pearson PL, Lewis KR, editors. Chromosomes Today, Vol. 5. Jerusalem: John Wiley.
18. Muller HJ, Klinger HP, Glasser M (1975). Chromosome polymorphism in a human newborn population. II. Potentials of polymorphic chromosome variants for characterizing the ideogram of an individual. Cytogenet Cell Genet. 15:239–55.
19. McKenzie WH, Lubs HA (1975). Human Q and C chromosomal variations: distribution and incidence. Cytogenet Cell Genet. 14:97–115.
20. Lin CC, Gideon MM, Griffith P, Smink WK, Newton DR, Wilkie Land Sewell LM (1976). Chromosome analysis on 930 consecutive newborn children using quinacrine fluorescent banding technique. Hum Genet. 31:315–28.
21. Paris Conference (1971). Standardization in Human Genetics. Birth Defects Original Article Series, Vol. 8, No. 7. New York: National Foundation, 1972.
22. Paris Conference Supplement (1975). Standardization in Human Genetics. Birth Defects Original Article Series, Vol. XI, No. 9. New York: National Foundation, 1975.
23. Bishop A, Blank CE, Hunter H (1962). Heritable variation in the length of the Y chromosome. Cytogenetics. 5:34–52.
24. Cohen MM, Shaw MW, MacCluer JW (1966). Racial differences in the length of the human Y chromosome. Cytogenetics. 5:34–52.
25. Makino S, Muramoto T (1964). Some observations on the variability of the human Y chromosome. Proc Jpn Acad. 40:757–61.
26. El-Alfi O (1970). A family with a large Y chromosome. J Med Genet. 7:37–40.
27. Bobrow M, Pearson PL, Pike MC, El-Alfi OS (1971). Length variations in the quinacrine-binding seg   ᵃt of human Y chromosomes of different sizes. Cytogenetics. 10:190–8.

28. Borgaonkar DS, Hollander DH (1971). Quinacrine fluorescence of the human Y chromosome. Nature. 230:52.
29. Laberge C, Gagne R (1971). Quinacrine mustard staining solves the length variations of the human Y chromosome. John Hopkins Med. J. 128:79–83.
30. Schnedl W (1971). Unterschiedliche Fluorescenz der beiden homologen Chromosoms beim Menschen. Hum Genet. 12:59–63 [German].
31. Schnedl W (1971). Fluorescenzuntersuchungen uber die Langenvaria-bilitat des Y Chromosoms beim Menschen. Hum Genet. 12:188–94 [German].
32. Borgoankar DS (1971). Non-fluorescent Y chromosome. Lancet. 1:1017.
33. Wahlstrom J (1971). Human chromosomes and fluorescence. Hum Genet. 12:77–8.
34. Lubs HA, Patil SR (1975). Mediterranean origin of long Y chromosome in Caucasians. American Society of Human Genetics, Baltimore, MD (8–11 October) (abstract).
35. Fogle TA, McKenzie WH (1980). Cytogenetic study of a large Black kindred: inversions, hetero-morphisms and segregation analysis. Hum Genet. 58:345–52.
36. Soudek D, Sroka H (1978). Inversion of "fluorescent" segment in chromosome 3: a polymorphic trait. Hum Genet. 44:109–15.
37. Mikelsaar A-V, Tuur SJ, Kaosaar ME (1973). Human karyotype polymorphism. I. Routine and fluorescence microscopic investigation of chromosomes in a normal adult population. Humangenetik. 20:89–101.
38. Mikelsaar AV, Viikmaa MH, Tuur SJ, Koasaar ME (1974). Human chromosome polymorphism. II. The distribution of individual s according to the presence of brilliant bands in chromosomes 3, 4, and 13 in a normal adult population. Humangenetik. 23:59–63.
39. Mikelsaar AV, Ilus T, Kivi S (1978). Variant chromosome 3 (inv3) in normal newborns and their parents, and in children with mental retardation. Hum Genet. 41:109–13.
40. Kuleshov NP, Kulieva LM (1979). [Frequency of chromosome variants in human populations]. Chastota khromosmnykh variantov v populiatsiiakh cheloveka. Genetika. 15:745–51 [Russian].
41. Belloni G, Benincasa A, Bosi A et al. (1983). Screening for cytogenetic polymorphisms in a random sample of live born infants from Italian population. Acta Anthropogenet. 7:205–17.
42. Potluri VR, Singh IP, Bhasin MK (1985). Chromosomal heteromorphisms in Delhi infants. III. Qualitative analysis of C-band inversion heteromorphisms of chromosomes 1, 9 and 16. J Hered. 76:55–8.
43. Potluri VR, Singh IP, Bhasin MK (1985). Human chromosomal heteromorphisms in Delhi new-borns. II. Analysis of C-band size heteromorphisms in chromosomes 1, 9 and 16. Hum Hered. 35:333–8.
44. Potluri VR, Singh IP, Bhasin MK (1985). Human chromosomal heteromorphisms in Delhi new-borns. VI. Inter-relationship between C-band size and inversion heteromorphisms. Cytobios. 44:149–52.
45. Verma RS, Dosik H, Lubs HA (1977). Size variation polymorphisms of the short arm of human acrocentric chromosomes determined by R-banding using acridine orange (RFA). Hum Genet. 38:231–4.
46. Verma RS, Dosik H, Lubs HA (1977). Frequency of RFA colour polymorphisms of human acro-centric chromosomes in Caucasians: inter-relationship with QFQ polymorphisms. Ann Hum Genet. 41:257–67.
47. Verma RS, Dosik H (1981). Human chromosomal heteromorphisms in American Blacks. III. Evidence for racial differences in RFA color and QFQ intensity heteromorphisms. Hum Genet. 56:329–37.
48. Olson SB, Magenis RE, Lovrien EW (1986). Human chromosome variation: the discriminatory power of Q-band heteromorphism (variant) analysis in distinguishing between individuals, with specific application to cases of questionable paternity. Am J Hum Genet. 38:235–52.

4
Heteromorphisms
in Clinical Populations

SHIVANAND R. PATIL AND HERMAN E. WYANDT

Several early studies suggested that variations in size of heterochromatic (C-banded) regions on human chromosomes might have deleterious effects [1–5]. In particular, studies by Lubs *et al.* [4,5] suggested an increased frequency of 9qh+ in retarded Black males. Tharapel and Summitt [6] studied 200 mentally retarded children and 200 normal adults by G-, Q- and C-banding techniques. They found an increased frequency of 9qh+ in Black but not in White subjects. No significant differences were seen for prominent or decreased size of short arms satellites of acrocentrics, 1qh, 9qh, 17ph, 17qh or for inversions of 9qh. Funderburk *et al.* [7] examined the frequency of minor variants in 1289 child psychiatric subjects with moderate retardation, autism or chronic behavior disorders. One-fourth had behavior problems and three-fourths had congenital abnormalities and severe mental retardation. Overall, they found an increased frequency of 9qh+. However, they also found only a random association with prominent qh regions, prominent satellites or long Y, although racial differences were evident as had been shown earlier. Matsuura *et al.* [8] studied Q-band heteromorphisms in 374 mentally retarded individuals from a variety of ethnic backgrounds, including Oriental, Filipino, Caucasian and Polynesian. Although differences were seen for 3cen, 13p and 14p, except for the size of the Y chromosome, none of these differences among the races was significant. 13cen and 13p11 were larger in a group with socio-familial retardation, significant at the 0.05 level, but because of the small size of the various groups, the observation was not considered to be important.

Soudek and Sroka [9] studied 100 Caucasian male patients with idiopathic mental retardation and 100 normal male controls by Q- and C-banding. Q-banding only was done on an additional 169 mentally retarded males and females who were not part of the controlled study [10]. Their results showed higher frequencies of 9qh−, 9qh+ and also of inv(3cen), and 16qh− in retarded individuals than in the control group. The differences were statistically significant for 9qh− and 16qh−, but were of borderline significance for 9qh+. A higher frequency of 9qh+ was found in the additional population studied by Q-banding, but no uniform phenotype

47

was associated, and risks appeared to be non-specific. Inversions of 9qh were found in controls, but not in patients. The ratio of brightly fluorescent 3cen was the same for both samples. Inversion of 3cen was increased in patients in the controlled study, but not increased in the additional patients without controls. Hence these authors were unable to confirm an effect of inv(3cen) on brain function. They also did not find differences in the length of the Y in the two populations. Studies by Mikelsaar *et al.* [11,12] also failed to find a significant increase in frequency of inv(3) associated with mental retardation.

Soudek *et al.* [9] give four attributes of heteromorphisms: (1) they contain repetitive satellite DNA; (2) they are inherited; (3) there is no syndrome associated; (4) possible phenotypic effects are (a) none or (b) an indirect selective effect. Based on a report by Barlow [13] they suggest that extra heterochromatin may affect birth weight, body weight, immunoglobulin levels and cell growth rate. They also point out the technical variables that make it difficult to compare different studies; namely, C bands contract less than the rest of the chromosome, and Q bands can vary depending on degree of photographic exposure [14]. Generally, there have been no adequately controlled studies to further suggest any role of variations in size of the common heteromorphisms directly on phenotype or in mental retardation.

4.1 VARIANTS IN SPONTANEOUS ABORTIONS AND REPRODUCTIVE FAILURE

Numerous studies have suggested indirect effects such as a higher incidence of spontaneous abortions associated with striking chromosomal variants such as a large Y or large satellites on acrocentric chromosomes. From the New Haven study of 4400 newborns, Patil and Lubs [15] determined that 50 mothers in the study had a history of three or more abortions. Twenty-nine of the newborns from these mothers were male and three of these (10.3%) had a long Y compared with 1.9% of infants of mothers with less than three abortions. This 5-fold difference was statistically significant. The proportion of pregnancies ending in prior abortion was also higher (33%) in mothers of infants with a long Y (2-fold over mothers in the overall study; 16%). Similar findings were reported by Genest [16].

Ford and Lester [17] studied the frequency of hyperdiploid cells in 10 fertile men, 10 subfertile men, 10 men with 9qh+ and 10 men with a pericentric inversion in 9qh (nine of these men were also subfertile). Three groups of females were also studied: a control group, five women with 9qh+, and six women with inv(9qh) (women were fertile but had histories of reproductive wastage). Fifty metaphases were examined from each group. The two male control groups did not differ from each other, whereas the two groups with variants had increased frequencies of hyperdiploid cells that were significant. Females showed similar results with significant differences from the control group. Aneuploidies involved C, D, E, F and G group chromosomes with no preference for any particular group.

Tsvetkova and Iankova [18] found no differences in the frequencies of routine variants between couples with reproductive failure and normal couples. Maes *et al.* [19] did a careful analysis on heterochromatin values in 15 couples with recurrent early abortion and 15 normal couples (Caucasian) and found no relationship between C heterochromatin lengths and recurrent abortions. Bobrow [20] attempted to critically review the literature on association of heterochromatic variants on reproductive failure manifesting as infertility or recurrent spontaneous abortions. Differences in methods made it difficult to interpret data, but the majority of evidence was against any significant effect of autosomal variants. Although conflicting reports occurred for the Y, he concluded that the effects of Yq− in infertility and Yq+ in recurrent abortion were mainly positive.

Eiben et al. [21] found a high frequency of 9qh+ (25% of patients) in teratozoospermic males with a significantly higher fraction of malformed spermatozoa in the 9qh+ group than in the chromosomally normal group. Rodriguez-Gomez et al. [22] examined heterochromatin length of 1, 9, 16 and Y on reproductive wastage in 100 couples with recurrent miscarriages and 106 normal couples. While Y/F index was increased in the test group, it did not reach significance. The mean C-band length for 1, 9 and 16 was lower than for the control group. Variants were not restricted to a specific chromosome. Their conclusion was that Y chromosome length as well as autosomal C-band size was not directly related to reproductive wastage. Krumina et al. [23] found a reduction in the amount of heterochromatin in couples with repeated spontaneous abortion. No differences were found for lengths of C bands on the Y chromosome. Del Porto et al. [24] suggest inv(9) as the only heteromorphism marginally related to recurrent miscarriages in an Italian population. Buretic-Tomljanovich et al. [25] studied couples with two or more miscarriages, couples with a stillborn child and couples with no history of miscarriages and at least two normal children. Results showed an increase in heterochromatin of chromosome 16 in couples with a stillborn or stillborn malformed child. The same couples had a significant increase in heterochromatin in potential zygotes. The Y/F index was lower in both groups. No increased heterochromatin was seen in couples with increased spontaneous abortions. Kuleshov and Kulieva [26] determined frequencies in 403 married couples with recurrent abortions, and in 113 couples with a history of congenital malformations in offspring. In the first group, excluding major chromosome abnormalities, 14.6% had extreme variants. This was compared with an overall frequency of 12.6% in 6000 newborns (see Chapter 3). In couples with history of congenital malformations in offspring, 13.3% had chromosome variants. In patients with Down syndrome (n = 139), 7.2% had variants (most frequent were Ds+, Dp+, Es+ and Yq+).

Podugol'nikov and Solonichenko [27] have suggested that the C-band heterochromatin is less in children with fetal alcohol syndrome and their parents, suggesting a possible susceptibility of these families to disturbances of developmental homeostasis.

4.2 NUCLEOLAR ORGANIZING REGIONS (NORs) AND NON-DISJUNCTION

Heritability of variations in the size or number of nucleolar organizing regions (NORs) in combination with Q-banding was first investigated in seven families by Mikelsaar et al. [28], and in two cases was used to determine parental origin of trisomy 21. Magenis *et al.* [29] and others have done extensive studies using heteromorphisms to determine parental and meiotic origin of trisomy 21 and of other chromosome abnormalities (see Chapter 5B) and have shown that the majority of trisomy 21 cases are maternal in origin and occur in the first meiotic division. Mikkelson *et al.* [30] studied NOR distribution in 110 families with trisomy 21; 76% of families were informative. Maternal meiosis I errors predominated in both high and low maternal ages. Paternal meiosis I non-disjunction errors were also more frequent than meiosis II errors.

A variety of mechanisms have been proposed for the cause of non-disjunction leading to trisomy 21 in Down syndrome. Aside from a parental age effect and determination of parental and meiotic origin, mechanisms causing non-disjunction have remained elusive. The most recent studies have suggested a reduction in meiotic recombination [31,32]. Others have suggested familial or genetic risks for increased rates of trisomy [33], while still others [34,35] have suggested at least three different categories of families at risk based on DNA polymorphism studies. Perhaps, however, the most persistent idea has been that of the influence of the heteromorphic regions themselves on non-disjunction.

Jackson-Cook *et al.* [36] first attempted to look at NOR variants in parents as a risk factor for Down syndrome. Parental origin of 41/50 cases of trisomy 21 was determined using Q band and NOR heteromorphisms. The addition of Q-banding in combination with NOR staining increased the informativeness of the variants with regard to parental origin of chromosome 21. Consistent with previous studies of parental origin of non-disjunction leading to trisomy 21 (see Chapter 5B), 69.3% were maternal errors and 30.7% were paternal errors. Also consistent with previous studies, meiosis I errors were more frequent: 72% in males and 93.2% in females. In 15 families an unusual NOR variant was observed – termed a "double NOR" (dNOR). All cells did not show dNORs. The frequency varied from 50% to 100%. The segregation ratio of dNORs did not differ from random. Although parental origin was not informative in all cases, and one case showed a dNOR in both parents, the frequency in informative parents of the Down cases was 13/41. Of the 9 indeterminate families, two had a dNOR in one parent. In only one of the 41 informative cases was the dNOR in the parent in whom normal meiosis occurred. None of the 50 normal control subjects had a dNOR.

The studies of Jackson-Cook have been controversial. Studies by other groups have not been able to confirm a role of dNORs in Down syndrome. Green *et al.* [37] studied the role of NOR size and frequency in 43 parents of Down children and 39 controls. The risk for having a child with trisomy 21 correlated with a higher frequency of associations and NORs per cell, but slightly lower NOR size. Although group differences were not statistically significant, specific types of NOR variants such as large NORs or dNORs appeared to be associated with an increased risk for trisomy 21 offspring. Results suggested NOR activity remained constant even though distribution of NOR regions varied. Others [38–40] also have been unable to confirm the finding of Jackson-Cook, regarding double NORs.

NORs have not generally been implicated in other chromosome abnormalities. However, at least one case has suggested a pathonomic role of dNOR leading to loss of an X chromosome in Turner syndrome [41].

Some of the problems in making the determination of whether NORs play a role in non-disjunction may be technical. Although variation in size or number of

NORs was often regarded to be heritable and fixed [42–44], NOR staining was early suggested to be a reflection of NOR activity [45–47], and the size of the NOR band was shown to correlate with the number of active rRNA clusters [48,49]. Balicek and colleagues [50,51] studied the intercalary fine structure of multiple satellites on acrocentrics and showed the light staining regions were heat-resistant and stained heavily with the RHG banding technique, indicating these regions were GC-rich. Such regions became extremely under-condensed when 5-azacytidine was added to cultures (Part II, Plates 39 and 40) and were felt to represent potentially active NOR sites that could show variably positive silver-staining anywhere along their length. Regions that were negatively silver-stained but RGH-positive were interpreted to be inactive NOR sites. Perez-Castillo et al. [52] report studies of a very long short arm on a chromosome 15 that was homogeneous in the proband, with up to four secondary constrictions in other sibs. Q and G bands stained similarly in four carriers but C-banding was more intense in three carriers than in the proband. DAPI staining showed only a proximal intense band. Silver staining revealed from none to four silver-positive regions. If only a single NOR was present it was usually the distal one. The distribution and number of NOR regions on different acrocentric chromosomes varied in each carrier. However, the mean number for all chromosomes was similar for the different carriers, suggesting an optimal threshold level of NOR activity. The exception was the index case that showed a mean value significantly higher than the other cases. Evidence for compensatory mechanisms in NOR activity has also been described by Nikolis and Kekic [53].

4.3 HETEROMORPHISM IN CANCER

Over the years a number of studies have suggested correlations of susceptibility to malignancy, both in solid tumors and in hematological disease, with increased heterochromatin length, striking size difference between homologs (asymmetry), or pericentric inversions in heterochromatic regions, especially in human chromosomes 1, 9 and 16.

4.3.1 Solid Tumors

The amount of heterochromatin in chromosome 1 and susceptibility for ovarian carcinoma was first suggested by Atkin [54]. Later in the same year Atkin and Baker [55,56] also reported the possible association of pericentric inversions of chromosome 1 with cancer, and subsequently suggested a higher frequency of asymmetry and inversions along with structural abnormalities of chromosome 1 in bladder cancer. Observations of variations in size, position and asymmetry of heterochromatin in chromosomes 1, 9 and 16 in patients with various malignant tumors (Table 4.1) were subsequently made by many groups [57–73]. Some studies, for example of colon cancer and pituitary adenoma, show differences for only the 9qh region [74–76]. Other studies show no differences in heteromorphisms between cancer patients and control groups [59,77–81].

Ovarian Cancer

Heteromorphism and abnormalities of chromosome 1 in ovarian cancer were first studied by Atkin and Pickhall [82], who found structural abnormalities in nine of

Table 4.1 Heteromorphisms associated with various forms of cancer and leukemia

Disease	Subjects		Controls		Chromosome and type	Ref.
	No.	Percent	No.	Percent		
A. Solid tumors						
1 Breast and ovarian	37		40		Q and C-band variants – no difference	77
2 Breast and ovarian	45		45		21 nor+	109
3 Breast and ovarian	33		180		C-banding variants – no difference	78
Breast and ovarian	71	80.3	35	31.4	C-band size variation and location	71
4 Breast	23		23		1qh variants	59
5 Breast			78		1qh+, 9qh+, 16qh+, inv(1), inv(9qh)	61
(a) Premenopausal					inv(9qh)	61
(b) Postmenopausal					inv(9qh)	61
(b) Familial					16qh+	61
(d) Sporadic					16qh−	61
6 Ovarian	14	64.3	9	67.0	Structural abnormalities of 1, inv(1qh)	82
7 Ovarian	13	43.8	7	19.5	1qh asymmetry	64
8 Ovarian	109		192		1qh asymmetry, inv(1qh)	69,70
9 Ovarian					Structural abnormalities of 1, inv(1qh)	73
10 (a) Cervical cancer	8	62.5			1qh variants more frequent than 9 or 16	58
(b) Cervical dysplasia	15	53.3		normal	1qh variants more frequent than 9 or 16	58
11 Cervical and uterine	38	72.9		32.2	Partial inversions	60
12 Endometrial cancer	23		5		Increased heterochromatin	72
13 Malignancy (non-spec.)	120		?		Variants of 1qh and 9qh; greater breakage	57
14 Malignancy (non-spec.)	128		111		1, 9 and 16qh asymmetry	110
15 Malignancy (non-spec.)	23		23		1qh in breast cancer	59
16 Malignancy (non-spec.)	90		91		1, 9 and 16qh asymmetry	62
17 (a) Epithelial	135	62.0	107	36.0	1qh asymmetry (62%), inv(1qh)(49%)	111
(b) Non-epithelial	67	49.0			1qh asymmetry (49%)	111
18 Squamous cell carcinoma	1		none		Structural abnormalities of 9qh	112
19 Child malignancy	38		42		9qh+; asymmetry in 1, 9 and 16qh	63
20 Solid tumors	101		85		inv(1qh)	65
21 (a) Testicular – less malignant	48		30		9qh+, ?16qh+	74
(b) Testidular – more malignant					9qh++, 16qh++ (borderline signif.)	74
22 Pituitary adenoma	100		30		inv(9qh)	76
23 Colon and rectal	23	37		21.8	inv(9qh)	75
24 Colon and rectal	62	62		18	inv(1qh), inv(9qh)	68
25 Bladder carcinoma	13	61.5	13	46.1	1qh+; inv(1qh); structural abnormalities of 1	55
26 Prostatic cancer	52		183		No differences	81
< age 70	56		56		1qh+ and 16qh+	81
27 Soft-tissue sarcomas	45		78		No differences	80

Table 4.1 Continued

Disease	Subjects		Controls		Chromosome and type	Ref.
	No.	Percent	No.	Percent		
B. *Hematological*						
1 NHL	55	90	50	44	inv(1qh), 1qh−, 9qh−	97
2 CML	15			controls	9qh−(+other), 9qh+ (−other), 1qh+	92
3 CML, PV and MDS					1, 9 and 16qh asymmetry	57
4 CML	56		?		1qh	88
CML	18				9qh same for leuk (PH1+) and non-leuk. cells	93
5 CML	50		50		None	94
6 CML	23		23		1qh−, asymmetry	90
7 Pre-leukemia	40	85	55	44	1qh+,1qh−	89
8 Pre-leukemia	11		11		none	90
9 Leukemia	50		50		Yqh+	85,95
10 AML	100		70		Excess sym 9qh; no age or sex difference	87
11 AML	19		?		1qh	84,88
12 AML	14		14		1qh−	90
13 ALL	45		?		1qh−	88
14 ALL	7		7		1qh−	90
15 Childhood ALL	67		50		1, 9 and 16qh−	113

14 tumors, possible abnormalities in three, and pericentric inversions of 1qh in the remaining two. Variations in size or inversion of 1qh were found in eight of the tumors. Constitutional variations in size and/or pericentric inversion of chromosome 1 were found in lymphocytes of six of the 14 patients. A German group [79], attempting to confirm the results of Atkin and Pickhall, studied 50 patients with ovarian cancer, 25 of whom had undergone treatment, and 25 controls, but were not convinced that variations in size in 1qh in the two groups were significant. However, studies by Naujouks and Weil [64] revealed a high frequency of asymmetry (size difference) in the 1qh region of homologs in 13 patients with ovarian cancer compared to seven controls. Kopf *et al.* [70] also found a high rate of asymmetry in 1qh in 109 patients with ovarian cancer compared to 192 healthy controls. This study was revisited by Islam *et al.* [73]: 99 of 111 ovarian cancer patients, which included many that had been studied up to 6 years earlier [70], had chromosomes 1 and 9 that each was heteromorphic by C- or G-banding in greater than 91% of patients. Heteromorphisms of chromosome 16 were present in 69%. Comparison was made of the frequency and types of chromosome abnormalities found in 33 surviving patients before and up to 6 years after cancer therapy. However, there is no mention of a comparison of heteromorphism frequency in this group.

Breast Cancer

Similar studies of amount, asymmetry or inversions in C-band heterochromatin were made for breast cancer [61,78,80]. Berger *et al.* [61] studied the patterns of heteromorphisms in the C-band-positive heterochromatin of human chromosomes 1, 9 and 16 in lymphocytes of 54 patients and 78 control individuals. An excess in the amount of C-band heterochromatin on chromosomes 1, 9 and 16, as well as a higher incidence of inversions in chromosomes 1 and 9, were observed in the breast cancer patients. Berger *et al.* [61] also noted a significant difference in C-band size on chromosome 16 between the familial and sporadic breast cancer patients. Heteromorphic differences were *not* noted in other breast cancer series by Atkin and Brito-Babapulle [60]. In a study of 33 female patients with ovarian or breast adenocarcinoma and 180 control women, Kivi and Mikelsaar [78] also found no causal association between the presence of C-band variants of chromosomes 1 or 9 or 16 and malignancy.

Soft-tissue Sarcomas

Forty-five patients with soft-tissue sarcomas and 78 control individuals were studied by Berger *et al.* [80] for patterns of heteromorphisms in the C-band-positive heterochromatin in lymphocytes. No consistent differences were found between these groups for relative size, symmetry–asymmetry between homologs or in the incidence of inversions in the heterochromatic regions of 1, 9 and 16.

Prostatic Cancer

Fifty-two prostatic cancer patients and 183 healthy controls studied by Lundgren *et al.* [81] showed no differences in C-band heteromorphisms on chromosomes 1, 9 and 16 regardless of the disease stage. However, younger patients (less than 70 years old) had significantly higher frequencies of large C bands on chromosome 1 and 16 compared to patients more than 70 years old. The investigators suggested that such differences could be age-related, but also speculated as to a possible relationship between the amount of constitutive heterochromatin on chromosome 1 and 16 and susceptibility to early development of prostatic cancer.

Laryngeal Cancer

Milan and Lamberti [83] did a case–control study of the C bands on chromosomes 1, 9 and 16 from PHA-stimulated lymphocytes in 16 individuals with laryngeal carcinoma and 13 normal controls. No significant difference with regard to heteromorphism size was observed between patients and controls. However, a significant difference was seen in the frequency of a partial pericentric inversion in chromosome 9 in the patients (56%), compared to controls (15%), suggesting that heteromorphism size could be a predisposing factor for the onset of laryngeal carcinoma. Fifty-two prostatic cancer patients and 183 healthy controls studied by Lundgren *et al.* [81] showed no differences in C-band heteromorphisms on chromosomes 1, 9 and 16 regardless of the disease stage. However, younger patients (less than 70 years old) had significantly higher frequencies of large C bands on chromosome 1 and 16 compared to patients more than 70 years old.

Nerve Tissue Cancers

C-banding studies were performed on blood samples from 100 patients with tumors of the nervous system (different grades of astrocytomas, meningiomas, pituitary adenomas, etc.) and 30 controls [76]. No significant differences in the frequency of C-band variants were seen between the patients and the controls.

An excess of pericentric inversion of 9qh region was found in some groups of tumor patients.

Head and Neck Cancers

Adhvaryu and colleagues [84,85] studied the variability of euchromatic and heterochromatic regions of Y chromosome in lymphocytes of patients with head and neck cancer as well as leukemic patients. The results were compared with similar data obtained in normal males. Based on the overall length of the Y chromosome in these three groups, they observed that the euchromatic region of the Y chromosome was shorter in patients with head and neck malignancies and the heterochromatic region was significantly larger in patients with leukemia.

Non-polyposis Colon Cancer

C-band heteromorphism was not seen in 17 unaffected or 12 affected individuals with inherited non-polyposis colon cancer [86].

4.3.2 Hematological Disorders

Several studies have also reported on C-band heteromorphisms in patients with hematological disorders (Table 4.1B).

Shabtai and Halbrecht [57] detected a higher frequency of chromosomes 1qh+ and 9qh+ variants in 30 patients with acute leukemia compared to controls. Le Coniat et al. [87] studied heterochromatin by C-banding in 100 acute non-lymphocytic patients (ANLL). No differences were found among patients related to age or sex. However, an excess of symmetrical distribution in 9qh was found compared to 70 healthy controls. Labal de Vinuesa et al. [88] studied 120 leukemic patients with CML, ALL and ANLL, and later [89] studied 40 preleukemic and 55 normal subjects for frequencies of heteromorphisms of chromosomes 1, 9 and 16. In the leukemic populations significant differences were found only for chromosome 1. In the preleukemic population a statistically higher frequency was found in the patient population (85%) compared to the normal controls (44%). Also, the latter patient population showed an increased incidence of size variation in chromosome 1 only, which the authors suggested was related to a high risk of leukemia and preleukemia. Based on densitometric measurements of C bands of chromosomes 1, 9, 16 and Y in 56 leukemic and preleukemic patients, Sampaio et al. [90] suggested a reduction in the amount of heterochromatin in the human genome could be more detrimental than an increase, and particularly could be a factor in hematological cancers. Petkovic et al. [91] studied 38 children with ALL and 90 control subjects. A longer C segment was observed on chromosomes 1, 9 and 16 in children with a three-fold higher frequency of homolog 9 heteromorphism compared to controls.

Rajasekariah and Garson [92] specifically studied translocations between 9 and 22 in chronic myelogenous leukemia (CML) in 15 patients. They reported translocations to randomly involve one chromosome 9 or the other. However, when 9qh was small, additional abnormalities in blast phase were seen, whereas when 9qh was larger, additional abnormalities were not found in blast transformation. Sadamori and Sandberg [93] made a similar observation in a study of

18 patients with CML. They also compared C-band polymorphism in the Ph1-positive cells and in normal PHA-stimulated lymphocytes and found no difference. Ph-positive cells were demonstrated to be clonal (i.e. to always involve the same chromosome 9 within a patient). Verma *et al.* [94] examined the length polymorphism of the Y chromosome in 50 males with CML and 50 normal males. No significance difference in the size of Y chromosome was noted between these two groups. Another study [95] of 44 CML patients and 44 controls found a significant increase in the length of C-band region in chromosomes 1, 9, 16 and pericentric inversions in CML patients compared to that in controls. Stuppia *et al.* [96] also noted a high frequency of C-band heteromorphisms in CML patients. However, they especially found an increased frequency of heteromorphisms in chromosome 16 using the Alu I digestion protocol Vs. the routine C-banding procedure.

In a study involving 50 patients with non-Hodgkin's lymphoma and 55 normal individuals, Labal de Vinuesa *et al.* [97] reported increased frequencies of inv(1), 1qh− and 9qh− variants in the lymphoma patients.

Ranni *et al.* [67] examined the incidence of heterochromatic variants in 26 patients with multiple myeloma (MM) and 55 controls. An increased frequency of heteromorphisms was seen in MM patients (92%) compared with controls (44%). The patients had a high incidence of inversions of 1qh (23% vs. 4% for controls) and 9qh (54% vs. 5% for controls). Overall, the heteromorphic variants most frequently involved were 1qh−, inv(1), inv(9) and 16qh−. The authors reported that the 1qh− was seen both in MM and in hematological malignancies, whereas 1qh−, inv(1), inv(9), and 16qh− variants are frequently present in MM, lymphomas and solid tumors.

A few studies have indicated that there are no differences among the different tissues of the same individual, indicating that the heteromorphic variants observed are constitutional in nature [58,89,93]. Recently, an acquired pericentric inversion of chromosome 9qh was reported in a patient with essential thrombocytopenia [98]. Chromosome analysis from PHA-stimulated cultures from a blood sample did not show the inversion. The significance of the inversion in the pathogenesis of essential thrombocytopenia in this case can only be speculated. However, the case raises an interesting point – namely, when an unusual heteromorphism is seen in the bone marrow sample of a patient with a hematological disorder it may be important to determine whether it is acquired or constitutional, rather than assuming the latter.

4.3.3 Overview

Association of various types of cancers and leukemias (Table 4.1) with higher heteromorphism frequencies, especially asymmetry (striking differences between homologs) is intriguing. In spite of the volume of reports suggesting such an association, the role, if any, of constitutive heterochromatin variation in the development of malignancies remains unclear. This association is even less clear for hematological disorders. Few studies have tried to differentiate variations that are *acquired* vs. those that are *constitutional* in nature, a distinction that may be important in determining whether observed differences are causal or a result of the neoplastic process. Secondly, studies of cancer patients have been small, and few have rigorously matched cancer patients and controls for age, ethnicity, race, etc. As aptly pointed out by Erdtmann [99] technical factors such as quality of preparations, criteria for scoring variants and variations in methodology between studies also do not allow direct comparisons of results from different studies, or definitive conclusions to be drawn from existing data. Thirdly, only a few studies have looked for mosaicism in cancer patients vs. normal controls. Mosaicism for C-band heteromorphism has been reported previously [100]. Doneda *et al.* [101] in a study of three families with a high incidence of cancer, reported C-band length mosaicism for chromosome 1 in lymphocytes from six cancer patients and from one normal individual from these families. However, it is not known how common such mosaicism is. A higher rate of mosaicism for the length differences of C-band heteromorphism might be expected, especially if unequal mitotic crossing-over contributes to an inherent chromosome instability in cancer patients vs. controls, as has been speculated [99].

A possible argument against heterochromatin involvement in cancer is the notable example of ICF syndrome, a rare autosomal recessive genetic condition that has the characteristic features of immunodeficiency, centromeric heterochromatin instability, and facial anomalies, but cancer is not associated. Frequent rosette formation and multiple copies of chromosome arms joined at their qh regions are suggested to be due to defective DNA methylation. Classical satellite 2 DNA in the pericentromeric regions of chromosomes 1 and 16 in leukocytes from ICF patients is hypomethylated compared to leukocytes from normal individuals [102,103]. On the other hand, Qu *et al.* [104] recently reported frequent hypomethylation of pericentromeric DNA in chromosomes 1 and 16 in Wilms tumors. They found a significant relationship between the loss of 16q and hypomethylation of 16qh satellite 2 DNA, suggesting that this hypomethylation is causally involved.

Finally, not all apparent variants involve only heterochromatin. Rearrangements in the pericentromeric region of chromosome 1 or 16, for example, frequent in several types of cancers, are now known to involve particular oncogenes that are close to the pericentromeric regions [105–108]. Inversions or insertions of these genes into heterochromatin regions could certainly play a role in turning such genes on or off by virtue of position effect.

References

1. Halbrecht I, Shabtay F (1976). Human chromosome polymorphism and congenital malformations. Clin Genet. 10:113–22.
2. Say B, Carpenter NJ, Lanier PR, Banez C, Jones K, Coldwell JG (1977). Chromosome variants in children with psychiatric disorders. Am J Psychiatry. 134:424–6.
3. Lubs HA, Ruddle FH (1971). Chromosome polymorphism in American negro and white populations. Nature. 233:134–6.
4. Lubs HA, Kimberling WJ, Hecht F *et al.* (1977). Racial differences in the frequency of Q and C chromosomal heteromorphisms. Nature. 268:631–3.
5. Lubs HA, Patil SR, Kimberling WJ *et al.* (1977). Q and C-banding polymorphisms in 7 and 8 year old children: racial differences and clinical significance. In: Hook E, Porter IH, editors. Population Cytogenetic Studies in Humans. New York: Academic Press, pp. 133–59.
6. Tharapel AT, Summitt RL (1978). Minor chromosome variations and selected heteromorphisms in 200 unclassifiable mentally retarded patients and 200 normal controls. Hum Genet. 41:121–30.
7. Funderburk SJ, Guthrie D, Lind RC, Muller HM, Sparkes RS, Westlake JR (1978). Minor chromosome variants in child psychiatric patients. Am J Med Genet. 1:301–8.

8. Matsuura JS, Mayer M, Jacobs PA (1979). A cytogenetic survey of an institution for the mentally retarded. III. Q-band chromosome heteromorphisms. Hum Genet. 523:203–10.

9. Soudek D, Sroka H (1979). Chromosomal variants in mentally retarded and normal men. Clin Genet. 16:109–16.

10. Soudek D, Sroka H (1978). Inversion of "fluorescent" segment in chromosome 3: a polymorphic trait. Hum Genet. 44:109–15.

11. Mikelsaar AV, Ilus T, Kivi S (1978). Variant chromosome 3 (inv3) in normal newborns and their parents, and in children with mental retardation. Hum Genet. 41:109–13.

12. Mikelsaar AV, Kaosaar ME, Tuur SJ, Viikmaa MH, Talvik TA, Laats J (1975). Human karyotype polymorphisms. III. Routine and fluorescence microscope investigation of chromosomes in normal adults and mentally retarded children. Humangenetik. 26:1–23.

13. Barlow P (1973). The influence of inactive chromosomes on human development. Hum Genet. 17:105–36.

14. Overton KM, Magenis RE, Brady T, Chamberlin J, Parks M (1976). Cytogenetic darkroom magic: now you see them, now you don't. Am J Hum Genet. 28:417–19.

15. Patil SR, Lubs HA (1977). A possible association of long Y chromosomes and fetal loss. Hum Genet. 35:233–5.

16. Genest P (1979). Chromosome variants and abnormalities in 51 married couples with repeated spontaneous abortions. Clin Genet. 16(6):387–9.

17. Ford JH, Lester P (1978). Chromosomal variants and nondisjunction. Cytogenet Cell Genet. 21:300–3.

18. Tsvetkova TG, Iankova MF (1979). [Human chromosome polymorphism and disordered reproductive function. I. Routine chromosome variants]. Genetika. 15:1858–69 [Russian].

19. Maes A, Stassen C, Hens L et al. (1983). C heterochromatin variation in couples with recurrent early abortions. J Med Genet. 20:350–6.

20. Bobrow M (1985). Heterochromatic chromosome variation and reproductive failure. [review]. Exp Clin Immunogenet. 2:97–105.

21. Eiben B, Leipoldt M, Rammelsberg O, Krause W, Engel W (1987). High incidence of minor chromosomal variants in teratozoospermic males. Andrologia. 19:684–7.

22. Rodriguez-Gomez MT, Martin-Sempere MJ, Abrisqueta JA (1987). C-band length variability and reproductive wastage. Hum Genet. 75:56–61.

23. Kruminia AR, Kroshkina VG, Voskoboinik NI, Reshetnikov AN (1987). [Quantitative analysis of C segments of chromosomes 1,9,16 and Y in couples with reproductive disorders]. Genetika. 23:540–3 [Russian].

24. Del Porto G, D'Alessandro E, Grammatico P et al. (1993). Chromosome heteromorphisms and early recurrent abortions. Hum Reprod. 8:755–8.

25. Buretic-Tomljanovic A, Rodojcic-Badovinac A, Vlastelic I, Randic LJ (1997). Quantitative analysis of constitutive heterochromatin in couples with fetal wastage. Am J Reprod Immun. 38:201–4.

26. Kuleshov NP, Kulieva LM (1979). [Frequency of chromosome variants in human populations]. Genetika. 15:745–51 [Russian].

27. Podugol'nikova OA, and Solonichenko VG (1994). [The C heterochromatin of chromosomes 1, 9, 16 and Y in patients with Noonan's syndrome]. Tsitol Genet. 28:85–8 [Russian].

28. Mikelsaar AV, Schwarzacher HG, Schnedl W, Wagenbichler P (1977). Inheritance of Ag-stainability of nucleolus organizer regions. Investigations in 7 families with trisomy 21. Hum Genet. 38:183–8.

29. Magenis RE, Overton KM, Chamberlin J, Brady T, Lovrien E (1977). Prental origin of the extra chromosome in Down's syndrome. Hum Genet. 37:7–16.

30. Mikkelsen M, Poulsen H, Grinsted J, Lange A (1980). Non-disjunction in trisomy 21: study of chromosomal heteromorphisms in 110 families. Ann Hum Genet. 44:17–28.

31. Warren AC, Chakravarti A, Wong C et al. (1987). Evidence for reduced recombination on the nondisjoined chromosomes 21 in Down syndrome. Science. 237:652–4.

32. Sherman SL, Takaesu N, Freeman SB et al. (1991). Trisomy 21: association between reduced recombination and nondisjunction. Am J Hum Genet. 49:608–20.

33. Hobbs CA, Sherman SL, Yi P et al. (2000). Polymorphisms in genes involved in folate metabolism as maternal risk factors for Down syndrome. Am J Hum Genet. 67:623–30.

34. Pangalos CG, Talbot CC Jr, Lewis JG et al. (1992). DNA polymorphism analysis in families with recurrence of free trisomy 21. Am J Hum Genet. 51:1015–27.

35. Pangalos C, Avramopoulos D, Blouin JL et al. (1994). Understanding the mechanism(s) of mosaic trisomy 21 by using DNA polymorphism analysis. Am J Hum Genet. 54:473–81.

36. Jackson-Cook CK, Flannery DB, Corey LA, Nance WE, Brown JA (1985). Nucleolar organizer region variants as a risk factor for Down syndrome. Am J Hum Genet. 37: 1049–61.
37. Green JE, Rosenbaum KN, Rapoport SI, Schapiro MB, and White BJ (1989). Variant nucleolar organizing regions and the risk of Down syndrome. Clin Genet. 35:243–50.
38. Serra A, Bova R (1990). Acrocentric chromosome double NOR is not a risk factor for Down syndrome. Am J Med Genet Suppl. 7:169–74.
39. Sheng WW, Perng CK, Wuu KD (1992). Double NOR is not a good indicator of risk for Down syndrome. Jpn J Hum Genet. 37:151–5.
40. Hassold T, Jacobs PA, Pettay D (1987). Analysis of nucleolar organizing regions in parents of trisomic spontaneous abortions. Hum Genet. 76:381–4.
41. Jones C, Ahmed I, Cummings MR, Rosenthal IM (1988). Association of double NOR variant with Turner syndrome. Am J Med Genet. 30:725–32.
42. Mikelsaar AV, Schwarzacher HG, Schnedl W, Wagenbichler P (1977). Inheritance of Ag-stainability of nucleolus organizer regions. Investigations in 7 families with trisomy 21. Hum Genet. 38:183–8.
43. Markovic VD, Worton RG, Berg JM (1978). Evidence for the inheritance of silver-stained nucleolus organizer regions. Hum Genet. 41:181–7.
44. Dev VG, Byrne J, Bunch G (1979). Partial translocation of NOR and its activity in a balanced carrier and in her cri-du-chat fetus. Hum Genet. 51:277–80.
45. Miller DA, Dev VG, Tantravahi R, Croce CM, Miller OJ (1978). Human tumor and rodent–human hybrid cells with an increased number of active human NORs. Cytogenet Cell Genet. 21:33–41.
46. Lau Y-F, Wertelecki W, Pfeiffer RA, Arrighi FE (1979). Cytological analyses of a 14p+ variant by means of N-banding and combinations of silver staining and chromosome bandings. Hum Genet. 46:75–82.
47. Bernstein R, Dawson B, Griffiths J (1981). Human inherited marker chromosome 22 short-arm enlargement: investigation of rDNA gene multiplicity, Ag-band size, and acrocentric association. Hum Genet. 58:135–9.
48. Warburton D, Atwood KC, Henderson AS (1976). Variation in the number of genes for rRNA among human acrocentric chromosomes: correlation with frequency of satellite association. Cytogenet Cell Genet. 17:221–30.
49. Miller DA, Tantravahi R, Dev VG, Miller OJ (1977). Frequency of satellite association of human chromosomes is correlated with amount of Ag-staining of the nucleolus organizer region. Am J Hum Genet. 29:490–502.
50. Balicek P, Zizka J (1980). Intercalar satellites of human acrocentric chromosomes as a cytological manifestation of polymorphisms in GC-rich material. Hum Genet. 54:343–7.
51. Balicek P, Zizka J, Skalska H (1982). RGH-band polymorphism of the short arms of human acrocentric chromosomes and relationship of variants to satellite association. Hum Genet. 62:237–9.
52. Perez-Castillo A, Martin-Lucas MA, Abrisqueta JA (1986). New insights into the effects of extra nucleolus organizer regions. Hum Genet. 72:80–2.
53. Nikolis J, Kekic V (1986). De novo 21/21 translocation Down syndrome. Studies of parental origin of the translocation and acrocentric associations in parents. Hum Genet. 73:127–9.
54. Atkin NB (1977). Chromosome 1 heteromorphism in patients with malignant disease: a constitutional marker for a high risk group? Br Med J. 1:358.
55. Atkin NB, Baker MC (1977). Pericentric inversion in chromosome 1: frequency and possible association with cancer. Cytogenet Cell Genet. 19:180–4.
56. Atkin NB, Baker MC (1977). Abnormal chromosomes and number 1 heterochromatin variants in C-banded preparations from 13 bladder carcinomas. Cytobios. 18:101–9.
57. Shabtai F, Halbrecht I (1979). Risk of malignancy and chromosomal polymorphism: a possible mechanism of association. Clin Genet. 15:73–7.
58. Heneen WK, Habib ZA, Rohme D (1980). Heteromorphism of constitutive heterochromatin in carcinoma and dysplasia of the uterine cervix. Eur J Obstet Gynecol Reprod Biol. 10:173–82.
59. Aguilar L, Lisker R, Ruiz L, Mutchinick O (1981). Constitutive heterochromatin polymorphisms in patients with malignant disease. Cancer. 47:2437–42.
60. Atkin NB, Brito-Babapulle V (1983). Chromosome 1 C-band heteromorphism in patients with carcinoma in situ and invasive carcinoma of the cervix uteri. Austr NZ J Obstet Gynaecol. 23:73–6.
61. Berger R, Bernheim A, Kristoffersson U, Mitelman F, Olsson H (1985). C-band heteromorphism in breast cancer patients. Cancer Genet Cytogenet. 18:37–42.

62. Petkovic I (1983). Constitutive heterochromatin of chromosomes 1, 9, and 16 in 90 patients with malignant disease and 91 controls. Cancer Genet Cytogenet. 10:151–8.
63. Petkovic I, Nakic M, Cepulic M, Tiefenbach A, Konja J (1985). Variability of chromosomes 1, 9 and 16 in children with malignant diseases. Cancer Genet Cytogenet. 16:169–73.
64. Naujoks H, Weil H (1985). Heterochromatic C-bands of chromosome 1 in ovarian cancer patients. Cancer Detect Prev. 8:151–3.
65. Suciu S (1986). Constitutive heterochromatin studies in patients with solid tumors. J Cancer Res Clin Oncol. 111:291–4.
66. Gosh PK, Shome D, Sahay S, Pa A, Gosh R (1986). Polymorphism of constitutive heterochromatin in cancer of cervix uteri. Indian J Med Res. 84:601–6.
67. Ranni NS, Labal de Vinuesa M, Mudry de Pargament M, Slavutsky I, Larripa I (1987). Heterochromatic variants and their association with neoplasias. III. Multiple myeloma. Cancer Genet Cytogenet. 28:101–5.
68. Labal de Vinuesa M, Mudry de Pargament M, Slavutsky I, Meiss R, Chopita N, Larripa I (1988). Heterochromatic variants and their association with neoplasias. IV. Colon adenomas and carcinomas. Cancer Genet Cytogenet. 31:171–4.
69. Kopf I, Islam MQ, Friberg LG, Levan G (1989). Familial occurrence of cancer and heteromorphism of the heterochromatic segment of chromosome 1. Hereditas. 110:79–83.
70. Kopf I, Strid KG, Islam MQ et al. (1990). Heterochromatin variants in 109 ovarian cancer patients and 192 healthy subjects. Hereditas. 113:7–16.
71. Adhvaryu SG, Rawal UM (1991). C-band heterochromatin variants in individuals with neoplastic disorders: carcinoma of breast and ovary. Neoplasma. 38:379–84.
72. Polishchuk LZ, Nesina IP (1993). [Polymorphism of the C-band segments of chromosomes 1, 9 and 16 in the peripheral blood lymphocytes of patients with endometrial cancer]. Tsitol Genet. 27:66–71 [Russian].
73. Islam MQ, Kopf I, Levan A, Granberg S, Friberg LG, Levan G (1993). Cytogenetic findings in 111 ovarian cancer patients: therapy-related chromosome aberrations and heterochromatic variants. Cancer Genet Cytogenet. 65:35–46.
74. Robson MK, Anderson JM, Garson OM, Matthews JP, Sandeman TF (1981). Constitutive heterochromatin (C-banding) studies in patients with testicular malignancies. Cancer Genet Cytogenet. 4:319–23.
75. Heim S, Berger R, Bernheim A, Mitelman F (1985). Constitutional C-band pattern in patients with adenomatosis of the colon and rectum. Cancer Genet Cytogenet. 18:31–5.
76. Rey JA, Bello J, de Campos JM, Benitez J, Valcarcel E, Castro PM (1985). C-banding studies in lymphocytes from patients with tumors of the nervous system. Cancer Genet Cytogenet. 15:129–36.
77. Kivi S, Mikelsaar AV (1980). Q- and C-band polymorphisms in patients with ovarian or breast carcinoma. Hum Genet. 56:111–14.
78. Kivi S, Mikelsaar AV (1987). C-band polymorphisms in lymphocytes of patients with ovarian or breast cancer. Cancer Genet Cytogenet. 28:77–85.
79. Adomat W, Weise W (1981). [Heterochromatin polymorphism of A1 chromosome in patients with ovarian carcinoma]. Zentralbl Gynakol. 103:865–73 [German].
80. Berger R, Berheim A, Mitelman F, Rydholm A (1983). C-band pattern in lymphocytes of patients with soft tissue sarcomas. Cancer Genet Cytogenet. 9:145–50.
81. Lundgren R, Berger R, Kristoffersson U (1991). Constitutive heterochromatin C-band polymorphism in prostatic cancer. Cancer Genet Cytogenet. 51:57–62.
82. Atkin NB, Pickhall VJ (1977). Chromosomes 1 in 14 ovarian cancers. Heterochromatin variants and structural changes. Hum Genet. 38:25–33.
83. Milan C, Lamberti L (1996). Study of C-polymorphisms of chromosomes 1, 9 and 16 in lymphocytes of patients with laryngeal carcinoma. Boll Soc Ital Biol Sper. 72:187–94.
84. Adhvaryu SG, Dave BJ, Trivedi AH, Rawal UM, Jani KH (1989). Variability of euchromatic and heterochromatic regions of Y chromosomes in different types of cancer patients. Tumori. 75:547–9.
85. Adhvaryu SG, Jani KH, Trivedi AH, Dave BJ, Rawal UM (1989). Y chromosome in leukemia patients. A study on the heteromorphic nature of its heterochromatic segment. Neoplasma. 36:343–7.
86. Lukeis R, Garson OM, Macrae FA, St John DJ, Whitehead RH (1987). Chromosome studies in inherited nonpolyposis colon cancer syndrome. Cancer Genet Cytogenet. 27:111–24.

87. Le Coniat M, Vecchione D, Bernheim A, Berger R (1982). C-banding studies in acute nonlymphocytic leukemia. Cancer Genet Cytogenet. 5:327–31.
88. Labal de Vinuesa M, Larripa I, Mudry de Pargament M, Brieux de Salum S (1984). Heterochromatic variants and their association with neoplasias. I. Chronic and acute leukemia. Cancer Genet Cytogenet. 13:297–302.
89. Labal de Vinuesa M, Larripa I, Mudry de Pargament M, Brieux de Salum S (1985). Heterochromatic variants and their association with neoplasias. II. Preleukem states. Cancer Genet Cytogenet. 14:31–5.
90. Sampaio DA, Mattevi MS, Cavalli IJ, Erdtmann B (1989). Densitometric measurements of C bands of chromosomes 1, 9, 16, and Y in leukemic and preleukemic disorders. Cancer Genet Cytogenet. 4:71–8.
91. Petkovic I, Nakic M, Konja J (1991). Heterochromatic variability in children with acute lymphoblastic leukemia. Cancer Genet Cytogenet. 54:67–9.
92. Rajasekariah P, Garson OM (1981). C-banding studies in patients with Ph1 + chronic granulocytic leukemia. Pathology. 13:197–203.
93. Sadamori N, Sandberg AA (1983). The clinical and cytogenetic significance of C-banding on chromosome #9 in patients with Ph1-positive chronic myeloid leukemia. Cancer Genet Cytogenet. 8:235–41.
94. Verma RS, Thomas S, Coleman M, Silver RT, Dosik H (1987). Length polymorphisms of the human Y chromosome in patients with chronic myelogenous leukemia. Cancer Genet Cytogenet. 24:295–7.
95. Adhvaryu SG, Dave BJ, Trivedi AH, Jani KH, Vyas RC (1987). Heteromorphism of C-band positive chromosomal regions in CML patients. Cancer Genet Cytogenet. 27:33–8.
96. Stuppia L, Guanciali Franchi P, Calabrese G, Di Virgilio C, Parruti G, Palka G (1989). Heterochromatic polymorphisms of chromosome 16 evidenced by Alu I endonuclease digestin in chronic myelogenous leukemia. Cancer Genet Cytogenet. 39:139–40.
97. Labal de Vinuesa M, Slavutsky I, Mudry de Pargament M, Larripa I (1988). Heterochromatic variants and their association with neoplasias. V. Non-Hodgkin's lymphomas. Cancer Genet Cytogenet. 31:175–8.
98. Wan TS, Ma SK, Chan LC (2000). Acquired pericentric inversion of chromosome 9 in essential thrombocythemia. Hum Genet. 106:669–70.
99. Erdtmann (1982). Aspects of evaluation, significance and evolution of human C-band heteromorphism. Hum Genet. 61:281–94.
100. Craig-Holmes AP, Moore FB, Shaw MW (1975). Polymorphism of human C-band heterochromatin. II. Family studies suggestive for somatic crossing over. Am J Hum Genet. 27:178–89.
101. Doneda L, Conti AF, Gualandri V, Larizza L (1987). Mosaicism in the C-banded region of chromosome 1 in cancer families. Cancer Genet Cytogenet. 27:261–8.
102. Jeanpierre M, Turleau C, Aurias A et al. (1993). An embryonic-like methylation pattern of classical satellite DNA is observed in ICF syndrome. Hum Mol Genet. 2:731–5.
103. Ji W, Hernandez R, Zhang XY et al. (1997). DNA demethylation and pericentromeric rearrangements of chromosome 1. Mut Res. 379:33–41.
104. Qu GZ, Grundy PE, Narayan A, Ehrlich M (1999). Frequent hypomethylation in Wilms tumors of pericentromeric DNA in chromosomes 1 and 16. Cancer Genet Cytogenet. 109:34–9.
105. Mugneret F, Dastugue N, Favre B et al. (1995). Der(16)t(1;16)(q11;q11) in myelodysplastic syndromes: a new non-random abnormality characterized by cytogenetic and fluorescence in situ hybridization studies. Br J Haematol. 90:119–24.
106. Tse W, Zhu W, Chen HS, Cohen A (1995). A novel gene, AF1q, fused to MLL in t(1;11) (q21;q23), is specifically expressed in leukemic and immature hematopoietic cells. Blood 85:650–6.
107. Cazzaniga G, Tosi S, Aloisi A et al. (1999). The tyrosine kinase abl-related gene ARG is fused to ETV6 in an AML-M4Eo patient with a t(1;12)(q25;p13): molecular cloning of both reciprocal transcripts. Blood. 94:4370–3.
108. Mercher T, Busson-Le Coniat M, Monni R et al. (2001). Involvement of a human gene related to the *Drosophila* spen gene in the recurrent t(1;22) translocation of acute megakaryocytic leukemia. Proc Natl Acad Sci USA. 98:5776–9.
109. Kivi S, Mikelsaar AV (1985). Polymorphism of Ag-stained nucleolus organizer regions in lymphocytes of patients with ovarian or breast adenocarcinoma. Hum Genet. 69:350–2.
110. Atkin NB, Brito-Babapulle V (1981). Heterochromatin polymorphism and human cancer. Cancer Genet Cytogenet. 3:261–72.

111. Atkin NB, Brito-Babapulle V (1985). Chromosome 1 heterochromatin variants and cancer: a reassessment. Cancer Genet Cytogenet. 18:325–31.
112. Sen P (1993). Chromosome 9 anomalies as the primary clonal alteration in a case of squamous cell carcinoma of the epiglottis. Cancer Genet Cytogenet. 66:23–7.
113. Tsezou A, Kitsiou-Tzeli S, Kosmidis H, Paidousi K, Katsouyanni K, Sinaniotis C (1993). Constitutive heterochromatin polymorphisms in children with acute lymphoblastic leukemia. Pediatr Hematol Oncol. 10:7–11.

5
Technical Variables and the Use of Heteromorphisms in the Study of Human Chromosomes

SUSAN BENNETT OLSON AND R. ELLEN MAGENIS

A. CHROMOSOME HETEROMORPHISMS IN PATERNITY TESTING

5.1 HISTORICAL PERSPECTIVE

Disputed parentage is not a problem unique to our modern society. One of the first recorded cases dating back to Biblical times actually involved disputed maternity. After considerable quarreling over who was the true mother of a child, two women took their complaints to King Solomon for resolution. Solomon offered to cut the child in half so that the two women could then share the child equally. The true mother dropped her claim in order to save the life of her child, thus allowing Solomon to make a fair judgement (Old Testament, I Kings 3:16–27). Equally creative methods, employing blood tests of sorts, are found in twelfth-century Japanese folklore. In situations where an individual was claiming to be the heir to an estate, his finger was pricked and the blood was allowed to drip onto the skeleton of the deceased. If the blood soaked in, a relationship was established. Another popular method for determining relationships was to allow drops of blood from each individual to fall into a basin of water. If the drops came together, the claim was upheld [1]. One of the most important events leading to the development of modern paternity testing was Landsteiner's discovery of the ABO blood group. In his 1901 paper Landsteiner suggested that the ABO system might be useful in blood transfusions and criminology. This breakthrough, coupled with the work done by Dunern and Hirszfeld in 1910 showing Mendelian inheritance of A, B and O, provided a foundation for paternity testing [2]. Until the late 1950s the only blood systems used were ABO, Rh and MN. In most cases a man could not expect much more than a 50/50 chance of being exonerated if falsely accused [1]. With the addition of at least 20 other red cell enzymes,

red cell antigens, and serum proteins, as well as HLA and chromosome heteromorphism analysis, a falsely accused man's chance of being excluded approached
100% by the mid-1980s. These technologies were for all practical purposes
replaced in the early 1990s by a more cost-effective DNA technology.

5.2 GENERAL ASPECTS OF PATERNITY TESTING

In paternity testing it is always assumed that the child's mother is its biological
mother. There are then two possibilities for exclusion of an alleged father at a
given locus. An allele cannot appear in a child unless present in one or both of its
parents (first-order exclusion). A man is also excluded if an allele which he must
transmit to the child is not present in that child (second-order exclusion).

The more genetic systems tested, the greater the chances of excluding a wrong-
fully accused man. Even if an alleged father is not excluded, there still exists a
chance that he is not the father. For this reason it is important to calculate some
measure of the degree to which the alleged father is likely to be the biological
father. Three basic statistics are used to describe this likelihood: (1) probability of
exclusion (measure of the ability of a given set of genetic systems to provide an
exclusion), (2) paternity index (ratio between the chance that the alleged father
contributed the paternal allele versus the chance that a random man passed it on)
and (3) probability of paternity (the paternity index expressed as a percentage).

In order for a genetic trait to be useful as a marker for distinguishing between
people it must fit certain criteria: (1) the marker must be inherited in a predictable
fashion as established through family and population studies; (2) the markers
should exhibit wide variation; (3) reliable techniques and accurate interpretation
of results must be available; and (4) there must be absence of effect of all other
variables on expression of the markers (i.e. environment, age, interaction with
other genes). Chromosome heteromorphisms fit these criteria [3–9].

5.3 CHROMOSOME HETEROMORPHISM ANALYSIS IN
PATERNITY TESTING

Use of chromosome heteromorphisms in cases of disputed paternity dates back to
1967 when de la Chapelle *et al.* [10] showed a discrepancy in the length of the
Y chromosome between alleged father and child. With the advent of C-banding
[11] and Q-banding [12], the greater variability in staining patterns between individuals in the population became apparent. This lent more power to the use of heteromorphisms in paternity cases. Gürtler and Niebuhr [13] reported the exclusion
of 178 of 591 alleged fathers based on the size of acrocentric short arm satellites,
juxtacentromeric bands, and 1qh and 9qh regions as delineated by Q-banding.

Olson *et al.* [14] demonstrated the utility of heteromorphism analysis in conjunction with routine paternity testing. An alleged father was not excluded following testing with red cell antigens, plasma proteins and red cell enzymes. The
probability of exclusion with the 21 systems was 98.19%; the probability of
paternity was only 93.90%. Quinacrine-stained heteromorphic regions for chromosomes 13, 14, 15, 21 and 22 were compared between the child, mother and

alleged father. Maternal origin was established for one of each of the acrocentric chromosomes. The other homolog, which should be from the father, did not match those of any of the acrocentrics from the alleged father. These findings led to exclusion of paternity.

The power of chromosome heteromorphism analysis relies on the great amount of population variation. Hauge *et al.* [15] compared 50 mother–fetus pairs. In the 10 sets of chromosomes examined, differences were found between six or more chromosomes in 56% of the comparisons. Olson *et al.* [16] performed extensive comparisons of quinacrine variants between 57 persons, 39 of whom were unrelated. The heteromorphisms analyzed were those on chromosomes 3, 4, 13, 14, 15, 21, 22 and Y (see Part IIA). In this study there were six or more differences in 51% of the comparisons and no less than two differences between individuals. In a subset of parent–child comparisons, 10 of 21 (48%) had six or more differences and none showed less than two. Chromosomes 15 and 22 were most often informative in attempts to distinguish between two persons, and chromosomes 3,

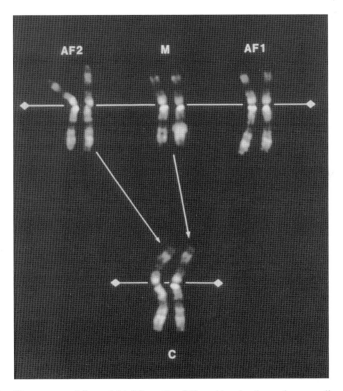

Fig. 5A.1 Chromosomes 3 from child (C), mother (M), and two brothers who were alleged fathers (AF1 and AF2). The child has one bright centromeric heteromorphism (variant) and one dull centromeric variant. Since the mother is homozygous for bright variants, one of these must have been contributed to the child (arrow). Therefore, the dull variant must be from the biological father. AF1 is homozygous for bright variants which excludes him. However, AF2 has one dull variant (homolog contribution indicated by the arrow). Contribution of AF2 variants to the child was consistent for all heteromorphisms examined

4 and Y were the least informative. The combined probability of exclusion for chromosomes 3, 4, 13, 14, 15, 21 and 22 approached 100%.

Exclusion of paternity has presented particular challenges when there is more than one alleged father who is related, or in cases where the mother and alleged father are related to each other. As a point of illustration we took several genetic families not involved in paternity disputes and created nonpaternity cases by replacing the biological father with a brother to see if he would be excluded, as he should be. Sixteen loci from the red cell enzyme, serum protein and red cell antigen systems were used. Out of 16 cases, only 68.75% of the brothers were excluded (unpublished). In a paternity case in which two brothers were the alleged fathers, neither of the brothers was excluded following red cell antigens, serum proteins, red cell enzymes and HLA testing. Both had a 99% probability of paternity. However, by examining Q-band heteromorphisms for chromosomes 3, 4, 13, 14, 15, 21 and 22, one of the brothers was excluded [17]. Figure 5A.1 illustrates exclusion based on the chromosome 3 variants.

References

1. American Association of Blood Banks (1978). Paternity Testing. Washington, DC: AABB.
2. Race RR, Sanger R (1975). Blood Groups in Man, 6th edn. Oxford: Blackwell Scientific Publications, p. 8.
3. Magenis RE, Chamberlin J, Overton K (1974). Sequential Q- and C-band variants: inheritance in four generations of a family. Thirteenth Annual Somatic Cell Genetics Conference, US Virgin Islands.
4. McKenzie WH, Lubs HA (1975). Human Q and C chromosomal variations: Distribution and incidence. Cytogenet Cell Genet. 14:97–115.
5. Müller HJ, Klinger HP, Glasser M (1975). Chromosome polymorphism in a human newborn population. II. Potentials for polymorphic chromosome variants for characterizing the ideogram of an individual. Cytogenet Cell Genet. 15:239–55.
6. Jacobs PA (1977). Human chromosome heteromorphism (variants). Prog Med Genet. 2:251–74.
7. Magenis E, Palmer CG, Wang L *et al.* (1977). Heritability of chromosome banding variants. In: Population Cytogenetics. New York: Academic Press, pp. 179–188.
8. Van Dyke DL, Palmer CG, Nance WE, Yu PL (1977). Chromosome polymorphism and twin zygosity. Am J Hum Genet. 29:431–47.
9. Verma RS, Dosik H (1980). Human chromosomal heteromorphisms: nature and clinical significance. Int Rev Cytol. 62:361–83.
10. De la Chapelle A, Fellman J, Unnerus V (1967). Determination of human paternity from the length of the Y chromosome. Ann Genet. 10:60–4.
11. Arrighi FE, Hjsu TC (1971). Localization of heterochromatin in human chromosomes. Cytogenetics. 10:81–6.
12. Caspersson T, Lomakka G, Zech L (1971). The 24 fluorescence patterns of human metaphase chromosomes – distinguishing characters and variability. Hereiditas. 67:89–102.
13. Gürtler H, Niebuhr E (1981). The use of chromosome variants in paternity cases. In: 9. Internationale Tagung der Gesellschaft fur forensisch Blutgruppenkund. Bern: Wurzburg, Schmitt & Meyer, pp. 597–601.
14. Olson SB, Magenis RE, Rowe SI, Lovrien EW (1983). Chromosome heteromorphism analysis in cases of disputed paternity. Am J Med Genet. 15:47–55.
15. Hauge M, Poulsen H, Halberg A, Mikkelsen M (1975). The value of fluorescence markers in the distinction between maternal and fetal chromosomes. Humangenetik. 26:187–91.
16. Olson SB, Magenis RE, Lovrien EW (1986). Human chromosome variation: The discriminatory power of Q-band heteromorphism (variant) analysis in distinguishing between individuals, with specific application to cases of questionable paternity. Am J Hum Genet. 38: 235–52.
17. Olson S, Magenis E, Lovrien E, Geyer J, Ryals L, Morrisey J (1984). Resolution of paternity disputes involving relatives as alleged fathers using chromosome heteromorphism analysis. Am J Hum Genet. 36:108S.

B. PARENTAL ORIGIN OF CHROMOSOME ABNORMALITIES

Because chromosome heteromorphisms are stable, highly variable and inherited in a predictable fashion, they are useful tools for establishing the parental origin of chromosomes. Although visible and sometimes distinguishable by routine G-banding, these variants are usually more informative when assessed following specialized staining such as Q-, C-, R- or G-11-banding, or through sequential staining using these methods. The Q-band heteromorphisms as a group are so variable in the population that no two people are expected to have the same set, unless identical twins [1]. Some of the chromosomes demonstrate such great variability that the chance for being informative in a parental origin study of that one chromosome is extremely high (see Part II, chromosomes 15 and 22). Such technical capabilities are still an important part of research in full service cytogenetic laboratories, as they may be valuable supplements to DNA marker analysis or may be the only approach available for a particular specimen or laboratory setting.

5.4 TRIPLOIDY*

Analysis of chromosome variants on chromosomes 1, 3, 4, 9, 13, 14, 15, 16, 21 and 22 have been used to establish the origin of the extra set of chromosomes in human triploids [2–5]. In the study by Jacobs *et al.* [4], 66% of triploids resulted from dispermy, 24% from fertilization of a haploid egg by a diploid sperm and 10% from fertilization of a diploid egg by a haploid sperm. Establishing the parental origin of the extra haploid set allowed observations to be made related to clinical outcome. An extra paternal set is associated with poor embryonic development and abundant placental tissue. An extra maternal set leads to severe embryonic growth retardation and a small, fibrotic placenta. These differences are presumably an effect of imprinting.

5.5 BENIGN OVARIAN TERATOMA AND COMPLETE HYDATIDIFORM MOLE

The karyotype of benign ovarian teratomas has long been known to be 46,XX [6,7]. In order to address the question of etiology, Linder *et al.* [8] analyzed five teratomas and their hosts for heteromorphisms on chromosomes 1, 3, 4, 9, 13, 14, 15, 16, 21 and 22. For many of the variant sites the hosts were heteromorphic; in other words, carried two distinguishable heteromorphisms. At each site where the

---

*In conflict with earlier data, several molecular studies of triploid fetuses suggested a predominance of digyny (material origin) of the extra haploid set of chromosomes [29]. However, Zaragoza *et al.* [30] recently studied 91 cases, which comprised 64 triploid from a consecutive series of spontaneous abortion at ≤ 20 weeks gestation and 27 cases of triploid spontaneous abortion ascertained for a variety of reasons. In agreement with earlier heteromorphism studies, dispermy was the most common mechanism (69%) overall. In analysis of results by gestational age a skewing toward a higher frequency of digyny was found mainly in early-gestation triploid abortuses (6 weeks or less) where later-gestation abortuses were heavily skewed for diandry.

host was heteromorphic the teratoma was homomorphic. These observations established the parthenogenetic origin of benign ovarian teratomas. In a similar approach, the origin of the 46,XX complete mole has been demonstrated to be the result of fertilization of an ovum lacking a nucleus by a 23,X sperm with subsequent duplication of the paternal genome [9].

5.6 TRISOMY 21

Several groups have investigated the origin of the extra chromosome in Down syndrome [10–16]. Using chromosome 21 quinacrine variants, it is possible not only to determine the parent of origin, but also the stage of meiosis at which the error occurred. Non-disjunction at the first meiotic division will result in the daughter cell receiving both chromosome 21 homologs with their different variants. Following the second meiotic division the mature gamete will contain two chromosomes 21 representing both parental homologs. With fertilization, a third chromosome 21 with its variant will be present. Should the non-disjunction event occur at the second meiotic division, two copies of the same chromosome 21 homolog with identical variants will be present in the mature gamete. Fertilization will introduce the third chromosome 21 with a differing variant (Fig. 5B.1a, b). In the summary by Magenis and Chamberlin [16], heteromorphism analysis demonstrated that approximately 80% of all trisomy 21 cases were attributed to a maternal error, in most cases in the first meiotic division. Where maternal cases were associated with advanced maternal age, trisomy 21 of paternal origin showed no age effect.

   In general, establishment of parental origin is useful in addressing questions regarding mechanisms and is, therefore, used only in the research setting. Parents naturally harbor feelings of guilt when a child is diagnosed with a chromosome

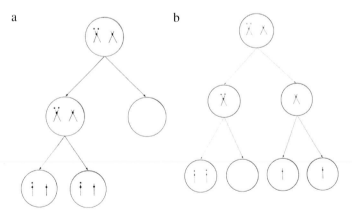

Fig. 5B.1 (a) Non-disjunction in meiosis I as followed by chromosome 21 heteromorphisms. Resulting gamete has two chromosomes 21 representative of both parental homologs. Variants are different. **(b)** Non-disjunction in meiosis II as followed by chromosome 21 heteromorphisms. Resulting gamete has two chromosomes 21, both representative of a single parental homolog. Variants are identical. (Reprinted from Magenis and Chamberlin (1981) Am J Med Genet. 35:333–49)

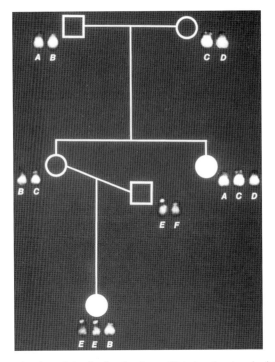

Fig. 5B.2 Pedigree showing origin of a female trisomy 21 to be of maternal origin (ACD) with an error in meiosis I, while her niece, also trisomy 21, resulted from an unrelated paternal meiosis II error (EEB). Letters distinguish chromosome 21 heteromorphisms. (Reprinted from Magenis *et al.* (1977). In: Population Cytogenetics. New York: Academic Press)

abnormality. Divulging the parent of origin adds to the anxiety. However, unique cases have presented for which sharing origin information with the family has been helpful. Figure 5B.2 illustrates the pedigree of a woman who came for genetic counseling to assess her risk for having a child with Down syndrome. She had grown up with a trisomy 21 sister. She was counseled that her risk was not elevated over her age-related risk. Her first child was trisomy 21. In analyzing the chromosome 21 variants in the patient, her husband and their offspring, it was clearly demonstrated that the extra chromosome 21 was paternal in origin and, therefore, an unrelated event.

5.7 STRUCTURAL CHROMOSOME ABNORMALITIES

The origins of *de-novo* structural rearrangements have been investigated with both Q-band (Fig. 5B.3) and C-band (Fig. 5B.4) heteromorphism analysis. In a compilation of new cases and cases then to date from the literature, Olson and Magenis [17] showed approximately 80% of these abnormalities to be paternal in origin and not associated with advanced age. A large group of these paternal

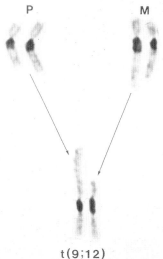

t(9;12)

Fig. 5B.3 C-banded paternal (P) and maternal (M) chromosomes 9, and derivative 9 with normal 9 in an offspring, demonstrating paternal origin of the child's *de-novo* rearrangement with smaller C-band positive block. (Reprinted from Olson and Magenis (1988). In: Daniel A, editor. The Cytogenetics of Mammalian Autosomal Rearrangements. New York: Alan R. Liss, pp. 583–599)

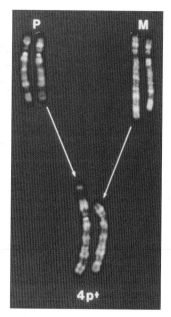

Fig. 5B.4 Q-banded paternal (P) and maternal (M) chromosomes 4, and an add(4p) and normal 4 in their offspring, demonstrating the abnormal 4 with bright juxtacentromeric heterochromatin to be of paternal origin. (Reprinted from Olson and Magenis (1988). In: Daniel A, editor. The Cytogenetics of Mammalian Autosomal Rearrangements. New York: Alan R. Liss, pp. 583–599)

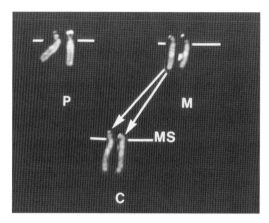

Fig. 5B.5 Q-banded chromosomes 15 from father (P), mother (M) and child with Prader-Willi syndrome (C). All chromosomes 15 appear structurally normal. However, the child has received both homologs from her mother as illustrated by the short arm heteromorphisms. Because they originate from the same maternal homolog, this represents maternal isodisomy. The syndrome has resulted from the absence of a paternal contribution

cases comprise the chromosome 15 deletion in Prader-Willi Syndrome [18–22]. In contrast, the origin of the apparently identical deleted chromosome 15 in Angelman syndrome patients was shown to be maternal [23–26]. In addition, unusual cases of both syndromes in which the chromosomes 15 appeared to be normal could be shown through parental origin studies to be due to uniparental disomy. For example, the Prader-Willi syndrome patient whose chromosomes are depicted in Fig. 5B.5 has two copies of one homolog from the mother and no chromosome 15 from the father. This imprinting phenomenon also holds true for chromosome 14, another chromosome with great Q-band heterochromatin variation. In fact, the chromosome 14 short arm heteromorphisms may prove informative when the available DNA polymorphisms fail to be. Additional staining techniques may be useful to further delineate the acrocentric heteromorphisms, such as R-banding to highlight differences in length and brilliance of the stalk region.

Structurally abnormal supernumerary chromosomes have also been investigated. As with trisomies, these chromosomes are primarily maternal and associated with advanced maternal age. By comparing short arm heteromorphisms from both ends of the extra pseudodicentric chromosome 15, preferential maternal origin has been demonstrated. In addition, differences in the variants on each arm show the abnormal chromosome to involve both maternal homologs [27]. With the realization that in fact two different chromosomes were involved in the structurally abnormal chromosome, the common descriptor of "inv dup (15)" was no longer appropriate. In a case of paternal origin, however, the extra bisatellited chromosome was shown to derive from a single chromosome 15 homolog (27). Similar preferential maternal origin involving both homologs has also been demonstrated for the extra bisatellited chromosome 22 (Fig. 5B.6).

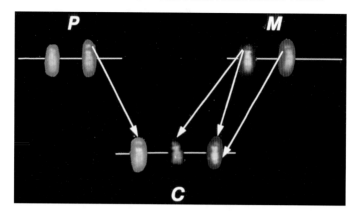

Fig. 5B.6   Q-banded paternal (P) and maternal (M) chromosomes 22, and deleted, bisatellited pseu-dodicentric and normal chromosomes 22, from child (C). The deleted and bisatellited chromosomes are maternal in origin as demonstrated by the heteromorphisms. The bisatellited chromosome comprises short arms of both maternal homologs

5.8   CONCLUSION

Chromosome heteromorphism analysis continues to be an important cytogenetics tool. Although establishment of the origin of a chromosome abnormality is most often useful in addressing questions of mechanism and etiology, there are scenarios in which this information is clinically relevant. In addition to the trisomy origin and uniparental disomy cases described above, establishment of parental origin of a structural balanced or unbalanced rearrangement may lead to further investigation of an apparently chromosomally normal parent to better assess recurrent risks. Opheim *et al.* [28] have reported the finding of low-level mosaicism for structural rearrangements in some parents of children originally thought to have *de-novo* rearrangements. These parents may appear chromosomally normal if only a directed or limited study, usually five to 10 metaphase cells analyzed, is carried out. By establishing parent of origin, the more extensive mosaicism study, which may involve skin biopsy for fibroblasts, may be directed to the specific parent rather than being carried out on both.

References

1. Olson SB, Magenis RE, Lovrien EW (1986). Human chromosome variation: the discriminatory power of Q-band heteromorphism (variant) analysis in distinguishing between individuals, with specific application to cases of questionable paternity. Am J Hum Genet. 38:235–52.
2. Jonasson J, Therkelsen AJ, Lauritsen JG, Lindsten J (1972). Origin of triploidy in human abortuses. Hereditas. 71:168–71.
3. Kajii T, Niikawa N (1977). Origin of triploidy and tetraploidy in man: 11 cases with chromosome markers. Cytogenet Cell Genet 18:109–25.
4. Jacobs PA, Angell RR, Buchanan IM, Hassold TJ, Matsuyama AM, Manuel B (1978). The origin of human triploids. Ann Hum Genet. 42:49–57.
5. Lauritsen JG, Bolund L, Friedrich U, Therkelsen AJ (1979). Origin of triploidy in spontaneous abortuses. Ann Hum Genet. 43:1–5.

6. Galton M, Benirschke K (1959). Forty-six chromosomes in an ovarian teratoma. Lancet. 2:761–2.
7. Corfman PA, Richart RM (1964). Chromosome number and morphology of benign ovarian cystic teratomas. N Engl J Med. 271:1241–4.
8. Linder D, McKaw BK, Hecht F (1975). Parthenogenic origin of benign ovarian teratomas. N Engl J Med. 292:63–6.
9. Kajii T, Ohama K (1977). Androgenetic origin of hydatidiform mole. Nature. 268:633–4.
10. Robinson JA (1973). Origin of extra chromosome in trisomy 21. Lancet. 1:131–3.
11. Uchida IA (1973). Paternal origin of the extra chromosome in Down's syndrome. Lancet. 2:1258.
12. Schmidt R, Dar H, Nitowsky HM (1975). Origin of extra 21 chromosome in patients with Down syndrome. Pediatr Res. 9:367a.
13. Wagenbichler P (1976). Origin of the supernumerary chromosome in Down's syndrome. ICS 397. V International Congress Hum Genet. Chicago: Excerpta Medica, p. 167a.
14. Magenis RE, Overton KM, Chamberlin J, Brady T, Lovrien E (1977). Parental origin of the extra chromosome in Down's syndrome. Hum Genet. 37:7–16.
15. Mikkelsen M, Poulsen H, Grinsted J, Lange A (1980). Non-disjunction in trisomy 21: study of chromosomal heteromorphisms in 110 families. Ann Hum Genet. 44:17.
16. Magenis RE, Chamberlin J (1981). Parental origin of nondisjunction. In: de la Cruz FF, Gerald PS, editors. Trisomy 21 (Down Syndrome): Research Perspectives. Baltimore: University Press, pp. 77–93.
17. Olson SB, Magenis RE (1988). Preferential paternal origin of *de novo* structural chromosome rearrangements. In: Daniel A, editor. The Cytogenetics of Mammalian Autosomal Rearrangements. New York: Alan R. Liss, pp. 583–599.
18. Butler MG, Palmer CG (1983). Parental origin of chromosome 15 deletion in Prader-Willi syndrome. Lancet. 1:1285–6.
19. Butler MG, Meany FJ, Palmer CG (1986). Clinical and cytogenetic survey of 39 individuals with Prader-Labhart-Willi syndrome. Am J Med Genet. 23:793–809.
20. Mattei JF, Mattei MG, Giraud F (1983). Prader-Willi syndrome and chromosome 15: a clinical discussion of 20 cases. Hum Genet. 64:356–61.
21. Nicholls RD, Knoll JH, Glatt K *et al.* (1989). Restriction fragment length polymorphism with proximal 15q and their use in molecular cytogenetics and the Prader-Willi syndrome. Am J Med Genet. 33:66–77.
22. Magenis RE, Toth-Fejel S, Allen LJ *et al.* (1990). Comparison of the 15q deletions in Prader-Willi and Angelman syndromes: specific regions, extent of deletions, parental origin, and clinical consequences. Am J Med Genet 35:333–49.
23. Donlon T (1988). Similar molecular deletions on chromosome 15q11.2 are encountered in both the Prader-Willi and Angelman syndromes. Hum Genet. 80:322–8.
24. Knoll JHM, Nicholls RD, Magenis RE, Graham JM Jr, Lalande M, Latt SA (1989). Angelman and Prader-Willi syndromes share a common chromosome deletion but differ in parental origin of the deletion. Am J Med Genet. 32:285–90.
25. Pembrey M, Fennell SJ, Van den Berghe J *et al.*(1989). The association of Angelman's syndrome with deletions within 15q11–13. J Med Genet. 26:73–7.
26. Williams CA, Gray BA, Hendrickson JE, Stone JW, Cantu ES (1989). Incidence of 15q deletions in the Angelman syndrome: a survey of 12 affected persons. Am J Med Genet. 32:339–45.
27. Maraschio P, Zuffardi O, Bernardi F *et al.* (1981). Preferential maternal derivation in inv dup(15): Analysis of eight new cases. Hum Genet. 57:345–50.
28. Opheim KE, Brittingham A, Chapman D, Norwood TH (1995). Balanced reciprocal translocation mosaicism: How frequent? Am J Med Genet. 57:601–4.
29. McFadden DE, Langlois S (1997). Meiotic origin of tripoidy. Med Genet Suppl. 9:525.
30. Zaragoza MV, Surti U, Redline RW, Millie E, Chakravarti A, Hassold T (2000). Parental origin and phenotype of triploidy in spontaneous abortions: predominance of diandry and association with partial hydatidiform mole. Am J Hum Genet. 66:1807–20.

6
Euchromatic Variants

S. M. JALAL AND R. P. KETTERLING

6.1 INTRODUCTION

The terms heterochromatin and euchromatin have evolved since their introduction in 1928 by Heitz (reviewed in ref. 1). This reference provides an excellent historical perspective of the conceptual changes of the two terms. Brown points out that Heitz proposed the term heterochromatin to refer to densely staining regions of chromosomes that remained "visible" for much of interphase. In contrast, euchromatin underwent a typical cycle of condensation and unraveling. Heitz therefore believed the heterochromatic regions to be genetically inert.

Two forms of heterochromatin (constitutive and facultative) were later recognized. Constitutive heterochromatin was expressed in a similar fashion on both paternal and maternal homologs during development. However, selective heterochromatization of a chromosome (e.g. human X in females) or a complete chromosome set (paternal in male mealy bug) occurred as facultative heterochromatization. Thus, facultative heterochromatization is a selective process due to suppression at the gene level. Brown [1] aptly pointed out that facultative heterochromatization was a "visible guide" to suppression of gene action.

By 1971 a technique (C-banding) became available to identify constitutive heterochromatin readily in mammals, especially humans [2,3]. It became evident that C-band-positive regions contained highly repetitive satellite DNA sequences [4,5]. The C-positive bands might have predominantly one type of repetitive sequence [3], or more commonly a multitude of repetitive DNA sequences [6]. However, exceptions do exist. The C-band-positive regions of sex chromosomes of Chinese hamster contain little, if any, repetitive DNA [7]. In addition, C-positive bands might not always be of the same intensity [8].

Most constitutive heterochromatin is late-replicating during the cell cycle, although not as late as facultative heterochromatin. However, exceptions do exist, such as in the mouse, *Mus musculus* [9]. Q-banding may also be helpful in distinguishing subtypes of C-band-positive regions. It is known that Q+C+ regions are AT-rich while Q−C+ regions are GC-rich. Based on these and other characteristics, Jalal *et al.* [9] describe 11 different categories of constitutive heterochromatin.

In summary, constitutive heterochromatin can therefore be considered as C-positive regions that are generally late replicating, rich in repetitive DNA sequences, and genetically inert. In contrast, facultative heterochromatin is a term used to describe selective DNA inactivation at the gene level.

There is a growing list of euchromatic duplications and deletions involving both G-positive and G-negative bands that seem to be phenotypically neutral. Since the term "heteromorphism" has been traditionally used to describe variations of constitutive heterochromatin, we have chosen to refer to the phenotypically neutral euchromatic anomalies as "variants". Herein, an effort is made to describe all currently identified euchromatic variants.

The C-band-negative regions are regarded as euchromatin that include both light and dark bands identified by G-banding. Historically, G-dark bands were regarded to be rich in middle repetitive DNA sequences [10]. It was subsequently discovered that G-dark bands could be as transcriptionally active as G-light bands [11]. It was also postulated that the G-dark bands involved in autosomal deletions associated with major malformations [12] might contain fewer active genes. However, it is difficult to judge what the phenotypic influence might be when only G-positive bands are involved in deletion or duplication. It is therefore imperative to regard all euchromatic duplications and deletions with suspicion until the issue for the band in question is resolved.

6.2   EUCHROMATIC VARIANTS DUE TO DUPLICATION EVENTS

The first case of a euchromatic variant was reported by Buckton *et al.* [13]. In a G-banded chromosome study of live-born infants, one child had an extra dark band in the 9 short arm (9p), proximal to the centromere, that was inherited from a normal mother. A similar extra G-positive band in 9p was subsequently described by Sutherland and Eyre (1981) [14]. This variant 9p was described in two families involving 11 members in three generations. All 11 individuals were normal except the probands who were referred for chromosomal analysis due to multiple dysmorphic features. These authors localized the additional dark band to the middle of 9p13. Following these first two reports, euchromatic variants due to duplications have been described for chromosomes 1, 2, 5, 8, 9, 15, 16 and 18 (Fig. 6.1). In addition, euchromatic variants based on molecular or molecular cytogenetic analysis have been described for chromosomes 2 and 15.

Chromosome 1

Bortotto *et al.* [15] described a duplication of sub-bands 1q42.11-q42.12 in a short-statured child and an asymptomatic mother. Zaslav *et al.* [16] reported a duplication involving 1p21-p31 in a fetus and normal mother (Part II, Plate 8). The amniocentesis was performed due to advanced maternal age. Use of a whole chromosome painting probe (wcp1) both for the fetus and the mother confirmed that the extra material was of chromosome 1 origin. The baby at 1, 2 and 3 months of age had normal physical examinations.

Chromosome 5

Shuan-Yow *et al.* [18] described a duplication of 5q15-q21 in a phenotypically normal father and in monozygotic twin daughters with different abnormal

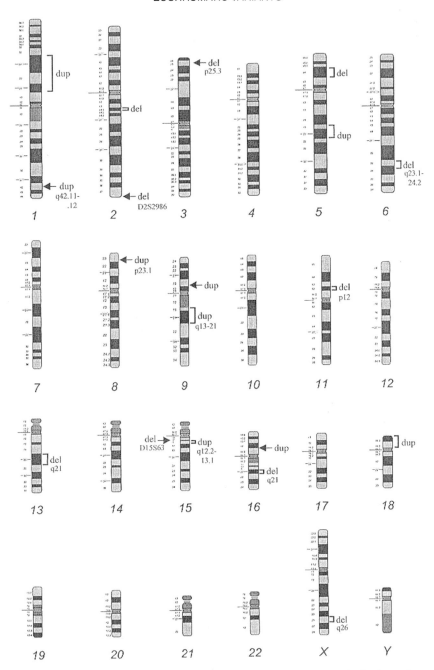

Fig. 6.1 An idiogram representing the reported euchromatic deletion and duplication variants. Deletion variants (del) involving chromosomes 2, 3, 5, 6, 11, 13, 15, 16 and X; and duplication variants (dup) involving chromosomes 1, 5, 8, 9, 15, 16 and 18 are indicated either by an arrow or the boundaries are demarcated by half-brackets.

phenotypes. The duplication was confirmed to be of chromosome 5 origin in all three by use of a whole chromosome painting probe (wcp5). The breakpoints were the same in the father and the twins as delineated by eight cosmid probes from the 5q13-23 region. The anomalies of the twin daughters were considered to be unrelated to the familial duplication.

Chromosome 8

Barber *et al.* [19] described duplication of band 8p23.1 in 18 individuals from seven families. In four of the seven families the duplication was transmitted from parents to children. The results were confirmed by use of a YAC that mapped to 8p23.1 and by chromosome painting with wcp8. The authors summarized all reported cases, from which they determined that 25 of 27 duplication carriers, including eight cases analyzed in the prenatal/neonatal time period, had no evidence of phenotypic anomalies. However, in two families the probands were dysmorphic. It is noteworthy that 8p23.1 is described at a resolution of 1250 band stage and is not recognized by ISCN. Engelen *et al.* [20] described a duplication of 8p23.1-p23.3 in an oligoasthenozoospermic male, a fertile brother, and their mother. The duplication was confirmed by reverse painting and band-specific FISH probes. Although the 8p23.1 duplication appeared to be a euchromatic variant, questions have been raised in a few cases with inconsistent anomalies. The importance of confirmation by parental chromosome studies was emphasized [21].

Chromosome 9

Structural variability of chromosome 9 is commonly observed due to variations in length of C-band-positive constitutive heterochromatin in the long arm adjacent to the centromere and in the short arm due to partial or complete pericentric inversions [22]. However, it should not be assumed that all such variants consist of heterochromatin. C-band-negative duplications in these regions can occur as a benign euchromatic variants.

Sutherland and Eyre [14] described two families with an extra G-positive band in the short arm of chromosome 9. The families were ascertained due to phenotypically abnormal children, but the extra G-positive band was present in normal members of both families, in three generations. In Family 1 the extra G-positive band was C-band positive. However, in Family 2 the extra G-positive band near the centromere was C-band negative. Hence, in these cases, Family 1 does not carry a euchromatic variant, while Family 2 carries a euchromatic variant.

Euchromatic variants are also reported as extra G-bands in the 9 long-arm. Verma *et al.* [23] elegantly demonstrate an extra G-positive band within the 9qh region that did not hybridize to satellite III probes, was not digested by Taq I endonuclease (digests the 9qh DNA repeats), but painted with wcp9 (Part II, Plate 28). Thus, the extra G-positive band was of euchromatic origin. They postulated that the *de-novo* extra band originated from the maternal 9p12 band because of a pairing disturbance between maternal homologous chromosomes caused by inversion of the large qh region to the 9p arm. The euchromatic band became "inactivated" when sandwiched within the heterochromatic 9qh region, because a phenotypically normal twin was born with the variant. The other twin was chromosomally and phenotypically normal. Roland *et al.* [24] also described a C-negative, Q-positive bright band within the 9qh region in two unrelated families, that appeared to be a normal variant. In the two families the variant band was transmitted from a normal father to a normal newborn daughter and to a normal fetus, respectively. However, it needs to be determined if such C-negative, Q-positive bands originate from DNA repeat sequences.

Jalal et al. [25] reported a duplication of 9q13-q21 (Part II, Plate 26f) in a phenotypically normal mother and a fetal hydrops. A similar variant was found by Knight et al. [26] in a phenotypically normal baby boy and his mother.

Wang and Miller [27] have correctly pointed out that, in addition to determining the C-band nature of chromosome 9 extra band variants, an effort should be made to identify those variants as either α-satellite- or β-satellite-positive. They cited cases of their own and of others, in which the extra band was C-negative and α-satellite-positive. However, the centromeric function of the α-satellite region was inactivated. These authors postulated the origin of such variants was either from unequal crossing over or from an inversion that split the centromere.

Chromosome 15

Losses involving the 15q11.2-q13 region have been of intense interest due to the association with Prader-Willi and Angelman syndromes. The critical region for each is distinct as defined by the two different hybridization sites with SNRP-N (Prader-Willi) and D15S10 (Angelman) DNA probes. It is noteworthy that duplications involving the Prader-Willi and Angelman syndromes' critical regions (15q11.2-q12) also result in abnormal phenotypes [30]. However, Ludowese et al. [28] reported 10 cases of 15q12.2-q13.1 duplication without adverse phenotypic expression. Jalal et al. [29] reported a similar finding (Part II, Plate 47 b–d) based on 15 cases from seven unrelated families. Whole chromosome 15 painting probes confirmed that the duplicated region was of chromosome 15 origin.

C-banding and molecular or FISH techniques are useful to determine the composition of the extra bands variants in the 15q12.2-q13.1 region. Rarely, however, "gaps" appear that are negative for most of the commonly available FISH probes but are positive by Ag-NOR staining. A case with such an insertion was observed in our laboratory at 15q11.2 (Part II, Plate 47a).

Chromosome 16

Thompson and Roberts [31] reported an additional C-band-negative segment in the proximal short arm of chromosome 16 that seemed to be a euchromatic variant. They observed the variant in four cases, two of which were detected prenatally. In the two prenatal cases a normal father also carried the variant. In one family, involving seven individuals, the variant was transmitted both maternally and paternally. Jalal et al. [32] reported a variant that increases the size of the 16p arm by about one-third (Part II, Plate 49b) in two infants with non-specific and unrelated abnormalities. The variant was present in the normal father and normal paternal grandmother in one case and in a mother with minor anomalies in the other case. Bryke et al. [33] reported a similar finding in a fetus and normal mother. They indicated that the C-band-negative region was not composed of α-satellite DNA. One case with a C-band-negative, α-satellite-positive region in 16qh was reported by Jalal et al. [34].

Chromosome 18

Wolff *et al.* [35] reported extra C-band negative material in the short arm of chromosome 18 in two generations without detectable phenotypic abnormalities. The 18p+ (complete duplication of the short arm) was detected prenatally and in the phenotypically normal mother. The pregnancy continued, and a normal female was born at 39 weeks. The authors confirmed that the duplicated material was of 18p origin by DNA dosage studies. The authors also compiled a summary of 14 reported cases of 18p duplications that seemed to result in either a normal phenotype or mild and inconsistent abnormalities. In view of the fact that 18p duplication was stably transmitted from the mother to the daughter and has been reported in many other cases, it does qualify as a euchromatic variant, but not necessarily an innocuous one.

6.3   EUCHROMATIC VARIANTS DUE TO DELETION EVENTS

In addition to duplications already described, euchromatic deletions at the cytogenetic level as well as finer deletions by molecular cytogenetics techniques have been described as variants for chromosomes 2, 3, 5, 6, 11, 13, 15, 16 and X (Fig. 6.1).

Chromosome 2

Sumption and Barber [17] reported an interstitial deletion involving band 2q14.1 (breakpoints at q13-q14.1) in a normal woman aged 38. The deletion was also present in her mother who was clinically normal. Chromosome analysis at the 600 band level failed to detect the deleted material elsewhere in the genome of either woman. This finding was confirmed by FISH analysis with a whole chromosome painting probe for chromosome 2 (wcp2). To exclude the possibility of an intrachromosomal insertion, eight YACs from this region were analyzed. Two YACs were missing, confirming a deletion in band 2q14.1. Thus, the deletion appeared to be a euchromatic variant.

Chromosome 3

A terminal deletion with a breakpoint at 3p25.3 was observed in a fetus and a phenotypically normal mother [36]. At term, a normal baby girl was born. The mother had a terminal deletion involving FISH probes for D3S1442, D3S1443 and D3S1444 that map between 3p26 and 3pter.

Chromosome 5

Walker *et al.* [37] reported an interstitial deletion of 5p13 to p15.1 in three children and in their mother. All had moderate mental retardation but inconsistent facial and other dysmorphic features. In an attempt to define the critical region for cri-du-chat syndrome, Overhauser *et al.* [38] identified a family with six individuals from three generations who had an interstitial deletion of band 5p14, but all were phenotypically normal. By quantitative blot hybridization experiments they demonstrated that these individuals were indeed deleted for 4–6 Mb of DNA. Keppen *et al.* [39] reported four individuals from three generations who had mental retardation and other inconsistent anomalies when the interstitial deletion was larger than the 5p14 band. In these individuals the deleted segment was 5p13.3-p14.3. The authors conclude that, from molecular comparisons of the deletion in this family of four, the clinical findings are due specifically to 5p13 deletions.

Recently, Hand *et al.* [40] reported a deletion of 5p14 (Part II, Plate 17) in a 19-year-old male with a peroxisomal disorder and a normal mother. It does seem that loss of a portion or complete loss of 5p14 has no adverse phenotypic effect. However, if the deletion extends to the 5p13 or 5p15 bands, dysmorphism including mental retardation results.

Chromosome 6

Kumar *et al.* [41] report a case of *de-novo* interstitial deletion of 6q23.3-q24.2 in a developmentally normal 3-year-old girl with very mild phenotypic anomalies. By use of microsatellite analysis involving 12 YAC clones, eight clones showed only one copy, and the deletion was estimated to be 4–5 Mb. By use of 15 markers the deletion was determined to be paternal in origin. Matkins *et al.* [42] reported a 2-year-old girl with an interstitial deletion of 6q23.1-q24.2. She had growth retardation (third centile) and multiple dysmorphic features quite unlike the features described in the case by Kumar *et al.* [41]. The authors contemplate that the differences may be either from the lack of a phenotype effect from haploinsufficiency of genes within 6q23.3-q24.2 or due to imprinting of paternal genes. Chromosome 6 imprinting has been implicated in neonatal diabetes mellitus [43]; therefore, the influence of imprinting in this case is a possibility. Confirmation of deletion of 6q23.1-q24.2 as a variant must await other reports, although the possibility raised by the present case is strong.

Chromosome 11

Interstitial deletion of the G-dark band at 11p12 has been reported in a fetus, a normal mother, and a normal son by Barber *et al.* [44]. At term a phenotypically normal female was born. Thus, a deletion variant involving 11p12 seems to exist.

Chromosome 13

Couturier *et al.* [45] reported the deletion of 13q21 band in a son and mother who were both phenotypically normal. Chromosome analysis was done due to a history of multiple miscarriages.

Chromosome 16

Naritomi *et al.* [46] reported a 1-year-old girl with growth retardation and multiple dysmorphic features to have a *de-novo* deletion (16)(q13q22). After a review of the literature they concluded that the critical region (smallest region of overlap) for the anomalies involving reported cases of 16q deletions was in 16q21. Witt *et al.* [47] contradicted this finding and reported three members of a two-generation family who were all normal and had a deletion of band 16q21. However, Callen *et al.* [48] rightly pointed out that standard cytogenetic analysis cannot resolve with precision the phenotype–genotype correlations involving varying degrees of 16q13q22 interstitial deletion. They indicated that, to establish such a relationship, the deletions need to be mapped by molecular analysis either using microsatellite repeats or DNA FISH probes that span the region or somatic cell hybrids that contain the deletions. Using somatic cell hybrids and FISH probes they confirmed the loss of 16q21 in one patient who was phenotypically normal. They also observed that all other reported deletions that include larger segments extending proximal or distal to 16q21 result in patients with phenotypic anomalies. Recently, Hand *et al.* [40] reported the deletion of 16q21 (Part II, Plate 49a) in a mother, son and newborn daughter, all of whom are phenotypically normal.

Chromosome X

A female infant with Down syndrome (+21) and her normal mother had an interstitial deletion of band Xq26 [49]. The finding was confirmed in the mother from leukocyte and fibroblast cultures as a non-mosaic deletion. This finding is of interest not only because Xq26 appears to be a haploinsufficiency variant in females, but it helps define the Xq deletion resulting in a variant of Uhrlich-Turner syndrome.

6.4   MOLECULAR DELETIONS AS EUCHROMATIC VARIANTS

Buiting *et al.* [50] describe a 28-kb deletion spanning the D15S63 locus in five different families. Since methylation analysis is often used with probe PW71 (D15S63) for Prader-Willi and Angelman syndromes, such a rare neutral variant can lead to false-positive results. The deletion, however, was not detected in 1000 unrelated controls so it must be quite rare.

Silverstein *et al.* [51] confirm the finding by Buiting *et al.* [50] in five unrelated individuals, each of whom had inherited the 28-kb deletion involving D15S63 locus from one of the parents. Three of the families were of Ashkenazi Jews, and the ancestry in the other two families was unknown. The frequency of the 28-kb deletion was 1/75 in Ashkenazi individuals and rarer in people of mixed origin. The authors recommend the use of SNRPN rather than D15S63 since the deletion of D15S63 as a normal variant can lead to misdiagnosis.

While using telomere-specific probes for couples with multiple miscarriages and individuals with non-specific dysmorphic features and normal karyotype, we encountered a deletion variant at a frequency of about 8% involving the locus D2S2986 (Part II, Plate 67) at 2qter [52]. The deletion was present when using the probe set of one company but was absent when the probe set of another company was used who did not use D2S2986. The deletion variant was also seen in a dysmorphic child and his phenotypically normal father.

6.5   ORIGIN OF EUCHROMATIC VARIANTS

The origin of euchromatic variants presumably involves the same mechanisms that result in disease-associated duplications and deletions. Duplications involving defined regions that do not involve more than two repeats can arise by unequal crossing over during meiosis, a two-break translocation event, or a three-break insertion event involving sister or non-sister chromatids. An inherited dup(18p) in a mother and daughter described by Wolff *et al.* [35] serves as a good example of this type of origin resulting from unequal crossing over, a two-break reciprocal translocation, or a three-break insertion. Another mechanism at a finer level that may be widely responsible for both deletions and duplications is misalignment of repeat sequences that mediate pairing between homologous chromosomes. An excellent example is the deletion or duplication of the same 1.5-Mb region from 17p11.2-p12 that results in hereditary neuropathy with liability to pressure palsies (HNPP) or Charcot-Marie-Tooth type 1A (CMT1A), respectively [53]. Based on the analysis of 76 CMT1A and 38 HNPP patients, a 12.9-kb restriction map was constructed involving proximal and distal CMT1A flanking repeat sequences. A hot spot of crossover breakpoints involving a 3.2-kb region was involved in 75% of the rearrangements from unequal crossing over.

Although the euchromatic variants are C-band-negative, can they still have certain amounts of the highly or moderately repetitive DNA sequences? In cases of duplicated segments the earlier evidence seems to be negative for alpha satellite for 16p variants [33] and negative for alpha satellite, satellite III, and ribosomal DNA for 9p variants [54]. Such observations may be generally true, but future studies of possible euchromatic variants should include these probes in questionable cases.

Recent evidence shows, however, that amplification of pseudogene cassettes may well be a common mechanism of duplicated euchromatic variants. This is an exciting mechanism which could account for many euchromatic variants. Barber *et al.* [55] provide evidence for the presence and amplification of non-functional immunoglobulin heavy chain and myosin heavy chain pseudogenes at 16p11.2. In addition to the pseudogenes for immunoglobulin heavy chain from 14q32 and myosin heavy chain from Xq28, minisatellite sequences from the telomeric region of 6p were also present in variant 16p11.2. These authors suggest that the immunoglobulin heavy chain locus was transposed to chromosome 14 about 7 million years ago, and the myosin heavy chain locus was transposed to chromosome 16 some 7–10 million years ago. The amplification (six to 12 copies) resulting in the 16p variant primarily involves these two loci. It is indeed fascinating that often the cytogenetically detectable variants may result from a relatively common process of genomic flux and subsequent amplification of the pseudogenes. Paralogous segments from Xq28 have been reported near the centromeres of 2p, 10p, 16p and 22q [56,57].

6.6 SUMMARY

Awareness of the euchromatic variants, either as duplications or deletions, is immensely important as the numbers grow (Fig. 6.1) at the cytogenetic as well as the molecular cytogenetic levels. All deletion variants mentioned, with the exception of Xq26, involve G-dark bands. Historically, G-dark bands have been regarded as rich in middle repetitive DNA sequences and genetically inert. Therefore, it is not surprising that deletion variants often involve the G-dark bands. The G-dark bands, however, can be as transcriptionally active as G-light bands and are often involved in autosomal deletions associated with malformations. The dark bands may well contain fewer active genes, and those involved in deletion variants may function normally even with haploinsufficiency. Deletion variants range from a loss of a locus (e.g. D2S2986) or even finer loss at molecular level to a relatively large band such as 5p14. It is noteworthy that, if the deletion extends to the proximal or distal band of 5p14, it results in phenotypic abnormality.

Duplication variants range from a repeat of sub-bands such as 8p23.1 to a complete duplication of an arm (e.g. 18p arm). In each of these cases the duplication variants have been reported in a relatively large number of individuals, have been passed on from parents to children, were associated with a normal phenotype, and the identity of the extra chromatin was confirmed by chromosome banding and molecular/molecular cytogenetic procedures. When euchromatic variants are encountered, they must be treated with concern until the issue of variant status is settled, and special care is warranted to determine precise deletion/duplication boundaries since the location is crucial in establishing phenotypic neutrality. In addition, chromosome analysis of parents/family members must be performed to confirm the variant state. The interpretation of the chromosomal anomaly may well be critical in prenatal counseling and in the management regimen for the patient.

References

1. Brown S (1966). Heterochromatin. Science. 151:417–25.
2. Arrighi FE, Hsu TC (1971). Localization of heterochromatin in human chromosomes. Cytogenetics. 10:81–6.
3. Pardue ML, Gall JG (1970). Chromosomal localization of mouse satellite DNA. Science. 168:1356–8.
4. Yunis JJ, Yasmineh WG (1971). Heterochromatin, satellite DNA, and cell function. Science. 174:1200–9.
5. Arrighi FE, Saunders GF (1973). The relationship between repetitious DNA and constitutive heterochromatin with special reference to man. Symp Medica-Hoechst 6:113–133. Stuttgart New York: Schattauer.
6. Hsu TC, Arrighi FE, Saunders GF (1972). Compositional heterogeneity of human heterochromatin. Proc Natl Acad Sci USA. 69:1464–6.
7. Arrighi FE, Hsu TC, Pathak S, Swada H (1974). The sex chromosomes of the Chinese hamster: constitutive heterochromatin deficient in repetitive DNA sequences. Cytogenet Cell Genet. 13:268–74.
8. Jalal SM, Pfeiffer RA, Pathak S, Hsu TC (1974). Subdivision of the human Y chromosome. Humangenetik. 24:59–65.
9. Jalal SM, Clark RW, Hsu TC, Pathak S (1974). Cytological differentiation of constitutive heterochromatin. Chromosome (Berl). 48:391–403.
10. Comings DE (1978). Mechanisms of chromosome banding and implications for chromosome structure. Annu Rev Genet. 12:25–46.
11. Holmquist G, Gray M, Porter T, Jordan J (1982). Characterization of Giemsa dark- and light-band DNA. Cel. 31:121–9.
12. Brewer C, Holloway S, Zawalaryski P, Schinzel A, Fitzpatrick D (1998). A chromosomal deletion map of human malformations. Am J Hum Genet. 63:1153–9.
13. Buckton KE, O'Riordan ML, Ratcliffe S, Slight J, Mitchell M (1980). A G-band study of chromosomes in liveborn infants. Ann Hum Genet Lond. 43:227–39.
14. Sutherland GR, Eyre H (1981). Two unusual G-band variants of the short arm of chromosome 9. Clin Genet. 19:331–4.
15. Bortotto L, Piovan E, Furlan R, Rivera H, Zuffardi O (1990). Chromosome imbalance, normal phenotype, and imprinting. J Med Genet. 27:582–7.
16. Zaslav AL, Blumenthal D, Fox JE, Thomson KA, Segraves R, Weinstein ME (1993). A rare inherited euchromatic heteromorphism on chromosome 1. Prenat Diagn. 13:569–73.
17. Sumption ND, Barber JCK (2001). A transmitted deletion of 2q13 to 2q14.1 causes no phenotypic abnormalities. J Med Genet. 38:125–6.

18. Shuan-Yow L, Gibson LH, Gomez K, Pober BR, Yang-Feng TL (1998). Familial dup(5)(q15q21) associated with normal and abnormal phenotypes. Am J Med Genet. 75:75–7.

19. Barber JCK, Joyce CA, Collinson MN *et al.* (1998). Duplication of 8p23.1: a cytogenetic anomaly with no established clinical significance. J Med Genet. 35:491–6.

20. Engelen JJM, Moog U, Evers JLH, Dassen H, Albrechts JCM, Hamers AJH (2000). Duplication of chromosome region 8p23.1 → p23.2: a benign variant? Am J Med Genet. 91:18–21.

21. Williams L, Larkins S, Roberts E, Davison EV (1996). Two further cases of variations in band 8p23.1. Not always a benign variant. J Med Genet. 33:S22.

22. Hansmann I (1976). Structural variability of human chromosome 9 in relation to its evolution. Hum Genet. 31:247–62.

23. Verma RS, Luke S, Brennan JP, Mathews T, Conte RA, Macera MJ (1993). Molecular topography of the secondary construction region (qh) of human chromosome 9 with an unusual euchromatic band. Am J Hum Genet. 52:981–6.

24. Roland B, Chernos JE, Cox DM (1992). 9qh+ variant band in two families. Am J Med Genet. 42:137–8.

25. Jalal SM, Kukolich MK, Garcia M, Day DW (1990). Euchromatic 9q+ heteromorphism in a family. Am J Med Genet. 37:155–6.

26. Knight LA, Soon GM, Tan M (1993). Extra G positive band on the long arm of chromosome 9. J Med Genet. 30:613.

27. Wang J-CC, Miller WA (1994). Molecular cytogenetic characterization of two types of chromosome 9 variants. Cytogenet Cell Genet. 67:190–2.

28. Ludowese CJ, Thompson KJ, Sekon GS, Pauli RM (1991). Absence of predictable phenotypic expression in proximal 15q duplications. Clin Genet. 40:194–201.

29. Jalal SM, Persons OL, Dewald GW (1994). Form of 15q proximal duplication appears to be a normal euchromatic variant. Am J Med Genet. 52:495–7.

30. Mao R, Jalal SM, Snow K, Michels VV, Szabo SM, Babovic-Vuksanovic D (2000). Characteristics of two cases with dup(15)(q11.2-12): one of maternal and one of paternal origin. Genet In Med. 2:131–5.

31. Thompson PW, Roberts SH (1987). A new variant of chromosome 16. Hum Genet. 76:100–1.

32. Jalal SM, Schneider NR, Kukolich MK, Wilson GN (1990). Euchromatic 16p+ heteromorphism: first report in North America. Am J Med Genet. 37:548–50(b).

33. Bryke CR, Breg WR, Potluri VR, Yang-Feng TL (1990). Duplication of euchromatin without phenotypic effects: a variant of chromosome 16. Am J Med Genet. 36:43–4.

34. Jalal SM, Law ME, Dewald GW (1993). Inverted duplication involving α satellite DNA resulting in a C-negative-band in the qh region of chromosome 16. Am J Med Genet. 46:351–2.

35. Wolff DJ, Raffel LJ, Ferre MM, Schwartz S (1991). Prenatal ascertainment of an inherited dup(18p) associated with an apparently normal phenotype. Am J Med Genet. 41:319–21.

36. Knight LA, Yong MH, Tan M, Ng ISL (1995). Del(3)(p25.3) without phenotypic effect. J Med Genet. 32:994–5.

37. Walker JL, Blank CE, Smith BAM (1984). Interstitial deletion of the short arm of chromosome 5 in a mother and three children. J Med Genet. 21:465–7.

38. Overhauser J, Golbus MS, Schonberg SA, Wasmuth JJ (1986). Molecular analysis of an unbalanced deletion of the short arm of chromosome 5 that produces no phenotype. Am J Hum Genet. 39:1–10.

39. Keppen LD, Gollin SM, Edwards D, Sawyer J, Wilson W, Overhauser J (1992). Clinical phenotype and molecular analysis of a three-generation family with an interstitial deletion of the short arm of chromosome 5. Am J Med Genet. 44:356–60.

40. Hand JL, Michels VV, Marinello MJ, Ketterling RP, Jalal SM (2000). Inherited interstitial deletion of chromosomes 5p and 16q without apparent phenotypic effect: further confirmation. Prenat Diagn. 20:144–8.

41. Kumar A, Cassidy SB, Romero L, Schwartz S (1999). Molecular cytogenetics of a de novo interstitial deletion of chromosome arm 6q in a developmentally normal girl. Am J Med Genet. 86:227–31.

42. Matkins SV, Meyer JE, Berry AC (1987). A child with partial monosomy 6q secondary to a maternal direct insertional event. J Med Genet. 24:227–9.

43. Christian SL, Rich BH, Loebl C *et al.* (1999). Significance of genetic testing for paternal uniparental disomy of chromosome 6 in neonatal diabetes mellitus. J Pediatr. 134:42–6.

44. Barber JCK, Mahl H, Portch J, Crawfurd MD'A (1991). Interstitial deletions without phenotypic effect: prenatal diagnosis of a new family and brief review. Prenat Diagn. 11:411–16.

45. Coutuier J, Morichon-Delvallez N, Dutrillaux B (1986). Deletion of band 13q21 is compatible with normal phenotype. Hum Genet. 70:87–91.
46. Naritomi K, Shiroma N, Izumikawa Y, Sameshima K, Ohdo S, Hirayama K (1988). 16q21 is critical for 16q deletion syndrome. Clin Genet. 33:372–5.
47. Witt DR, Lew SP, Mann J (1988). Heritable deletion of band 16q21 with normal phenotype: relationship to late replicating DNA. Am J Hum Genet. 43:A127.
48. Callen DF, Eyre H, Lane S *et al.* (1993). High resolution mapping of interstitial long arm deletions of chromosome 16: relationship to phenotype. J Med Genet. 30:828–32.
49. Taysi K (1983). Del(X) (q26) in a phenotypically normal woman and her daughter who also has trisomy 21. Am J Med Genet. 14:367–72.
50. Buiting K, Dittrich B *et al.* (1999). A 28-kb deletion spanning D15S63 (PW71) in five families: a rare neutral variant? Am J Hum Genet. 65:1588–94.
51. Silverstein S, Lerer I, Buiting K, Abeliovich D (2001). The 28-kb deletion spanning D15S63 is a polymorphic variant in the Ashkenazi Jewish population. Am J Hum Genet. 68:261–3.
52. Jalal SM, Harwood A, Anderson M *et al.* (2000). Screening for subtle structural anomalies by use of subtelomeric specific probe set. Am J Hum Genet. A770.
53. Lopes J, LeGuern E, Gouider R *et al.* and the French CMT Collaborative Research Group (1996). Recombination hot spot in a 3.2-kb region of the Charcot-Marie-Tooth type 1A repeat sequences: new tools for molecular diagnosis of hereditary neuropathy with liability to pressure palsies and of Charcot-Marie-Tooth type 1A. Am J Hum Genet. 58:1223–30.
54. Webb GC, Krumins EJM, Eichenbaum SZ, Voullaire LE, Earle E, Choo KH (1989). Non C-banding variants in some normal families might be homogeneously staining regions. Hum Genet. 82:59–62.
55. Barber JCK, Reed CJ, Dahoun SP, Joyce CA (1999). Amplification of a pseudogene cassette underlies euchromatic variation of 16p at the cytogenetic level. Hum Genet. 104:211–18.
56. Eichler EE, Lu F, Shen Y *et al.* (1996). Duplication of a gene-rich cluster between 16p11.1 and Xq28: a novel pericentromeric-directed mechanism for paralogous genome evaluation. Hum Mod Genet. 5:899–913.
57. Eichler EE, Budarf ML, Rocchi M *et al.* (1997). Interchromosomal duplications of the adrenoleukodystrophy locus: a phenomenon of pericentromeric plasticity. Hum Mol Genet. 6:991–1002.

7
FISH Technologies

HERMAN WYANDT AND VIJAY TONK

7.1 INTRODUCTION

Fluorescence in-situ hybridization (FISH) is the latest technology for studying specific sequences on whole chromosomes. Discussing all ramifications and applications is beyond the scope of this book. However, FISH methodologies hold unlimited promise as a means to more accurately identify and characterize chromosomal variants. In principle, any piece of DNA can be cloned, sequenced, characterized, amplified, labeled and hybridized to intact chromosomes or nuclei and detected. These cloned DNA segments, called probes, are prepared by a variety of techniques including: (1) synthesis of cDNAs from mRNAs by reverse transcriptase [1]; (2) isolation of specific sequences by PCR amplification and/or gel electrophoresis [2,3]; (3) propagation of larger DNA fragments in bacteria or yeast by insertion into cloning vectors such as plasmids, phage, cosmids, BACS, or YACS [4,5]; (4) isolation and cloning of partial or complete DNA libraries from specific chromosome regions or entire chromosomes by microdissection [6,7] or chromosome sorting [8,9]. Whatever the source, labeling is usually completed by nick translation or random priming with nucleotides that either have fluorescent label attached directly or combined with a ligand that is recognized by a fluorescent-tagged protein [10,11].

The principal components and steps of in-situ hybridization procedures [10,11] are: (1) the probe, (2) the target DNA, (3) denaturation of probe and target DNA sequences to single strands, (4) incubation of probe and target under conditions that allow specific association (hybridization) of labeled probe DNA to complementary target sequences, (5) washing away non-hybridized probe, and (6) detection of hybridized sequences in target cells. The rate of hybridization of probe in solution to complementary DNA targets bound on the glass slide follows first-order kinetics [11]. This rate is dependent upon the labeled probe concentration in solution (number of copies of a specific sequence per unit volume) at a given time. If the ratio of labeled probe to unlabeled target is too low, insufficient labeled sequence will anneal to the target to permit subsequent detection. If the ratio is too high, precipitation of probe or non-specific hybridization to imperfect complements may result in false-positive signals. Typical ratios of probe to target DNA are on the order of 100 : 1.

Other factors controlling rates and specificity of hybridization are salt and formamide concentrations and temperature, in both the hybridization and subsequent wash steps [10]. The melting or denaturation temperature (T^m) of DNA is 90–100°C. Such high temperatures applied to intact cells or chromosomes destroy their morphology and integrity. Formamide is used to lower the melting temperature of the DNA so that it does not unduly damage the target cells. A standard denaturation temperature in 50% formamide in 2 × SSC is about 70°C.

Reassociation is done at temperatures 16–33°C lower than the melting temperature, in most laboratories at 37°C. Divalent cations such as Ca^{++} and Mg^{++} strongly stabilize double-stranded DNA so that EDTA is typically added to the reaction mixtures to bind them. Monovalent sodium ions decrease electrostatic repulsion between DNA strands above 0.4 M. Concentrations less than 0.4 M have considerable effect on reassociation and on T^m. A standard salt concentration (SSC) is 0.15 M NaCl, 0.015 sodium citrate and 20 mM phosphate. Hybridization reactions are typically done in 2 × SSC. Excess probe is removed by washing, usually at formamide and SSC concentrations equivalent to about 15°C below the melting temperature. Lower sodium concentrations attained by lowering the concentration of SSC in conjunction with variations in wash temperatures are typically used to optimize hybridization stringency. Hybridization to closely related sequences, which show as little as 70% homology, can occur at low stringency. At high-stringency wash the specificity of hybridization can exceed 99% [10,11].

Aside from the above conditions that effect hybridization kinetics and stringency, probe selection and preparation are the most important factors in obtaining optimal hybridization results. A single-copy sequence that hybridizes to a single genomic site is ideal. The disadvantage of such a probe is that it is generally small (1–5 kb) with a high signal-to-noise ratio that makes it difficult to detect except under the most ideal hybridization conditions. In practice, probes of 50 kb and larger that contain the specific sequence of interest are more commonly used. These include cosmids, BACS and YACS. However, such probes contain not only the sequence being probed, but also a high proportion of repeated sequences that are labeled along with the sequence of interest. These labeled repeat sequences, if hybridized using the principles we have discussed, will anneal throughout the genome and will be indistinguishable from the sequence of interest. Single-copy sequences are actually in a minority in the human genome. Therefore, an excess of unlabeled fragmented human DNA, or DNA enriched in repeated sequences (so-called Cot DNA), is added to the labeled probe and the entire mixture is denatured and allowed to reassociate for a specified time in solution before applying the probe to the target. Reassociation in solution follows second-order kinetics [12]. Repeated sequences (labeled and non-labeled) reassociate at a faster rate in solution, leaving mainly unique sequences in single-stranded form. Hence, non-specific hybridization of the repeated sequences is minimized when the probe solution is finally hybridized with the target.

The advantage of a longer probe is a longer hybridized sequence with a larger signal that is easier to detect in the target area. The disadvantage is that unique sequences other than the specific sequence of interest are likely to be present.

7.2 TYPES OF FISH PROBES

FISH is rapidly becoming the technique of choice to detect chromosome abnormalities that are either too complex to be interpretable by banding or are below the resolution of standard chromosome banding techniques. Several types of probes are commonly in use. These include:

1. *Satellite probes*: these are probes that are homologous to repeated sequences around the centromeres of chromosomes, the qh regions of 1, 9 and 16, the satellites and short arms of acrocentric chromosomes, and the distal end of the Y chromosome. Chapters 8 and 9 are devoted to the description of these sequences and how they have evolved. Probes specific for sequences that are unique to nearly all of the centromeric regions of individual human chromosomes are commercially available.
2. *Painting probes*: these are libraries of probes that are specific for unique sequences isolated throughout the entire chromosome. Such libraries usually have repeated sequences repressed or removed and label the entire chromosome, except for the repetitive centromeric regions and large blocks of heterochromatin in the qh regions and distal end of the Y. Paints specific for each human chromosome are commercially available.
3. *Locus-specific probes*: microdeletions that involve loss of segments of chromosomes less than a few megabases are usually not detectable by banding but are detectable by FISH when the appropriate probe is available. Several criteria must be met for such a probe to be useful: (a) it must be specific for a gene region associated with disease; (b) it must have been tested on enough cases to confirm specificity (frequency of association with the disease in question) and sensitivity (frequency of false-positive and/or false-negative results) [13]; (c) the laboratory using the probe should establish that it is at least as reliable as reported in a peer-reviewed publication. Commercially available probes exist for about a dozen microdeletion syndromes and for a number of chromosome regions involving oncogenes in cancer or leukemia.
4. *Subtelomeric probes*: these are probes for sequences 70–300 kb in length that are immediately adjacent to the telomeres themselves and are specific for each chromosome arm [14]. Forty-one different probes are available commercially and are used as a panel to rule out subtle structural deletions or rearrangements involving the ends of all of the chromosome arms except the short arms of the acrocentric chromosomes.
5. *Telomeric probe sequence*: one specific repeated sequence, (TTAGGG)n, is present at the end of every chromosome arm [15]. The number of repeats (n) for each arm varies from 400 to 1000. A critical number of repeats on each arm are necessary for the chromosome to be stable and for DNA replication of both strands to be completed without gradual loss of DNA over time.

7.3 APPLICATIONS

A number of variations in the application of in-situ hybridization techniques have been developed. The principles as outlined above are the same for all of them. Only the combinations of probes used, and their targets, are changed. With increasing complexity of the technology, detection and data analysis is typically augmented by special computer software.

1. *Dual-colored probes*: in the case of microdeletions or other locus-specific probes, a control probe of a different color is typically included in the probe mixture and hybridized at the same time. Detection can either be with a triple bandpass filter that allows detection of three different wavelengths (three different colors) simultaneously, or with three different single bandpass filters that allow detection of only a single color at a time. In the latter case individually collected digitized images are typically superimposed by computer software designed to generate a single three-colored image [16,17].
2. *Multiple-colored probes*: several systems are now available that allow visualization of the entire genome in multiple colors. Multiple colors are accomplished by labeling DNA representing a particular chromosome in three or more colors and combining these colors in different ratios to give a different color for each chromosome [18]. Such combinatorial labeling can be achieved by superimposing narrow bandpass filter images that allow distinction of the various color ratios (so-called M-FISH) [19] or by quantitatively measuring the pixel value of each color and assigning a new color for each of the ratios (so-called SKY-FISH) [20,21]. A third more esoteric method combines color ratio labeling of individual orangutan chromosomes and inter-species hybridization of the multicolored orangutan DNA to human metaphases with a resultant multicolored banding pattern on the human chromosomes representing rearrangement of the orangutan genome in its evolution to the human karyotype (so-called Rx-FISH) [22].
3. *Comparative genomic hybridization*: this method of hybridization has been used mainly to characterize complex multiple chromosome abnormalities in tumor cell lines [23–25]. DNA from the tumor line is extracted and labeled with a green fluorescent tag such as FITC and is mixed in equal molar amounts with DNA extracted from a normal cell line that has been labeled with a red fluorescent tag such as Texas red or rhodamine. The probe mixture is then hybridized to metaphases prepared from normal cells. Segments of chromosomes or entire chromosomes that are either in excess or deleted will have more or fewer green- vs. red-labeled sequences competing for complementary sites on the normal chromosomes. A segment that is in excess will have more green than red fragments ($3:2$ ratio) and produce a signal on the target chromosome that is correspondingly more green; conversely, a segment that is deleted will have more red than green fragments ($2:1$ ratio) and produce a signal that is correspondingly more red. Normal diploid segments have equal numbers ($1:1$ ratio) of red- and green-labeled fragments in the probe mixture and hence produce a yellow signal over chromosome regions that are not lost or gained. Such differences in ratios, affected by mosaicism or stability of the chromosome imbalance, may not be seen easily by eye and so are typically

measured spectrophotometrically. Target sites that differ by more than one copy from normal are detected more readily.

7.4 STUDIES OF HETEROMORPHISMS BY FISH

The dissection of heteromorphisms at the molecular level is alluded to in various sections of this book. Chapter 8 deals directly with the molecular characterization, particularly of the satellite DNAs that make up the most visible, structurally variable regions of the human genome. Such studies, for the most part, are based on results from a few cases and do not attempt to correlate molecular and cytological findings in any significant population of normal individuals. With one or two exceptions [26,27], the characterization of heteromorphisms at the molecular level is more anecdotal than systematic. However, it is also apparent that, just as banding techniques dramatically increased the number of heteromorphisms that could be detected microscopically, molecular cytogenetic techniques have similar potential for increasing this number still further. FISH techniques allow identification of specific segments of DNA in ways that are not possible with any of the standard ways of studying chromosomes by conventional banding techniques. At the same time they raise the possibility for detecting new forms of heteromorphism in the human genome that were not detectable by previous methods. One of the drawbacks of the new FISH technologies is that variation in signal size, or the apparent lack of a signal with a probe that is associated with a certain diseases, could be reflecting normal variability instead of a disease-associated modification. Therefore, great care must be taken in the application and interpretation of results when a new probe is used or the disease has not been well characterized [13]. It is also important to realize that differences in signal size by FISH are more qualitative than quantitative. The smaller the signal, the more it may vary in size and frequency of detection. A second feature of the most variable regions studied by FISH, revealed in Chapter 9, is that regions most easily detected by FISH are often the most heterogeneous. The larger the size of the region, the greater the diversity in the repeated sequences is likely to be.

A handful of variants have been characterized by FISH analysis. The main impediments are: (1) the expense of developing and characterizing probes that are not necessarily disease-related and (2) the application to sufficiently large populations to establish variant frequencies. The following is a discussion of some of the more commonly recognized variants (see Part II of this volume for examples).

7.5 FISH RESULTS WITH ALPHOID REPEATS

Chromosomes 13 and 21

Alpha satellite probes were initially used for rapid detection of aneuploidy in uncultured amniotic fluid cells. Verlinsky *et al.* [28] reported three false-negative results and one false-positive in 516 prenatal cases, using alpha satellite probe for chromosomes 13 and 21. False-negatives were interpreted to be due either to failure of hybridization or to polymorphism. A diminished signal size in the chromosome 13 centromeric region of occasional individuals had also been previously reported by Weier and Gray [29] and Lapdot-Lifson *et al.* [30], who recommended caution in interpreting interphase FISH results to diagnose aneuploidy. Bossuyt *et al.* [26] gave a similar warning in a report of diminished signal intensity in four of 101 cases. The false-positive case of Verlinsky *et al.* [28] was due to cross-hybridization of the centromeric probe for 13 and 21 with a chromosome 22. Similar cross-hybridization with chromosome 22 also occurred in the mother. Tardy and Toth [31] reported similar cross-hybridization to the chromosome 22 of a 4-year-old boy with mild mental retardation and dysmorphism, and of his unaffected father. Hybridization with unique probes for 14 and 22 failed to reveal a translocation between 13 or 21 and 14 or 22. Therefore, the investigators interpreted this cross-hybridization to represent a normal polymorphism. Such polymorphism is also supported by molecular studies. Vissel and Choo [32] reported four distinct alpha-satellite subfamilies shared by chromosomes 13, 14 and 21.

Chromosome 14

Earl *et al.* [34] found absence of satellite III DNA in the centromere and proximal long arm of a 14p− variant, but retention of the centromeric region. These results demonstrated that satellite III was not an essential component of centromere function but this does not exclude the possibility that satellite DNA enhances and/or protects centromeric function (see Chapter 9).

Chromosome 15

The cross-hybridization between 13/21 alpha satellite and chromosome 22 received considerable attention because of interest in probes to prenatally detect trisomy 21. However, other satellite sequences have also shown cross-hybridization. Two distinct classes of satellite DNA are found on chromosome 15 [34]: alpha satellite and classical satellite. The classical satellite sequence, corresponding to satellite III and DA/DAPI-positive regions on the short arm of chromosome 15 reportedly cross-hybridizes with short arm regions of other acrocentrics with a frequency of about 10%. Stergianou *et al.* [27] found cross-hybridization in 12 of 100 randomly selected individuals studied. This was consistent with a study by Smeets *et al.* [35] using non-fluorescent immunoperoxidase detection of alphoid sequences specific for chromosome 15. They found hybridization corresponding to DA/DAPI-positive regions on acrocentric chromosomes other than 15 in seven of 127 individuals studied. In a FISH analysis of a case with 15p− [36] (see Plate 44), classical satellite D15Z1 (Vysis) was absent. However, alpha satellite D15Z4 (Vysis), specific for the centromeric region, was present. In another case being tested for Prader-Willi syndrome, from this same study (Plate 69), both chromosome 14 homologs showed a signal with D15Z1.

Chromosome 18 and Other Rare Variants

Bonfatti *et al.* [37] found individual variations in pericentromeric regions of chromosome 18 with alpha satellite probe that were almost undetectable by C-banding. In addition to the above cases, a number of alpha-satellite variants are included in the present volume, including variants of chromosomes 11, 13, 14, 15, 18 and 20.

Table 7.1 Subtelomeric polymorphisms and cross-hybridizations revealed by FISH

	Probe(s) used
Polymorphism ID (Blake et al.) [38]	
ish add(1)(qter)(13qtel+)	PAC 163C9
ish del(2)(q37.3q37.3)mat or pat*	PAC 1011017, P1 21OE14
ish del(9)(p34p34)pat	PAC 43N6
ish del(X)(p22.3p22.3)pat	Cosmid CY29
Cross-hybridizations (Knight and Feint) [14]	
5p with acrocentric p arms	114j1B (BAC)
5q with acrocentric cen	B22n4 (cosmid)
8p with 1p	2205n2 (cosmid)
1p with 17p	2209n2 (cosmid)
12p with 6p and 20q	496z11 (PAC)

*Deletions of PAC 1011017 but not of P1 21OE14 were found in 8/8 cases.

7.6 SUBTELOMERIC DELETIONS: NORMAL VARIATION OR CHROMOSOME ABNORMALITY

Apparently normal variants have also been reported using the panel of 41 subtelomeric probes specific for the subterminal regions of each chromosome arm except the acrocentric short arms. Such probes are used to detect cryptic or semi-cryptic rearrangements involving the exchange, loss or duplication of the ends of chromosome arms associated with idiopathic developmental delay and mental retardation. A number of cases with a subtle deletion, however, have revealed a similar deletion in an unaffected parent of the affected proband.

Probes used for these studies have been tested through two generations of development. The first generation showed a high frequency of cross-hybridization [14] with other chromosome regions, indicating that varying degrees of sequence homology exist between different chromosomes (Table 7.1). A second generation of probes has shown less cross-hybridization and more reliable detection of subtle rearrangement and deletion. However, all such deletions should be confirmed by parental or family studies or other forms of molecular characterization where possible. Blake *et al.* [38] report a list of chromosome deletions that were determined, in some cases through parental studies, to be normal chromosome variants. The most frequent of these were 2q deletions (Table 7.1).

References

1. Efstratiadis A, Kafatos FC, Mazam AM, Maniatis T (1976). Enzymztic *in vitro* synthesis of globin genes. Cell. 7:279–88.
2. White TJ, Arnheim N, Erlich HA (1989). The polymerase chain reaction. Trends Genet. 5:185–9.
3. Sambrook J *et al.* (1989). Molecular Cloning: A Laboratory Manual. Cold Spring Harbor: Cold Spring Harbor Laboratory.
4. Shero JH, McCormick MK, Antonarakis SE, Hieter P (1991). Yeast artificial chromosome vectors for efficient clone manipulation and mapping. Genomics. 10:505–8.
5. Monaco AP, Larin Z (1994). YACs, BACs and MACs: artificial chromosomes as research tools. Trends Biotechnol. 12:280–6.

6. Ludecke HJ, Senger G, Claussen U, Horsthemke B (1989). Cloning defined regions of the human genome by microdissection of banded chromosomes and enzymatic amplification. Nature. 338:348–50.
7. Kao F-T, Yu J-W (1991). Chromosome microdissection and cloning in human genome and genetic disease analysis. Proc Natl Acad Sci USA. 88:1844–8.
8. Harris P, Boyd E, Ferguson-Smith MA (1985). Optimizing human chromosome separation for the production of chromosome-specific DNA libraries by flow sorting. Hum Genet. 70:59–65.
9. Deaven LL, van Dilla MA, Bartholdi MF et al. (1986). Construction of human chromosome-specific DNA libraries from flow-sorted chromosomes. Cold Spring Harb Symp Quant Biol. 51:159–67.
10. Hopman AHN, Raap AK, Landegent JE, Wiegant J, Boerman RH, Van der Ploeg M (1988). Non radioactive in situ hybridization. In: Van Leeuwen FW, et al., editors. Molecular Neuroanatomy Amsterdam: Elvesier, pp. 43–68.
11. Lichter P, Ried T (1994). Molecular analysis of chromosome aberrations. In situ hybridization. In: Gosden JR, editor. Methods in Molecular Biology. Chromosome Analysis Protocols. Totowa, NJ: Humana Press, pp. 449–78.
12. Britten RJ, Kohne DE (1968). Repeated sequences in DNA. Science. 161:529–40.
13. American College of Medical Genetics (1999). Standards and Guidelines for Clinical Genetics Laboratories, 2nd edn. Bethesda, MD: ACMG.
14. Knight SJ, Flint J (2000). Perfect endings: a review of subtelomeric probes and their use in clinical diagnosis. J Med Genet. 57:401–9.
15. Moyzis RK, Buckingham JM, Cram LS et al. (1988). A highly conserved repetitive sequence (TTAGGG)$_n$, present at the telomeres of human chromosomes. Proc Natl Acad Sci USA. 85:6622–6.
16. Nederlof PM, Robinson D, Abuknesh R et al. (1989). Three-color fluorescence in situ hybridization for the simultaneous detection of multiple nucleic acid sequences. Cytometry. 10:20–7.
17. Lichter P, Tang CJ, Call K et al. (1990). High resolution mapping of human chromosome 11 by in situ hybridization with cosmid clones. Science. 247:64–9.
18. Dauwerse JG, Wiegant J, Raap AK, Breuning MH, van Ommen GJ (1992). Multiple colors by fluorescence in situ hybridization using ratio-labelled DNA probes create a molecular karyotype. Hum Mol Genet. 1:593–8.
19. Spiecher MR, Ballard S, Ward, DC (1996). Karyotyping human chromosomes by combinatorial multifluor FISH. Nat Genet. 12:368–75.
20. Schrock E, Veldman T, Padilla-Nash H et al. (1997). Spectral karyotyping refines cytogenetic diagnsotic of constitutional chromosomal abnormalities. Hum Genet. 101:255–62.
21. Bayani J, Squire JA (2001). Advances in the detection of chromosomal aberrations using spectral karyotyping. Clin Genet. 59:65–73.
22. Muller S, O'Brien PC, Feguson-Smith MA, Weinberg J (1998). Cross-species colour segmenting: a novel tool in human karyotype analysis. Cytometry. 33:445–52.
23. Kallioniemi A, Kallioniemi OP, Sudar D et al. (1992). Comparative genomic hybridization for molecular cytogenetic analysis of solid tumors. Science. 258:818–21.
24. Kallioniemi OP, Kallioniemi A, Piper J et al. (1994). Optimizing comparative genomic hybridization for analysis of DNA sequence copy number changes in solid tumors. Genes Chromosomes Cancer. 10:231–4.
25. Levy B, Dunn TM, Kaffe S, Kardon N, Hirschhorn K (1998). Clinical applications of comparative genomic hybridization. Genet Med. 1:4–12.
26. Bossuyt PJ, Van Tienen MN, De Gruyter L, Smets V, Dumon J, Wauters JG (1995). Incidence of low-fluorescence alpha-satellite region on chromosome 21 escaping detection of aneuploidy at interphase by FISH. Cytogenet Cell Genet. 68:203–6.
27. Stergianou K, Gould CP, Waters JJ, Hulten MA (1993). A DA/DAPI positive human 14p heteromorphism defined by fluorescent in situ hybridization using chromosome 15-specific probes D15Z1 Satellite III) and p-TRA-25 (alphoid). Hereditas. 119:105–10.
28. Verlinsky Y, Ginsberg N, Chmura M et al. (1995). Cross-hybridization of the chromosome 13/21 alpha satellite DNA probe to chromosome 22 in the prenatal screening of common chromosomal aneuploidies by FISH. Prenat Diagn. 15:831–4.
29. Weir HU, Gray JW (1992). A degenerate alpha satellite probe, detecting a centromeric deletion on chromosome 21 in an apparently normal human male shows limitations of the use of satellite DNA probes for interphase ploidy analysis. Anal Cell Pathol. 4:81–6.

30. Lapidot-Lifson Y, Lebo RV, Flandermeyer R, Chung J-H, Golbus MS (1991). Rapid aneuploid diagnosis of high risk cases by fluorescence in situ hybridization. Am J Obstet Gynecol. 174:886–90.

31. Tardy EP, Totu A (1997). Letters to the Editor. Cross-hybridization of the chromosome 13/21 alpha satellite DNA to chromosome 22 or a rare polymorphism. Prenat Diagn. 17:487–90.

32. Vissel B, Choo KHA (1991). Four distinct alpha satellite subfamilies shared by human chromosomes 13, 14 and 21. Nucl Acids Res. 19:271–7.

33. Choo KH, Earl E, Vissel B, Filby RG (1990). Identification of two distinct subfamilies of alpha satellite DNA that are highly specific for chromosome 15. Genomics. 7:517–23.

34. Earle E, Voullaire L, Hills L, Stlate H, Choo KHA (1992). Absence of satellite III DNA in the centromere and the proximal long-arm region of human chromosome 14: analysis of a 14p- variant. Cytogenet Cell Genet. 61:78–80.

35. Smeets DFCM, Merkx GFM, Hopman HM (1991). Frequent occurrence of translocations of the short arm of chromosome 15 to other D-group chromosomes. Hum Genet. 87:45–8.

36. Shim SH, Pan A, Huang XL, Tonk VS, Wyandt HE (2002). FISH variants with D15Z1 in clinical cases. Am J Hum Genet. 71:307A.

37. Bonfatti A, Giunta C, Sensi A, Gruppioni R, Rubini M, Fontana F (1993). Heteromorphism of human chromosome 18 detected by fluorescent in situ hybridization. J Histochem. 37:149–54.

38. Blake C, Kashork CD, Shaffer KG (2000). The promise and pitfalls of telomere region-specific probes. J Am Hum Genet. 67: 1356–9.

8
Molecular Dissection of Heteromorphic Regions

BRYNN LEVY AND PETER E. WARBURTON

8.1 INTRODUCTION

The human genome project has provided detailed knowledge of the human DNA sequence and revealed its complexity. Genes and gene-related sequences (promotors, introns, etc.) account for about 25% of the 3300 Mb of DNA and only about 3% of the genome represents coding sequence. Repetitive sequences form a large part of our genome and are the basis of the polymorphisms detected at the molecular level and of the heteromorphisms observed at the chromosomal level. Repetitive DNA sequences are found either as individual repeat units *interspersed* throughout the genome, or as *tandemly repeated units* or motifs in various chromosomal locations. Three main types of tandemly repeated DNA sequences, classified by the length of the individual repeated motif and by the total size of the repeated units, are *satellite*, *minisatellite* and *microsatellite*. This chapter describes only tandemly repeated sequences, as these play a more significant role in chromosomal heteromorphisms.

8.2 SATELLITE DNA

Satellite DNA is composed of large arrays of tandemly repeated DNA elements, found mainly as heterochromatic blocks in the centromeric regions of human chromosomes. The many different families of satellite DNA comprise as much as 10% of the human DNA [1,2]. Classical satellites 1, 2 and 3 are found primarily in the large qh regions of human chromosomes [3–5]. Alpha satellite DNA found at the centromere of every human chromosome may have a functional role. Other satellite families include beta and gamma satellite DNAs [6–8]. Evolutionary processes acting on satellite DNA have played a role in shaping our chromosomes, leading to large arrays of highly homologous repeat units at particular chromosomal locations. Chromosome-specific satellite DNA repeats are routinely utilized as FISH probes for chromosome identification and/or enumeration,

97

and for pre- and post-natal identification of cytogenetic abnormalities such as trisomies or supernumerary marker chromosomes. ICF (immunodeficiency, centromere instability, facial abnormalities) [9] and Roberts syndromes [10] are rare disorders that manifest as distinct chromosome abnormalities involving the satellite DNA-containing heterochromatin.

Satellite DNA Families

Satellite DNA was historically defined as genomic DNA fractions that had different buoyant densities, on CsCl (cesium chloride) [11] or CsSO$_4$ (cesium sulfate) gradients, from the bulk of genomic DNA [12–14]. Several human "satellite" fractions consisting of heterogeneous mixtures of repetitive DNA sequences were identified and are referred to as *classical satellites I, II and III* [15,16]. In-situ hybridization of these different fractions to human chromosomes showed several large distinct blocks at specific chromosomal locations in the pericentromeric regions of human chromosomes 1, 9, 16 and Y [16–19]. These locations correspond to heterochromatin that is readily visualized by its relatively intense staining with the fluorescent dyes DAPI and distamycin or by staining with Giemsa 11. Other major locations for satellite DNA include the short arms of acrocentric chromosomes 13, 14, 15, 21 and 22, both proximal and distal to the rDNA (ribosomal DNA) arrays.

Restriction enzyme analysis of these different satellite DNA fractions revealed several patterns consisting of ladders of repetitive units, some of which are specific to certain chromosomes. DNA sequencing led to the identification of three specific predominant repeats, called satellites 1, 2 and 3. The separate classification of satellites 1, 2 and 3 indicates their enrichment in the density gradient fractions, but distinguishes them from satellites I, II and III [3]. Satellite 1 contains a 42 bp repeat consisting of alternating 17 bp (ACATAAAATAT$^C/_G$AAAGT) and 25 bp (ACCCAAAT$^A/_G$T$^A/_G$TATTATATACTGT) units. Satellite 2 is identified as poorly conserved ATTCCATTCG repeats. Satellite 3 is defined as ATTCC repeats occasionally interspersed with A$^T/_C$TCGGGTTG.

By in-situ hybridization, satellite 1 is localized to the pericentromeric regions of chromosomes 3 and 4, and the short arms of the acrocentric chromosomes in regions both proximal and distal to the rDNA arrays. Satellite 2 is localized to the large heterochromatic regions of chromosomes 1 and 16, with less prominent domains in the pericentromeric regions of chromosomes 2 and 10. Satellite 3 is localized to the variable heterochromatic regions of chromosome 1 and 9, the long arm of the Y chromosome, and the short arms of the acrocentric chromosomes proximal to the rDNA arrays [3]. Molecular approaches to map these satellite DNA domains have confirmed these localizations and uncovered additional small domains such as satellite III in the pericentromeric region of chromosome 10 [20].

Alpha satellite DNA has been found at the centromere of every normal primate chromosome examined. It was first identified as a highly repetitive DNA fraction from the African Green Monkey [21] and is the most extensively studied of all human satellite DNA families. Its hierarchical repeat unit organization serves as a conceptual framework for the organization of tandemly repeated satellite DNAs. The fundamental repeat unit of alpha satellite DNA is a monomeric repeat unit (~171 bp) which displays up to 40% divergence. The monomers are tandemly organized into distinct linear arrangements called higher-order repeat units (HORs) ranging from two to over 30 monomers [22,23]. At the centromeres of each homologous chromosome pair a particular HOR is in turn tandemly repeated up to several hundred times to form an array as large as several million base pairs. For example, on chromosome 17 a 2.7 kb 16 monomer subunit is repeated approximately 1000 times to form an array of approximately 3000 kb. HORs from a particular centromere are generally less than 5% diverged from each other, and thus can be used as a specific FISH probe to identify an individual chromosome. Alpha satellite DNA also contains a 9 bp degenerate motif in a subset of its monomers that serves as the binding site for a centromeric protein called centromere protein B (CENP-B) [24], found in most mammalian centromeres.

Several additional families of satellite DNA have been described and they are also found at the chromosomal locations typical of satellite DNA, e.g. centromeric regions, the short arms of acrocentrics and the Y chromosome. *Beta satellite* DNA is based on a 68 bp monomer, and individual subsets have been shown to be chromosome specific by FISH [6]. *Gamma satellite* DNA is based on a 220 bp monomer and has thus far been observed at the centromeres of chromosomes 8 and X [25]. Additional families include a 48 bp satellite DNA, found on acrocentric chromosomes, and the Sn5 satellite family [26] which can be found in the pericentromeric regions of chromosome 2, and the acrocentric chromosomes.

Satellite DNA and Centromere Function

Centromeres are functionally defined as the chromosomal region responsible for ensuring the proper segregation of replicated sister chromatids during mitosis and meiosis. The use of human artificial chromosomes in gene therapy is an appealing approach for delivering normal genes into target cells. However, a better understanding of the requirements for centromere function is necessary before human artificial chromosomes for use as autonomous gene therapy vectors can be readily constructed. All mammalian chromosomes contain satellite DNA at their centromeres, and alpha satellite DNA is the only satellite DNA family found at the centromere of every normal primate chromosome [23]. The following experimental data support its role in centromere function: (1) transfection of alpha satellite DNA into human fibrosarcoma HT1080 cells has resulted in small mitotically stable artificial chromosomes that contain *de novo* centromeres [27,28]; (2) immunoprecipitation of human CENP-A, a centromere-specific histone H3 homologue, resulted in isolation of a subset of alpha satellite DNA that is found in a specialized centromeric nucleosome [29]; (3) the alpha satellite DNA binding protein CENP-B is remarkably well conserved, being found at most mammalian centromeres [24,30]. Interestingly, the centromeric satellite DNAs of other mammalian chromosomes, e.g. the 120 bp mouse minor satellite DNA, do not share sequence homology with alpha satellite DNA, except for the 9 bp CENP-B binding site.

The analysis of variant human centromeres provides considerable caveats to the importance of satellite DNA and CENP-B to the functioning of centromeres, and suggests that epigenetic factors, in addition to the primary sequence, are important for centromere formation. Stable dicentric chromosomes contain one active centromere and one inactive centromere and both contain normal arrays of alpha satellite DNA and CENP-B [31]. This suggests that the presence of alpha satellite DNA and CENP-B alone is not sufficient for centromere function. Furthermore, mammalian Y chromosomes contain neither CENP-B nor its binding sites, and experimentally generated homozygous CENP-B null mice exhibit normal centromere function in mitosis and meiosis [30]. Finally, neocentromeres, a rare class of newly formed fully functional centromeres found on rearranged chromosomes, do not contain alpha or any other satellite DNA, thus providing examples of centromere function in the absence of satellite DNA [32–34]. Indeed, the functional role of satellite DNA at mammalian centromeres remains an active area of investigation.

Satellite DNA and Chromosome Evolution

The evolution of satellite DNAs is inextricably linked to the structure of mammalian chromosomes. The large arrays of satellite DNA found on human chromosomes are shaped by evolutionary processes such as unequal crossing over and gene conversion. Such processes lead to homogenization of repeat units and expansion of arrays within a species or particular chromosomal location. Satellite DNAs are thought to accumulate at centromeres because these regions are transcriptionally inert. Crossing over and recombination events in these regions, therefore, will have no adverse effect on the organism. A similar situation exists for the Y chromosome, which contains few genes and has also accumulated satellite DNAs. The alpha satellite DNA binding protein CENP-B has been observed to share homology with the tigger family of ancient transposases, prompting theories that remnant 3' nicking activity of CENP-B may accelerate the expansion and homogenization of alpha satellite DNA arrays that contain the CENP-B binding site [30].

The effect of satellite DNA evolution on chromosome structure will depend on the relative rates of exchange between sister chromatids, homologous chromosomes and non-homologous chromosomes. In the case of human alpha satellite DNA, the homogenization of repeat units at specific centromeres of each chromosome suggests a relatively high frequency of intrachromosomal exchanges. A notable exception are the shared alpha satellite sequences on subsets of human acrocentric chromosome pairs, e.g. the 13/21 and the 14/22 acrocentric chromosome pairs, likely due to the fact that exchanges between the centromeres of these chromosomes would result only in exchange of homologous rDNA arrays. Indeed, the abundance of satellite DNAs on human acrocentric chromosomes is likely to be due to a relatively high frequency of short arm exchanges that occurs freely with no observable negative effect.

Syndromes Associated with Satellite DNA

Two rare clinical syndromes are associated with typical morphological changes of satellite DNA in regions of human chromosomes. In cultured lymphocytes of patients with ICF syndrome (immunodeficiency, centromere instability, facial abnormalities), the heterochromatic regions of chromosomes 1, 9 and 16 have an elongated and threadlike appearance which is associated with the formation of complex multiradial chromosomes and extrusion into micronuclei [9]. These patients usually succumb to severe immunodeficiency early in life. Recently, this syndrome has been shown to be due to a homozygous mutation in a DNA methyl-transferase gene (Dnmt3B), which leads to almost complete demethylation of the normally heavily methylated heterochromatic regions. Robert's syndrome is a rare recessively inherited disorder characterized by growth retardation, limb reductions and craniofacial abnormalities [10]. Mitotic cells from affected individuals display a puffing and repulsion of heterochromatic regions near the centromeres, and this is especially evident on chromosomes 1, 9 and 16. In addi-tion, the acrocentric chromosomes and distal Yq show a splaying of the short arms and there is an increased number of lagging and missegregated chromo-somes. The gene for this syndrome has not yet been identified, but is likely to be involved in human mitosis.

In conclusion, satellite DNA represents a significant portion of the human genome. Once regarded as useless "junk" DNA, satellite DNA is now recognized to play a key role in shaping our genome, and may also have a functional role at the centromeres. Its high copy number and high homology have made it of great utility for use as FISH probes in molecular cytogenetics.

8.3 MINISATELLITE DNA

Minisatellites are a class of tandemly repeated sequences that are generally GC-rich [36]. There are many different minisatellite loci which vary not only in the size of the individual repeat motif (6 to ~100 bp) but also in their total length (100 bp to several kilobases). The extreme repeat copy number variation at these loci (also called VNTRs for variable number of tandem repeats) has made them a useful tool in forensic science for individual identification by DNA fingerprint-ing. These loci also provided the first highly polymorphic, multiallelic markers for linkage studies [37] and were remarkably useful at the onset of the human genome project.

AT-Rich Minisatellites

While most minisatellites are GC-rich, five AT-rich minisatellites have been described in humans which are remarkably different from the GC-rich minisatel-lites, ApoB [38,39], COL2A [40], FRA16B [41], FRA10B [42] and the Y-specific minisatellite MSY1 [43]. The common features of these alleles include a pre-dicted tendency to form hairpin structures, and a domain organization, with sim-ilar variant repeats commonly existing as blocks within arrays [36]. These loci may also share some mechanisms of mutation, with transiently single-stranded DNA forming stable secondary structures which promote inter-strand misalign-ment and subsequent expansions or contractions in repeat number [43]. Telomeres are a special subset of minisatellites.

Minisatellite DNA and their Effects

The greater majority of hypervariable minisatellite DNA sequences are not transcribed; however, some have been shown to cause disease by influencing gene expression, modifying coding sequences within genes or generating fragile sites [36]. An example of the regulatory effect of a minisatellite is the insulin-linked polymorphic region (ILPR, also known as IDDM2) which is one of the loci responsible for genetic susceptibility to insulin-dependent diabetes mellitus (IDDM) [44]. ILPR is located in the 5-prime flanking region of the human insulin gene and consists of VNTRs of a 14-bp motif [45,46]. An intriguing feature of ILPR is its capacity to form unusual DNA structures *in vitro*. Lew *et al.* [47] demonstrated that both inter- and intramolecular G-quartet formation in ILPR can influence transcriptional activity of the insulin gene and, as a result, may contribute to that portion of diabetes susceptibility attributed to the ILPR/IDDM2 locus. Minisatellites are also known to exist within the coding sequence of genes. For example, the D4 dopamine receptor (D4DR) contains a VNTR in the coding sequence which affects its ligand binding affinity [48,49]. Altered expression of D4DR, as a result of polymorphisms in this region, has been associated with cognitive and emotional disorders, particularly when it results in high-level expression in the limbic areas of the brain [50–52]. Altered gene expression may also occur in genes that have minisatellites located within their introns. The human interferon-inducible 6–16 gene contains a partially expressed minisatellite consisting of 26 tandemly repeated dodecanucleotides. The core motif (CAGGTAAGGGTG) is similar to the mammalian splice donor consensus sequence [(A/C)AGGT(A/G) AGT], the presence of which can interfere with gene splicing mechanisms by providing new functional splice donor sites [53].

8.4   SATELLITE DNA FISH PROBES IN MOLECULAR CYTOGENETICS

FISH probes comprised of satellite DNA have found great utility in cytogenetic laboratories by providing a rapid means of chromosome identification and enumeration. A single cloned repeat unit will often have several thousand highly homologous repeats in a particular chromosomal location. This provides a target locus in the genome of up to several million base pairs, and when labeled with a fluorescent tag results in a very strong, bright hybridization signal under fluorescence microscopy. Such probes have been developed commercially for identification of every human chromosome. The majority of these are chromosome-specific centromeric, alpha satellite DNA subsets. Other classical satellite probes are also used, particularly when a specific alpha satellite subset is not available or the array size is relatively small and yields a weak hybridization signal. The human genome mapping project has given these satellite DNA loci a Z number to indicate their repetitiveness. The Z number designation reflects the historical order of description of the particular satellite array. For example, D18Z1 indicates the chromosome 18-specific alpha satellite DNA subset, D15Z1 identifies a classical satellite 3 array in the short arm of chromosome 15, and D15Z4 identifies a chromosome 15-specific alpha satellite DNA subset. These chromosome-specific satellite DNAs may be labeled with different fluorescent colors and used as FISH probes to pre- or postnatally identify particular chromosome abnormalities (see Chapter 7).

References

1. Waye JS, Creeper LA, Willard HF (1987). Organization and evolution of alpha satellite DNA from human chromosome 11. Chromosoma. 95:182–8.
2. Choo KHA, Vissel B, Earle E (1989). Evolution of alpha satellite DNA on human acrocentric chromosomes. Genomics. 5:332–44.
3. Prosser J, Frommer M, Paul C, Vincent PC (1986). Sequence relationships of three human satellite DNAs. J Mol Biol. 187:145–55.
4. Tagarro I, Wiegant J, Raap AK, Gonzalez-Aguilera JJ, Fernandez-Peralta AM (1994). Assignment of human satellite 1 DNA as revealed by fluorescent in situ hybridization with oligonucleotides. Hum Genet. 93:125–8.
5. Jeanpierre M (1994). Human satellites 2 and 3. Ann Genet. 37:63–71.
6. Waye JS, Willard HF (1989). Human beta satellite DNA: genomic organization and sequence definition of a class of highly repetitive tandem DNA. Proc Natl Acad Sci USA. 86:6250–4.
7. Vissel B, Choo KH (1989). Mouse major (gamma) satellite DNA is highly conserved and organized into extremely long tandem arrays: implications for recombination between non-homologous chromosomes. Genomics. 5:407–14.
8. Wier HU, Zitzelsberger HF, Gray JW (1992). Differential staining of human and murine chromatin in situ by hybridization with species-specific satellite DNA probes. Biochem Biophys Res Commun. 182:1313–19.
9. Sawyer JR, Swanson CM, Wheeler G, Cunniff C (1995). Chromosome instability in ICF syndrome: formation of micronuclei from multibranched chromosomes 1 demonstrated by fluorescence in situ hybridization. Am J Med Genet. 56:203–9.
10. Barbosa AC, Otto PA, Vanna-Morgante AM (2000). Replication timing of homologous alpha satelllite DNA in Roberts syndrome. Chromosome Res. 8:645–50.
11. Schildkraut CL, Marmur J, Doty P (1962). Determination of the base composition of deoxyribonucleic acid from its buoyant density in CsCl. J Mol Biol. 4:430–43.
12. Corneo G, Ginelli E, Polli E (1968). Isolation of the complementary strands of human satellite DNA. J Mol Biol. 33:331–5.
13. Corneo G, Ginelli E, Polli E (1970). Repeated sequences in human DNA. J Mol Biol. 48:319–27.
14. Ginelli E, Corneo G (1976). The organization of repeated DNA sequences in the human genome. Chromosoma. 56:55–68.
15. Jones KW, Prosser J, Corneo G, Ginnelli E, Bobrow M (1973). Satellite DNA, constitutive heterochromatin and human evolution. In: Pfeiffer RA, editor. Modern Aspects of Cytogenetics: Constitutive Heterochromatin in Man. Stuttgart: F.K. Schattauer Verlag, pp. 54–61.
16. Miklos GLB, John B (1979). Heterochromatin and satellite DNA in man: properties and progress. Am J Hum Genet. 31:264–80.
17. Jones KW, Prosser J, Corneo G, Ginelli E (1973). The chromosomal location of human satellite DNA III. Chromosoma. 42:445–51.
18. Jones KW, Purdom LF, Prosser J, Corneo G (1974). The chromosomal location of human satellite DNA I. Chromosoma. 49:161–71.
19. Gosden JR, Mitchell AR, Buckland RA, Clayton RP, Evans HJ (1975). The location of four human satellite DNAs on human chromosomes. Exp Cell Res. 92:148–58.
20. Jackson MS, Mole SE, Ponder BA (1992). Characterization of a boundary between satellite III and alphoid sequences on human chromosome 10. Nucl Acids Res. 20:4781–7.
21. Madhani HD, Leadon SA, Smith CA, Hanawalt PC (1986). Alpha DNA in African green monkey cells organized into extremely long tandem arrays. J Biol Chem. 261:2314–18.
22. Wu JC, Manuelidis L (1980). Sequence definition and organization of a human repeated DNA. J Mol Biol. 142:363–8.
23. Willard HF (1991). Evolution of alpha satellite DNA. Curr Opin Genet Devel. 1:509–14.
24. Sullivan KF, Glass CA (1991). CENP-B is a highly conserved mammalian centromere protein with homology to the helix–loop–helix family of proteins. Chromosoma. 100:360–70.
25. Lee C, Li X, Jabs EW, Court D, Lin CC (1995). Human gamma X satellite DNA: an X chromosome specific centromeric DNA sequences. Chromosoma. 104:103–12.
26. Johnson DH, Kroisel PM, Klapper HJ, Rosenkranz W (1992). Microdissection of a human marker chromosome reveals its origin and a new family of centromeric repetitive DNA. Hum Mol Genet. 1:741–7.

27. Harrington JJ, Bokkelen GV, Mays RW, Gustashaw K, Willard HF (1997). Formation of de novo centromeres and construction of first-generation human artificial microchromosomes. Nat Genet. 15:345–55.

28. Henning KA, Novotny EA, Compton ST, Guan XY, Liu PP, Ashlock MA (1999). Human artificial chromosomes generated by modification of a yeast artificial chromosome containing both human alpha satellite DNA and single-copy DNA sequences. Proc Natl Acad Sci USA. 96:592–7.

29. Warburton PE, Cooke CA, Bourassa S et al. (1997). Immunolocalization of CENP-A suggests a distinct nucleosome structure at the inner kinetophore plate of active centromeres. Curr Biol. 7:901–4.

30. Sullivan BA, Schwartz S (1995). Identification of centromeric antigens in dicentric Robertsonian translocations: CENP-C and CENP-E are necessary components of functional centromeres. Hum Mol Genet. 4:2189–97.

31. Kipling D, Warburton PE (1997). Centromeres, CENP-B and Tigger too. Trends Genet. 13:141–5.

32. Choo KHA (1997). Centromere DNA dynamics: latent centromeres and neocentromere formation. Am J Hum Genet. 61:1225–33.

33. Depinet TW, Zackowski JL, Earnshaw WC et al. (1997). Characterization of neo-centromere in marker chromosomes lacking detectable alpha-satellite DNA. Hum Mol Genet. 6:1195–204.

34. Warburton PE, Dolled M, Mahmood R et al. (2000). Molecular cytogenetic analysis of eight inversion duplications of human chromosome 13q that each contain a neocentromere. Am J Hum Genet. 66:1794–806.

35. Amar DJ, Choo KH (2002). Neocentromeres: role in human disease, evolution and centromere study. Am J Hum Genet. 7:695–714.

36. Bosi PR, Grant GR, Jeffreys AJ (2002). Minisatellites show rare and simple intra-allelic instability in the mouse germ line. Genomics. 80:2–4.

37. Nakamura Y, Leppert M, O'Connell P et al. (1987). Variable number of tandem repeat (VNTR) markers for human gene mapping. Science. 235:1616–22.

38. Desmarais E, Vigneron S, Buresi C, Cambien F, Cambou JP, Roizes G (1993). Variant mapping of the Apo(B) AT rich minisatellite. Dependence on nucleotide sequence of the copy number variations. Instability of the non-canonical alleles. Nucl Acids Res. 21:2179–84.

39. Buresi C, Desmarais E, Vigneron S et al. (1996). Structural analysis of the minisatellite present at the 3' end of the human apolipoprotein B gene: new definition of the alleles and evolutionary implications. Hum Mol Genet. 5:61–8.

40. Berg K (1986). DNA polymorphism at the apolipoprotein B locus is associated with lipoprotein level. Clin Genet. 30:515–20.

41. Yu S, Mangelsdorf M, Hewett D et al. (1997). Human chromosomal fragile site FRA16B is an amplified AT-rich minisatellite repeat. Cell. 88:367–74.

42. Hewett DR, Handt O, Hobson L et al. (1998). FRA10B structure reveals common elements in repeat expansion and chromosomal fragile site genesis. Mol Cell. 1:773–81.

43. Jobling MA, Bouzekri N, Taylor PG (1998). Hypervariable digital DNA codes for human paternal lineages: MVR-PCR at the Y-specific minisatellite, MSY1(DYF155S1). Hum Mol Genet. 7:643–53.

44. Bennett ST, Lucassen AM, Gough SC et al. (1995). Susceptibility to human type 1 diabetes at IDDM2 is determined by tandem repeat variation at the insulin gene minisatellite locus. Nat Genet. 9:284–92.

45. Bell GI, Karam JH, Rutter WJ (1981). Polymorphic DNA region adjacent to the 5' end of the human insulin gene. Proc Natl Acad Sci USA. 78:5759–63.

46. Bell GI, Selby MJ, Rutter WJ (1982). The highly polymorphic region near the human insulin gene is composed of simple tandemly repeating elements. Nature. 295:31–5.

47. Lew A, Rutter WJ, Kenedy GC (2000). Unusual DNA structure of the diabetes susceptibility locus IDDM2 and its effect on transcription by the insulin promoter factor Pur-1/MAZ. Proc Natl Acad Sci USA. 97:12508–12.

48. Van Tol HH, Wu CM, Guan HC et al. (1992). Multiple dopamine D4 receptor variants in the human population. Nature. 358:149–52.

49. Lichter JB, Barr CL, Kennedy JL, Van Tol HH, Kidd KK, Livak KJ (1993). A hypervariable segment in the human dopamine receptor D4 (DRD4) gene. Hum Mol Genet. 2:767–73.

50. Benjamin J, Li L, Patterson C, Greenberg BD, Murphy DL, Hamer DH (1996). Population and familial association between the D4 dopamine receptor gene and measures of novelty seeking. Nat Genet. 12:81–4.

51. Ebstein RP, Segman R, Benjamin J, Osher Y, Nemanov L, Belmaker RH (1997). 5-HT2C (HTR2C) serotonin receptor gene polymorphism associated with the human personality trait of reward dependence: interaction with dopamine D4 receptor (D4DR) and dopamine D3 receptor (D3DR) polymorphisms. Am J Med Genet. 74:65–72.

52. Benjamin J, Ebstein RP, Belmaker RH (1997). Personality genetics. Isr J Psychiatry Relat Sci. 34:270–80.

53. Turri MG, Cuin KA, Porter AC (1995). Characteristics of a novel minisatellite that provides multiple splice donor sites in an interferon-induced transcript. Nucl Acids Res. 23:1854–6.

9

Evolution of Human Alpha Satellite Sequences Comprising Variant Centromeric Chromosome Regions

WILLMAR PATINO, MAURICIO ARCOS-BURGOS
AND ROGER V. LEBO

SUMMARY

This chapter addresses the origin of the alpha satellite repeat arrays comprising variable-size human centromeric chromosome regions. These repeats, which share a basic 171 bp monomeric unit, usually attach head-to-tail in extremely long arrays and have their own taxonomic nomenclature [15]. The emergence and function of these highly repeated sequences in higher primates has been the subject of considerable investigation in the past two decades. By-products of these investigations include the recent development of human artificial chromosomes with and without alpha satellite repeats [16,54–56] and the characterization of centromere-associated proteins [57]. This chapter describes a method for identifying 12,039 of the most homologous alpha satellite sequences in the current human genome database using BLAST and a 470 bp cloned sequence reported to hybridize to all human centromeres [22]. These data and three published sequences were used to identify the single most homologous sequence for each of 27 higher primate chromosomes. One highly homologous sequence was identified that is present in orangutan, gorilla, and chimpanzee. PAUP and Phylip computer analyses derived multiple similar parsimonious evolutionary trees based upon multiple algorithms that each included all 27 sequences. The PAUP-derived single heuristic evolutionary tree also defined a consensus sequence that represents the probable progenitor alpha satellite sequence common to all higher primate sequences analyzed. These results are consistent with initial dispersion of ancestral 171 bp repeat sequences to each human chromosome, followed by sequence divergence prior to and during duplication along with occasional inversion of larger numbers of tandem repeat sequences (higher order repeat; HOR). Our results are consistent with prior computer modeling results that suggested greater variability would be found near the euchromatic gene-carrying regions flanking the chromosome centromere, sites where ancestral sequences could be modified prior to generation of the current higher-order arrays. These higher-order arrays comprise the characterized centromeres that vary substantially, resulting in the microscopically visible size differences described in other chapters. These most homologous sequence repeats within the derived PAUP heuristic tree have been modified from the ancestral sequence by all the mechanisms that account for molecular and microscopic polymorphisms: inversion, insertion, deletion, translocation, base pair substitution, and duplication (by reciprocal translocation or concerted evolution).

9.1   INTRODUCTION

The centromere is a *cis*-acting chromosome region to which proteins and spindle microtubules bind prior to pulling each chromatid via the spindle apparatus into a cellular domain that becomes one of two daughter cell nuclei. Alpha satellite DNA sequences are reported to be sufficient but not necessary to confer centromere activity. Tandem alpha satellite repeats also exist in chromosome regions without active centromeres [1–3]. The repeated alpha satellite DNA sequences comprising the human chromosome centromeres were derived from a common 171 bp ancestral sequence [4] that existed in a hominid ancestor predating divergence of gorilla, chimpanzee, and human [5].

Results of the Human Genome Project include most unique gene region sequences and a portion of the repetitive sequence blocks that comprise up to 10% of the total human genome. Two categories of human repeated sequences have been reported: interspersed repeat sequences and tandem repeats [6]. Initially tandem repeats were purified from bulk genomic DNA by ultracentrifugation as "satellite" fractions based upon buoyant density differences. Several fractions consisting of heterogeneous mixtures of repetitive DNA were referred to as classical satellites I, II, III and IV [7]. Subsequent restriction enzyme analysis revealed several groups of different tandem repeats including a class of non-coding DNA comprising the family of centromeric alphoid repetitive DNA [8].

Alpha satellite DNA, the most abundant class of repetitive DNA, constitutes 3–5% of the human genome and is found only in higher primate centromeric regions [5,9,10]. The fundamental unit of selected human centromeric repeats is a 171 bp monomeric consensus unit with 10–40% sequence divergence between different monomers [4,8,12–15]. These units are reported to consist of two to 40 tandem monomers, designated as higher-order repeat units (HORs). Unique probes hybridize to arrays of HORs up to several thousand long that are found on one or more pairs of homologous chromosomes [6,16–19].

The organization of the relatively large number of alpha satellite sequences that hybridize specifically to one or more chromosome types can be complex. The alpha satellite repeats have been assigned to different suprachromosomal families according to the number and distribution of HORs. Three basic patterns of distribution of these chromosomal families have been reported. In the first pattern a repeat family is specific for a unique chromosome. In the second, two or more chromosomes are in the same family. In the third pattern unique and shared family sequences coexist on a single chromosome [12]. The origin of this complex organization is proposed to involve intra- and interchromosomal exchange and homogenization by the individual mechanisms of deletion, insertion, recombination, unequal crossing over, sequence conversion and translocation [12,15]. The complete 450 kb human X chromosome centromeric sequence has been characterized thoroughly from one individual [20]. The extent of variability in different individuals remains to be addressed.

This chapter reports the construction of evolutionary trees by both the PAUP and Phylip computer programs (Fig. 9.1) that include the most highly homologous sequences mapped to all the human chromosome centromeres and three selected centromeric sequences from chimpanzee, gorilla and orangutan. These trees were derived based upon principles used to characterize the relationship among 24 intronic repeats of the HLA DQA gene by PAUP analysis [21]. Because the applied multiple algorithms derived very similar trees, these results further validate each other. When compared individually to both published consensus monomers, the representative sequences selected from our most homologous 24 human centromeric cloned DNAs showed significantly greater variation in the 3' terminal portion of selected monomers in a majority of the compared sequences. Because the 171 bp repeat length is preserved in spite of substantial nucleotide substitutions throughout the 33 bp 3' terminal region, this highly variable region appears to act as a space holder to maintain the same distance between 171 bp repeats. Thus constructed phylogenetic trees showed additional evolutionary divergence within these variable regions. These terminal variable regions modify inter- and intrachromosomal patterns that may be preserved to minimize nonhomologous chromosome recombination.

9.2   RESULTS

A 470 bp sequence designated *Homo sapiens* centromeric alphoid repeat region has homologous sequences in all human chromosomal centromeres and in chromosome bands 2q21 and 9q31 (Fig. 9.2A) [22]. When compared to the previously reported 171 bp monomeric consensus sequences [4,13], this sequence was found to have an incomplete trimeric repeat with individual repeat sequence homologies exceeding 80%. When the BLAST feature of the genome database was used to search for other homologous sequences, 12,039 repeat sequence loci were found in the human genome database.

Each of the first 250 sequences of the 12,039 identified had an expected likelihood of finding the sequences randomly of less than $7e^{-21}$. From among these 250 identified sequences were selected the most homologous individual sequences for 21 of the 24 human chromosomes as well as individual sequences for *Pongo pygmaeus* (orangutan), *Pan troglodytes* (chimpanzee) and *Gorilla gorilla* (Table 9.1). In contrast, alpha satellite sequences mapped to human chromosome 1, 9 and 16 centromeres were found by searching the literature and comparing the published sequences to the 470 bp common centromeric alphoid repeat. The likelihood of randomly finding the same match between the chromosome 1, 9, or 16 centromeric sequences when compared to the common alpha satellite was individually less than e^{-39} (Table 9.1).

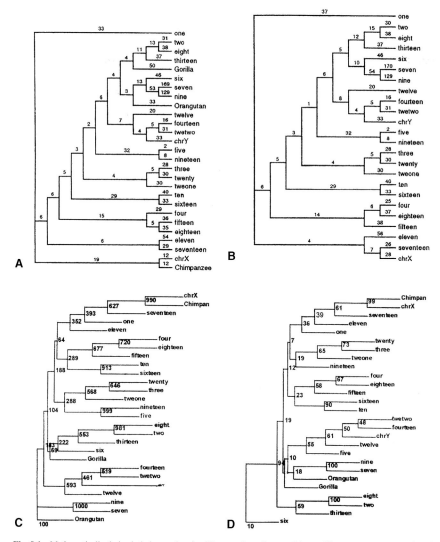

Fig. 9.1 Mathematically derived phylogenetic trees. The most homologous alpha satellite sequences were analyzed with the PAUP 4.0 Beta program written by David Swofford [58] or the PHYLIP program [52]. Modeltest version 3.06 [53] was used to select an adequate evolutionary inference model according to our data. Maximum-likelihood, neighbor joining, UPGMA, branch and bound, bootstrap and heuristic methods were used to construct evolutionary trees and selected results are described below. Results are illustrated from the most homologous 470 bp alpha satellite sequences from 21 human chromosomes and three selected primate chromosomes plus the most homologous 171 bp sequences written in tandem from three human chromosomes (Fig. 1A–D). **A**. Rectangular cladogram of the most homologous 470 bp alpha satellite sequences from 21 human chromosomes and three selected primate chromosomes plus the most homologous 171 bp sequences from three human chromosomes were analyzed using the PAUP program's heuristic methods. Tree length = 1304, consistency index = 0.592, relation index = 0.432. **B**: Rectangular cladogram analysis of all the human centromeric regions from Fig. 1A were analyzed using the PAUP program's heuristic methods. Observe that chromosome X is now closer to chromosomes 11 and 17 as previously reported. Tree length = 1203, consistency index = 0.619 and relation Index = 0.438. **C**: Phylogram generated by the Phylip neighbor joining program from 24 human centromeric sequences and 3 selected chimpanzee, gorilla, and orangutan sequences using orangutan as the outgroup. Branch numbers represent the number of replicates in the same location out of 1000 replicates. **D**: Phylogram generated by the Phylip neighbor joining program from 24 human centromeric sequences and three selected sequences from chimpanzee, gorilla, and orangutan, with the human chromosome 6 sequence as the outgroup. Branch numbers represent the number of replicates in the same location out of 100 replicates. Observe that the gorilla centromeric sequence is now closer to an individual human centromeric sequence

A
```
Alphoid:    gt.....................a......c..g..............a......tc 60
Ancestor1:  --attcaactcacagagttgaacattccttttgatagagcagttttgaaactctcttct 60
Ancestor2:  --...............................................a......t. 60

Alphoid:    g...g...............t.....tg......g.cc...g.......ga...a.... 120
Ancestor1:  ctagaatctgcaagtggatatgtggacctctttgaagatttcattggaaacgggattatc 120
Ancestor2:  g...............t...............g.........a.... 120

Alphoid:    ...............g..g..................t.......g..a...... 180
Ancestor1:  ttcacataaaaactaaacagaagcattctcagaaactactttgtgatgtttgcattcaac 180
Ancestor2:  ........................t................. 180

Alphoid:    ..t..........gc..t..a..g.........t.......a..cg.............. 240
Ancestor1:  tcccagagttgaacattccttttcatagagcagctttgaaacactcttttgtagaatct 240
Ancestor2:  ..a.................................t................. 240

Alphoid:    ..c..............a...g..a....ac......................... 300
Ancestor1:  gcaagtggacatttggagcgctttgaggcctgtggtggaaaaggaaatatcttcacataa 300
Ancestor2:  .......................c...................... 300

Alphoid:    ....c.....c...ag...................c.t...............a.... 360
Ancestor1:  aaactagacagaagcattctcagaaacttctttgtgatgattgcattcaactcacggagt 360
Ancestor2:  .............................................a.... 360

Alphoid:    ......ca......c............t...g..g.....tc........g....... 418
Ancestor1:  tgaacattccttttgatagagcagtttggaaacactctttctgtagaatctgcaagtg 418
Ancestor2:  ................................................ 418
```

B
```
Cons C :    1     cattctsagaaacttctttgtgatgtktgcattcaactcacagagttgaacmttyctttt 60
                  |||||| ||||||||||||||||||||||||||||||||||||||||||||||||
Cons W :    1     agcattctcagaaacttctttgtgatgtktgyattcaactcacagagttgaacmttyctttt 62
Ances1 :    1                        ......................a..c.... 30
Ances1 :    140   .......c.........a..........t..t.......c.........a..c.... 201
Ances1 :    311   .......c..............at...........g.........a..c.... 372

Cons C :    61    satwgagcagtttkgaaacactcttttgtagaatctgcaagtggatatttggasckctt 120
                  ||| ||||||||||||||||||||||||||||||||||||||||||| ||||||||||||
Cons W :    63    satagagcagtttkgaaacactcttttgtagaatctgcaagtggayatttggasckctt 122
Ances1 :    31    g..a.........t....t......c.c...............g....c.t... 90
Ances1 :    202   c..a.....c..t.................................c......g.g... 261
Ances1 :    373   g..a.........g...........c................. 418

Cons C :    121   tgaggcctwygktggaaamggraatatcttcayataaaaactagacagaag 171
                  ||||| ||||||||||||||||||||||||||||||||||||| |||||
Cons W :    123   tgaggmytwygktggaaamggraatatcttcayataaaaactaracaga 171
Ances1 :    91    ...a.at.tcat......c..g.t........c..........a....... 141
Ances1 :    262   .......gt.g.....a..a.........c............. 312
```

```
r= a, g      m= a, c       k= g, t      s= c, g
w= a, t      n= a,c,t,g    y= c,t       .= Match
```

Fig. 9.2 Comparison of derived ancestral sequences. **A**: Alignment and homology between the Alphoid DNA sequence of Meneveri and Ginelli, derived Ancestor 1, and derived Ancestor 2 using the Blastn service available at http://www.ncbi.nlm.nih.gov/ BLAST/. Ancestor 1: derived ancestor sequence from 24 human centromeric sequences and three sequences from chimpanzee, gorilla and orangutan (Fig. 9.1A). Ancestor 2: derived ancestor from 24 human centromeric regions excluding other apes sequences (Fig. 9.1B). Both ancestors were derived after rooting the consensus tree and then reconstructing the nodes using the PAUP program's heuristic method. The negative symbol (−) represents a missing nucleotide sequence. **B**: Comparison of derived Ancestor 1 sequence to published 171 bp consensus sequences. Ances 1: derived ancestral sequence from 24 human centromeric sequences and tree selected sequences from chimpanzee, gorilla and orangutan. Cons C: consensus sequence from Choo [4]. Cons W: consensus sequences from Waye and Willard [14]. Derived Ancestor 1 differed by 13% from the consensus sequences from Choo [4] and from Waye and Willard [14]. Cons C and Cons W shared 95% identical sequences

Table 9.1   The most homologous available sequences listed for each chromosome were derived by comparison to an alpha satellite sequence [22] using the Standard Nucleotide-Nucleotide BLAST [Blastn] program [51] provided through NCBI at website http://www.ncbi.nlm.nih.gov/blast/ bl2seq/bl2.html

Chromosome[1]	Designation[2]	Score	e-Value	Reference
1*	pSD-1	192	e^{-100}	Willard and Waye J 1987 [14]
2	Alpha satellite DNA	163	$1e^{-37}$	Haaf and Willard 1992 [34]
3	BAC clone RP11-557B13 from 3	492	e^{-136}	Sulston and Waterson 1998 [28]
4	Alpha satellite DNA	117	$7e^{-24}$	Mashkova *et al.* 1994 [35]
5	Alpha satellite, Clone CEPH-YAC 783-G-7	291	$2e^{-71}$	Puechberty *et al.* 1999 [36]
6	BamHI repeat region, alphoid DNA	165	$3e^{-38}$	Sugimoto *et al.* 1997 [37]
7	Alphoid DNA[3]	289	$8e^{-76}$	Dela-Puente *et al.* 1997 [38]
8	D8Z2 gene[3]	165	$3e^{-38}$	Ge *et al.* [14]
9*	Alpha satellite DNA	169	$1e^{-39}$	Rocchi *et al.* 1991 [40]
10	Alpha satellite DNA	137	$7e^{-30}$	Alexandrov *et al.* 1993 [41]
11	Alpha satellite DNA, clone pLC11A	119	$2e^{-24}$	Waye and Willard 1987 [13]
12	12 BAC RP11-496H24[3]	307	$4e^{-81}$	Worley 2001 (direct submission)
13	Alphoid DNA, clone alpha-RI[680]13-74-I-1	109	$2e^{-21}$	Joergensen *et al.* 1987 [42]
14	BAC R-146E13 of library RPCI-11[3]	331	$2e^{-88}$	Heilig *et al.* 2001 [43]
15	Alpha Satellite DNA	171	$5e^{-40}$	O'Keefe and Matera 2000 [44]
16*	Alpha satellite DNA, clone pSE16-2	260	$8e^{-67}$	Greig *et al.* 1989 [45]
17	Alpha satellite DNA, clone 14A-16MER (75)	246	$1e^{-62}$	Waburton *et al.* 1993 [46]
18	Alpha satellite DNA, clone pYAM 9–60	165	$3e^{-38}$	Alexandrov *et al.* 1991 [24]
19	Alpha satellite DNA	260	$2e^{-67}$	Puechberty *et al.* 1999 [36]
20	Alphoid DNA	412	e^{-113}	Bassi *et al.* 2000 [47]
21	Alphoid DNA, segment HS21C002[3]	442	e^{-122}	Hattori *et al.* 2000 (direct submission)
22	Alpha satellite DNA	147	$8e^{-33}$	McDermid *et al.* 1986 [48]
X	Alphoid DNA	285	$1e^{-74}$	Laursen *et al.* 1992 [49]
Y	Alpha satellite DNA	214	$4e^{-53}$	Tyler-Smith and Brown 1987 [27]
Pongo pygmaeus (orangutan)	Alpha satellite DNA, clone PPY3-1	240	$7e^{-61}$	Haaf and Willard 1998 [50]
Gorilla gorilla	Alphoid DNA, chromosome X	232	$2e^{-58}$	Laursen *et al.* 1992 [49]
Pan troglodytes (chimpanzee)	Alphoid DNA, chromosome X	262	$2e^{-67}$	Laursen *et al.* 1992 [49]

This table lists the designation, blastn score (score) and expected value (e-value) of centromeric sequences from each chromosome with the highest homology to the 470 bp alphoid DNA [22]. The expected value is a parameter that describes the number of "expected" chance hits observed when searching any database of the same size. This decreases exponentially with the score (S) that is assigned to a match between two sequences. Essentially, the e-value quantifies the random background noise for sequence matches. Literature searches were completed using PubMed at website http://www.ncbi.nlm.nih.gov/PubMed/ and referenced articles obtained from the Library of Congress, Washington, DC.
*Sequences obtained from PubMed: [1]chromosome source available at the Genome Database or PubMed; [2]original names or genome database designations; [3]unpublished; direct submission to the genome database.

9.2.1 Comparison of the Entire 420 bp Sequence

Comparison of the Blastn alignments for these 27 selected sequences revealed multiple base-pair gaps on either end of each aligned sequence. Thus these sequences were arbitrarily truncated to 420 bp to obtain homologous sequences that could be compared without introducing gaps that confounded the mathematical analysis. In the case of chromosomes 9, 13 and 22 the only sequences identified were shorter than 420 bp. Each of these shorter sequences was written arbitrarily as 420 bp long tandem copies in order to compare these more objectively to all the other sequences by both PAUP and Phylip. Modeltest [55] showed the Kimura two-parameter approach to be an appropriate evolutionary inference method with a calculated log-likelihood score of 6092.3179. Penny–parsimony (branch and bound) and compatibility methods were performed using 100 replicates. Maximum-likelihood, neighbor joining, UPGMA, bootstrap, and heuristic algorithms were performed using 1000 replicates. Significant clustering was observed in the trees generated by all mathematical methods of the human and chimpanzee X chromosome alpha satellites, as well as human alpha satellites from chromosomes 7 and 9, 10 and 16, 4 and 18, and 8 and 2 (Fig. 9.1). These clustering patterns are not related to the previously reported suprachromosomal families [23,24] consistent with dispersion of these sequences to individual chromosomes prior to higher primate speciation.

The chromosome locations on these multiple trees were also compared to the specificities of the 17 human chromosome-specific centromeric probes, which hybridize uniquely to individual human chromosome centromeres at high stringency (CEP Probes, Vysis, Downers Grove, IL). In contrast, cross-hybridization of the same probe to two different chromosomes was reported for chromosomes 14 and 22, chromosomes 5 and 19, and chromosomes 13 and 21. Fluorescence in-situ hybridization of three cloned centromeric probes each detects one of these pairs of chromosome centromeres. Independently of the mathematical method or the evolutive model considered, the PAUP and Phylip programs consistently place alpha satellites from the chromosome 14 and 22 pair, and from the chromosome 5 and 19 pair, in adjacent branches with the number of replicates ≥ 501 of 1000 and ≥ 999 of 1000 respectively (Fig. 9.1C). In contrast, the most homologous centromeric 13 and 21 sequences diverged more substantially according to the mathematical analysis of the entire 420 bp sequence, even though a prior attempt to distinguish these target sequences by selecting different repeat regions for FISH probes met with only limited success [25,26]. These results suggest that subsequent recombination between chromosomes 13 and 21 enhanced by their close proximity in the nucleolar organizing region may account for the current high degree of hybridization homology between the centromeres of these two chromosomes. No significant change in the relationship between the human centromeric sequences was observed when the trees were derived with or without higher nonhuman primate sequences for comparison. In this case the human chromosome X alpha satellite formed a new group with those of chromosomes 11 and 17 (Fig. 9.1B vs. Fig. 9.1A), according to the previous report of a common pentameric unit shared by these chromosomes [14].

Trees derived using the neighbor joining method, after selecting the orangutan as the outgroup, revealed the gorilla and the chimpanzee to be more similar to human chromosomes 6 and X, respectively, than to the orangutan sequence (Fig. 9.1C). To test whether the orangutan sequence was more similar to a human chromosome or belonged near the root of the tree, different sequences including nodes and chromosomes 6 and 1 were used as the outgroup for comparison. Gorilla and orangutan were both more similar to human chromosomes 7 and 9 than to the derived ancestral sequence in each instance (Fig. 9.1D). Together these results indicate that a common ancestral centromeric sequence existed on these chromosomes prior to the divergence of orangutan from the remaining primate lineage (gorilla, chimpanzee, and human) between 3 and 10 million years ago.

These trees were rooted and the node sequences were reconstructed to derive a likely ancestral sequence for the 27 centromeric regions from human and selected higher ape chromosomes. A second likely ancestral sequence was derived for the 24 human centromeric regions. Comparison of these two derived ancestors found 86% of the basepairs in these sequences were identical and 14% different when compared to the alphoid sequence by Meneveri and Ginelli, while 87% were identical and 13% different from both the Choo and the Waye and Willard consensus sequences (Fig. 9.2A and 9.2B). These derived ancestral sequences predict that a single highly homologous probe to the common ancestral sequence would hybridize to all human centromeres. In fact, Mitchell et al. [6] did report a sequence that hybridized to all human centromeres.

9.2.2 Increased Variability in the 3′ Region of the 171 bp Repeats

The number of sequences with significant variation from the fundamental 171 bp alpha satellite monomers was compared to Choo's previously reported 171 bp consensus sequences from each of the most homologous 24 different human chromosome centromeric sites selected from the database. For the most part, alignments obtained for each sequence were highly conserved, with lengths within 171 ± 10 bp (differing by less than 5.8%) and $\geq 80\%$ identity when compared to both consensus sequences (Fig 9.3, left; Table 9.2). In fact, the first 138 bp exhibited an 85% average sequence identity when comparing all repeats. In contrast, non-periodical variations were found in some monomers that exhibited considerable variability in size and constitution at the 3′ terminal portion of these sequences with an average of only 66.6% sequence identity (Fig. 9.3, right; Fig. 9.4, shaded arrowheads; Table 9.2). Closer inspection reveals that some of these sequences, like chromosomes 1, 22 and Y, are highly conserved, while others like chromosome 6 are modified substantially. Still others, like the chromosome 14 repeat that is 18 bp shorter, have terminal deletions. Chromosomes 2, 3, 4, 5, 6, 7, 8, 9, 10, 11, 15, 16, 17, 18, 19, 20, and X (17 of the 24) exhibited significantly higher variability in the terminal region than in the first 138 bp (Table 9.2).

The PAUP program was used to analyze shorter 171 bp centromeric repeat alignments representing each of the 24 unique human chromosomes. Modeltest found the Kimura two-parameter approach to be an appropriate inference model to complete this phylogenetic analysis. Heuristic algorithms were applied to obtain a rectangular cladogram relating these sequences. The derived phylogenetic trees differed significantly from the previously derived tree based on longer 420 bp sequences (Fig. 9.1) because the highly variable terminal region contributes more

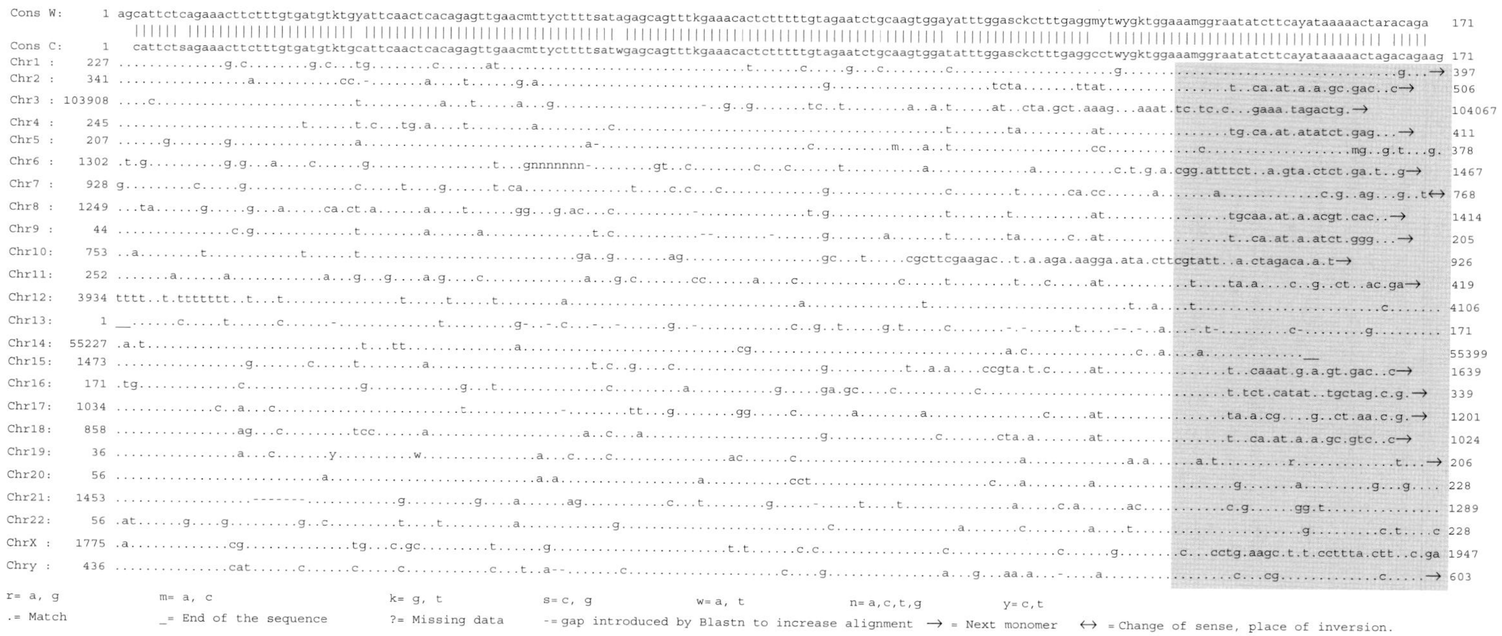

Fig. 9.3 Comparison of 171 bp consensus sequences. Comparison between both previously reported consensus sequences from Waye and Willard 1987 [18], and Choo et al. 1991 [4], and selected alpha satellite monomeric sequences from 24 different human centromeric regions. Notice the higher variation rate in last 30–40bp with respect to the first 120–130bp. Both consensus sequences showed an identity greater than 95% between them (vertical bars indicate match). These sequences were compared simultaneously to the 24 representative human centromeric regions. The majority of the alignments obtained showed significant variation at the terminal region of the sequence. The boundary of this region was selected arbitrarily and the sequences shaded with a gray rectangle. Note that the Blast program introduced some gaps (−) representing deleted basepairs to maximize the homology of the sequences being compared. Sequences within alpha satellite repeats cloned from chromosomes 7 and 21 were found to be inverted

Table 9.2 Number (N), frequency (F), and distribution of variations at the selected alpha satellite monomers from 24 different human centromeric regions compared in Fig. 9.1

Chromosone designation	Length (bp)	N^1	F^1	N^2 out of the first 138 bp	F^2 at the first 138 bp	N^3 at the last portion	F^3 at the last portion
1	171	16	9.3	15	10.87	[a]1/33[b]	3
2	167	30	18	17	12.32	13/29	44.8
3	161	47	29.2	31	22.46	16/23	69.6
4	167	29	17.4	14	10.14	15/29	51.7
5	173	17	9.8	11	7.97	6/35	17.14
6	168	50	29.8	29	21.01	21/30	70
7	171	28	16.4	21	15.22	7/33	21.2
8	166	40	24.1	25	18.11	15/28	53.6
9	167	31	18.6	18	13.04	13/29	44.8
10	159	56	35.2	40	28.98	16/21	76.2
11	168	33	19.6	21	15.22	12/30	40
12	173	34	19.6	32	23.19	2/35	5.7
13	173	32	18.5	26	18.84	6/35	17.1
14	155	13	8.4	12	8.69	1/17	5.9
15	167	35	21	21	15.22	14/29	48.3
16	169	32	19	15	10.87	17/31	54.8
17	169	28	16.6	16	11.59	12/31	38.7
18	167	31	18.6	18	13.04	13/29	44.8
19	171	17	10	13	9.42	4/33	12.1
20	173	14	8.1	10	7.25	4/35	11.4
21	173	28	16.2	23	16.6	5/35	14.3
22	173	19	11	15	10.87	4/35	11.4
X	173	40	23.1	17	12.32	23/35	65.7
Y	171	25	14.6	21	15.22	4/33	12.1
Ave:	168.5	30.2	18	20.04	14.52	10.2/30.5	33.4

Observe the significant difference of number and frequency of variations for 17 of the 24 sequences when the first 138 bp are compared to the last portion of the sequences. For the other seven sequences no significant difference between the initial and the terminal portions was found.
N^1 and F^1: number and frequency of variations within the entire monomer. N^2 and F^2: number and frequency of variations within the first 138 bp of the monomer. N^3 and F^3: number and frequency of variations within the last portion of the monomer. a/b: number of variations at the last portion/length of the last portion.

substantially to the total variability within an individual repeat. Most significantly, a common root was *not* derived mathematically for these 171 bp sequences consistent with earlier reports of multiple centromeric families. This is in contrast to the tree derived from the longer 420 bp sequences that are individually the most highly conserved centromeric region repeat locus for each chromosome found in the genome database.

This result raises the question: "Would a tree derived with the most homologous first 138 bp from the previously tested 27 sequences, plus derived Ancestor 1, differ substantially from the trees derived with the longer 420 bp sequences that included the variable 3′ repeats (Fig. 9.1A–D)?" In fact, a single tree of 138 bp sequences was derived using the neighbor joining method (Fig. 9.4; compare Fig. 9.1C) that preserved all major centromeric groups. This derived tree can be described using the same words as the trees derived in Fig. 9.1A–D (see above). Only chromosome 6 has moved to an immediately adjacent major branch. These

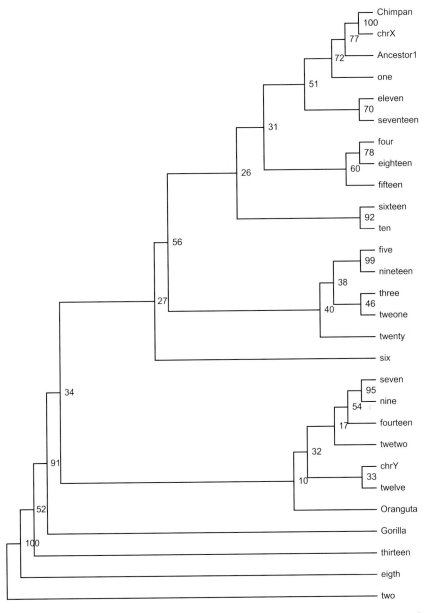

Fig. 9.4 Phylogram of the most homologous 138 bp sequences selected from 24 human centromeric sequences; three selected sequences from chimpanzee, gorilla, and orangutan; and Ancestor 1 derived using the Phylip neighbor joining method. Branch numbers represent the number of replicates in the same location out of 100 replicates. Observe that this rectangular cladogram is very similar to that derived in Fig. 1C by the same method, so that overall the longer 420 bp and shorter 138 bp sequences revealed the same evolutionary relationships

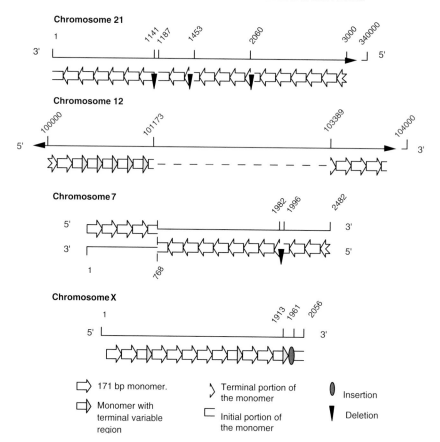

Fig. 9.5 Variability found at four selected loci in the most homologous sequences. Different mechanisms of evolution contribute to the divergence of the alpha satellite repeats in different chromosomes. Other families of repeats can be interposed within alpha satellite monomers as observed in chromosome 12. Nonperiodical deletions result in significant variation that confers specific hybridization patterns to specific alpha satellite families (chromosomes 21 and 7). Recombination contributes to homogenization of repeat sequences, but also introduces variability as seen in the inversion of alphoid DNA in chromosome 7. Insertion of DNA was also identified at the terminal variable region of one monomer in chromosome X

highly complementary results predict that the relationship among the centromeric repeat families will remain substantially unchanged as entire analyses of all the centromeric regions of individual chromosomes are completed.

In order to determine the number of adjacent substantially conserved repeats for each single most highly homologous cloned chromosome site available for each chromosome, the variability and number of tandem repeats was analyzed in longer cloned chromosome-specific sequences from which these single 171 bp sequences were selected (listed in Table 9.2). In fact, considerable variability was found among the numbers of adjacent 171 bp repeats conserved throughout the 3′ and 5′ sequences that were interrupted by 171 bp repeats with highly variable

3′ terminal regions as illustrated for four selected chromosome-specific segments (Fig. 9.5). For example, the 3 kb sequence analyzed from the 340 kb chromosome 21 cloned sequence (Fig. 9.5, top) has small deletions in three different terminal 171 bp repeat regions while the intervening number of highly conserved 171 bp repeats adjacent to these deletions are >6, 1, 3 and >5. This non-periodical variability in the number of 171 bp repeat sequences is typical of each of the chromosome sequences for which sufficient numbers of repeats could be compared in the database clones selected for highest homology: chromosomes 2, 3, 6, 7, 8, 10, 15, 17, 18 and X. Because the clones carrying the most homologous cloned sequence to the derived common ancestral sequence have different human DNA insert lengths, only the 10 aforementioned clones had a sufficient number of 171 bp repeats for this analysis. These results indicate that the initial divergence of dispersed alpha centromeric repeats can be explained by recombination between the homologous 171 bp repeats that are not at specific repeat intervals. At the same time the distance between the initial 138 bp of each homologous repeat is maintained in most structures even though content of the terminal 33–35 bp varies unpredictably. These data are entirely consistent with selection for the 171 bp repeat unit *length* along with a more stringent requirement for the initial 138 bp repeat *sequence*.

The human Y chromosome centromere is unique because it does not take part in meiotic recombination with a homologous sister chromosome. Comparison of variability within Y chromosome centromeric repeats to centromeric repeat variability on chromosomes where recombination has been reported on both sides of the centromere is anticipated to reflect the contribution of meiotic events to chromosome centromeric variability. The most homologous Y chromosome repeat alpha satellite sequence selected initially [27] consisted of only one terminal region in 14 repeats that was modified significantly from the 171 bp consensus sequence. To complete a more substantial sequence comparison, an additional Y chromosome-specific BAC clone was selected and analyzed with 89 alpha satellite monomers homologous to the 171 bp consensus monomer (RP11-160K17) [28]. Only four of 89 (4.5%) of these monomers had terminal variation exceeding 10 basepairs. These data are consistent with the hypothesis that meiosis contributes to a substantial proportion of the centromeric repeat sequence variability because the frequency of modifications is significantly less within the observed Y chromosome repeats.

Inversion, yet another means to modify alpha satellite small repeat sequences, was observed in two of these 24 most homologous human chromosome sequences: chromosomes 7 and Y. In the chromosome 7 centromeric repeat clone, two 171 bp fragments recombined to orient eight repeats in the opposite direction (Fig. 9.5, example 3). Additional analysis of the Y chromosome-specific BAC clone (previous paragraph) found 36 of the 89 repeat monomers inverted as a single group. Thus, while not as common as duplication, inversion belongs in the list of molecular rearrangements resulting in individual chromosome-specific cloned DNA sequences. Different length gaps from 1 bp to 2216 bp within and between 171 bp repeats were observed in the 24 clones containing the most homologous centromeric sequences. Typically the 1 bp to 18 bp sequences deleted from the 171 bp repeats representing each chromosome would not be considered to alter the repeat function, as a frameshift mutation would change a gene coding sequence. At the same time any three-dimensional structure formed by denaturing and annealing of adjacent 171 bp repeats could require conservation of similar-size repeats.

Further inspection revealed that the relatively large insertion sequences of 285 bp in the chromosome 15 clone and 2216 bp in the chromosome 12 clone (Fig. 9.5, example 2) consist of nonhomologous repeat units interposed within these two different alpha satellite repeats. The 2216 bp inserted sequence on chromosome 12 spans 1473 bp and 622 bp L1PA2 repeat sequences that are both members of the LINE/L1 repeat family. Other segments homologous to this 2216 bp insert were also found throughout this 160 kb chromosome 12 cloned sequence (12 BAC RP11-496H24). When BLAST was applied to the genome database the same repeat sequence was found at variable lengths and intervals in the same and reverse orientation among other reported centromeric alpha satellite repeat sequences and throughout the genome [53]. A 72 bp retroposon was identified in the terminal region of the 1473 bp repeat, suggesting the mechanism by which the L1 repeat sequences were introduced into this location. Furthermore, a clone found in chimpanzee (*Pan troglodytes* clone RP43-89H17, Ayele *et al.*) also has homologous centromeric alpha satellite sequences, sequences homologous to the inserted L1 repeat sequence, and multiple other homologous sequence elements. Taken together, these results in separate homologous clones from two closely related higher primates indicate that the L1 inserted repeat in the human chromosome 12 sequence is genetically transmitted in both species and cannot be dismissed as a cloning artifact.

In summary, these findings from the most highly homologous cloned sequences demonstrate that evolution of the alpha centromeric repeats include all the larger chromosome rearrangement categories that occurred on a molecular scale in other alpha satellite sequences. Namely, unequal recombination between sister chromatids and exchanges between homologous chromosomes resulted in: (1) inversion, (2) deletion of a few basepairs to entire 171 bp alpha satellite repeats, (3) insertion of nonhomologous sequences into 171 bp repeat arrays, and (4) duplication. Our observations can be explained best by initial sequence dispersion of the most homologous alpha satellite sequences to all the centromeric chromosome regions, followed by additional duplications and rearrangements that continue to occur in these ancestral repeats as well as in other longer tandem repeats generated by subsequent duplication.

9.3 DISCUSSION

By using the most homologous 420 bp alpha satellite sequences in the human genome database, a single parsimonious tree was derived by multiple methods that defines the most likely common ancestral sequence for all these primate sequences (Fig. 9.1). Mathematical analysis of DNA sequence homology is most effective when the sequences are sufficiently similar to identify the degree of homology between all the sequences analyzed and yet sufficiently different to distinguish the relative relationships among the items. The sequence most homologous to the common alphoid sequence found for each human chromosome fit these requirements when the longer 470 bp sequences were analyzed but not when the 171 bp shorter repeat sequences were tested. This most likely progenitor sequence, and the single nodes of the tree from which it was derived, can be used to compare the divergence of sequences along entire individual chromosome centromeres or between entire centromeres of different individuals. Thus one goal defined by Willard [15] has been addressed: namely, to define the likely alpha satellite ancestral sequence of the higher primate species (Ancestor 1) by mathematically deriving it from a single tree (Fig. 9.1A), hence providing a basis to measure rates of sequence divergence, spread, and fixation over defined periods of time within and between chromosome-specific centromeric arrays.

As Choo [31] suggested, because all the acrocentric satellites tend to be part of the nucleolar organizing region, tangling and recombination of individual acrocentric chromosome strands might have resulted in illegitimate recombination that would initiate selection or random assortment to result in closer current centromeric homology. Some unique chromosome-specific centromeric probes hybridize to two different chromosomes like probe D21Z1/D13Z1 to chromosomes 21 and 13 and probe D14Z1/D22Z1 to 14 and 22 [29] (also Hattori *et al.*, direct submission, 2000). The derived tree reflects a close relationship for the progenitor chromosome 14 and 22 alpha satellite repeats but not for the progenitor chromosome 13 and 21 sequences. Our derived tree is consistent with the hypothesis that recombination between heterologous pairs on chromosomes 13 and 21 adjacent to the analyzed sequences exchanged centromeric sequences more recently in evolutionary time since these progenitor sequences dispersed to the chromosome sites. For instance, we reported that recombination had moved a chromosome 13 centromere to another D-group chromosome so that FISH with a chromosome 13/21 probe revealed five signals in a 46, XX normal female karyotype instead of the usual four [30]. Given a reproductively successful individual carrying a block of centromeric sequence of either chromosome 13 or 21 that was translocated to the other chromosome and an evolutionary bottleneck that randomly selected for centromeres that were identical, this common centromere could have become fixed randomly. Alternatively, a common centromere could have been selected because a larger number of repeats assured more reliable chromosome segregation.

Because the most homologous sequences existed when all progenitor sequences were dispersed to centromeric chromosome regions and have since had time to diverge, the most highly homologous sequences in this group have undergone all of the same kinds of modifications reported for all of the centromeric alpha satellite repeats: (1) inversion, (2) duplication by illegitimate intra- and interchromosomal recombination or concerted evolution, (3) small and large deletion, (4) small and large insertion of homologous and nonhomologous sequences, and (5) basepair substitution. Together, these mechanisms generated inter- and intraspecies divergence and differentiation. Although detectable recombination rarely occurs between [30] or within [32,33] the centromeric domains, evolutionary time is sufficient to allow such events to occur multiple times.

The fact that these sequences were selected following dispersion to all chromosome centromeric regions that not only remain but were amplified to megabase tandem arrays indicates that the 171 bp repeat length serves an important function. At the same time, monomeric 171 bp centromeric sequences selected from the 24 human chromosome sequences revealed significantly greater variability in the 3′ terminal monomeric region. The average frequency of non-identity within the 3′ terminal variable regions was 33.4%, while the average frequency of nonidentity within the initial conserved 138 bp of these monomers was 14.5%. Within the same cloned sequence the 171 bp repeats with the most highly variable 3′ regions were separated by an unpredictable number of interspersed 171 bp repeat sequences with conserved 3′ sequences. These data indicate that

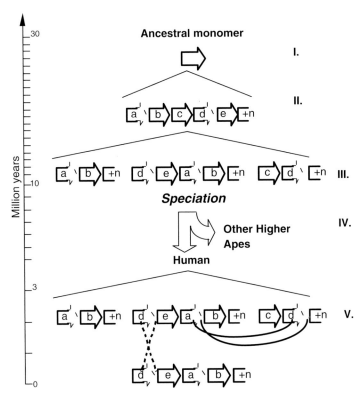

Fig. 9.6 Evolution of alpha satellite centromeric repeats. An ancestral monomer of approximately 171 bp long appeared more than 30 million years ago (I). This monomer evolved by tandem duplication forming short repeat units that were then disbursed to all the human chromosome centromeres (II). Subsequently these repeat units diverged appreciably and then formed higher-order repeat units and extensive individual chromosome arrays. In this process the monomers have evolved by duplication, recombination, translocation, insertion, mutation, deletion, unequal crossing over and transposition to accumulate significant variation, particularly in the terminal portion of some monomers (open arrowheads), suggesting conservation of the 5′ regions to maintain function (III). Speciation between human and other higher apes occurred 3–10 million years ago (IV). Since then species-specific homogenization within different suprachromosomal families, common to one or more chromosomes, has conferred diversity and specificity as observed following hybridization under high stringency conditions. However, under lower stringency conditions some cross-hybridization between species has been observed, further supporting the existence of a common progenitor. Sequence homogenization of the suprachromomal families continues to occur within species by the intra- and interchromosomal mechanisms described above between homologous and nonhomologous chromosomes (V). This results in substantial variability in the size of centromeric heteromorphisms (see text for discussion)

not only the 171 bp unit length but also the 5' sequences within this unit are more important to centromeric function than the 3' sequences.

In conclusion, the existing long alpha satellite arrays at each human centromere were all derived from a common ancestral sequence with a small number of 171 bp repeats that were very similar to the ancestral sequence derived mathematically from the 420 bp tree in this report (Ancestor 1, Figs 9.1, 9.2). This ancestral sequence with its small number of repeats was initially dispersed to all the human centromeric chromosome regions (Fig. 9.6). Subsequent unequal recombination, concerted evolution, and selection over evolutionary time are the most important mechanisms that generated the very long functional variable-length arrays found at each human chromosome centromere. Together these processes explain the source of the substantial variability in length of these centromeric heteromorphisms among normal individuals.

ACKNOWLEDGEMENTS

We thank the Charcot-Marie-Tooth Association, the Wilson Genetic Center at George Washington University, and the Children's Hospital Medical Center of Akron for supporting this work.

References

1. Earnshaw WC, Ratrie H 3rd, Stetten G (1989). Visualization of centromere proteins CENP-B and CENP-C on a stable dicentric chromosome in cytological spreads. Chromosoma. 98:1–12.
2. Page SL, Earnshaw WC, Choo KH, Shaffer LG (1995). Further evidence that CENP-C is a necessary component of active centromeres: studies of a dic(X;15) with simultaneous immunofluorescence and FISH. Hum Mol Genet. 4:89–294.
3. Sullivan BA, Schwartz S (1995). Identification of centromeric antigens in dicentric Robertsonian translocations: CENP-C and CENP-E are necessary components of functional centromeres. Hum Mol Genet. 4:2189–97.
4. Choo KHA, Vissel B, Nagy A, Earle E, Kalistis P (1991). A survey of the genomic distribution of alpha satellite DNA on all the human chromosomes, and derivation of a new consensus sequence. Nucl Acids Res. 19:1179–82.
5. Alexandrov I, Kazakov A, Tumeneva I, Shepelev V, Yurov Y (2001). Alpha-satellite DNA of primates: old and new families. Chromosoma. 2001 110:253–66.
6. Mitchell AR, Gosden JR, Miller DA (1985). A cloned sequence, p82H, of the alphoid repeated DNA family found at the centromeres of all human Chromosomes. Chromosoma (Berl.). 92:369–77.
7. Gosden JR, Mitchell AR, Buckland RA, Clayton RP, Evans HJ (1975). The location of four human satellite DNAs on human chromosomes. Exp Cell Res. 92:148–58.
8. Wu JC, Manuelidis L (1980). Sequence definition and organization of a human repeated DNA. J Mol Biol. 142:363–86.
9. Choo KHA, Vissel B, Earle E (1989). Evolution of alpha satellite DNA on human acrocentric chromosomes. Genomics. 5:332–44.
10. Waye JS, Creeper LA, Willard HF (1987). Organization and evolution of alpha satellite DNA from human chromosome 11. Chromosoma. 95:182–8.
11. Tatusova TA, Madden TL (1999). Blast 2 sequences – a new tool for comparing protein and nucleotide sequences. FEMS Microbiol Lett. 174:247–50.
12. Choo KH, Vissel B (1987). Human alpha satellite DNA-consensus sequence and conserved regions. Nucl Acids Res. 15:6751–2.
13. Waye JS, Willard HF (1987). Nucleotide sequence heterogeneity of alpha satellite repetitive DNA: a survey of alphoid sequences from different human chromosomes. Nucl Acids Res. 15:7549–69.

14. Willard HF, Waye JS (1987). Chromosome-specific subsets of human alpha satellite DNA: analysis of sequence divergence within and between chromosomal subsets and evidence for an ancestral Pentameric Repeat. J Mol Evol. 25:207–14.
15. Willard HF (1991). Evolution of alpha satellite. Curr Opin Genet Devel. 1:509–14.
16. Choo KHA (1997). The Centromere. Oxford: Oxford University Press.
17. Jorgensen L, Bostock CJ, and Leth-Bak A (1986). Chromosome-specific subfamilies within human alphoid repetitive DNA. J Mol Biol. 187:185–96.
18. Waye JS, Willard HF (1989). Concerted evolution of alpha satellite DNA: evidence for species specificity and general lack of sequence conservation among alphoid sequences of higher primates. Chromosoma (Berl.). 98:273–9.
19. Willard HF (1985). Chromosome-specific organization of human alpha satellite DNA. Am J Hum Genet. 37:524–32.
20. Schueler MG, Higgins AW, Rudd MK, Gustashaw K, Willard HF (2001). Genomic and genetic definition of a functional human centromere. Science. 294:30–1.
21. McGinnis MD, Lebo RV, Quinn DL, Malcolm JS (1994). Ancient, highly polymorphic human major histocompatibility complex DQA1 intron sequences. Am J Med Genet. 52:438–44.
22. Meneveri R, Ginelli E. (1999) Genome database direct submission, 02-Nov-1999.
23. Alexandrov IA, Mitkevich SP, and Yurov YB (1988). The phylogeny of human chromosome specific alpha satellites. Chromosoma. 96:443–53.
24. Alexandrov IA, Mashkova TD, Akopian TA et al. (1991) Chromosome specific-alpha satellite: two distinct families on human chromosome 18. Genomics. 11:15–23.
25. Jabs EW, Warren AC, Taylor EW, Colyer CR, Meyers DA, Antonarakis SE (1991). Alphoid DNA polymorphisms for chromosome 21 can be distinguished from those of chromosome 13 using probes homologous to both. Genomics. 9:141–6.
26. Lebo RV, Flandermeyer RR, Lynch ED, Lepercq JA, Diukman R, Golbus M (1992). Prenatal diagnosis with repetitive in situ hybridization probes. Am J Med Genet. 43: 848–54.
27. Tyler-Smith C, and Brown WRA (1987). Structure of the major block of alphoid DNA on the human Y chromosome. J Mol Biol. 195:457–70.
28. Sulston JE, Waterson R (1998). Toward a complete human genome sequence. Genome Res. 8:1097–108.
29. Han JY, Choo KH, Shaffer LG (1994). Molecular cytogenetic characterization of 17 rob(13q;14q) Robertsonian translocations by FISH, narrowing the region containing the breakpoints. Am J Hum Genet. 55:960–7.
30. Lapidot-Lifson Y, Lebo RV, Flandermeyer R, Chung J-H, Golbus MS (1996). Rapid aneuploid diagnosis of high risk cases by fluorescence in situ hybridization. Am J Obstet Gynecol. 174:886–90.
31. Choo KH (1990). Role of acrocentric cen-pter satellite DNA in Robertsonian translocations and chromosomal non-disjunction. Mol Biol Med. 7:437–49.
32. Trask B, Van den Engh G, Mayall B, Gray JW (1989). Chromosome heteromorphism quantified by high-resolution bivariate flow karyotyping. Am J Hum Genet. 45:739–52.
33. Trask B, Van den Engh G, Gray JW (1989). Inheritance of chromosome heteromorphisms analyzed by high-resolution bivariate flow karyotyping. Am J Hum Genet. 45:753–60.
34. Haaf T, Willard HF (1992). Organization, polymorphism, and molecular cytogenetics of chromosome-specific alpha satellite DNA from the centromere of chromosome 2. Genomics. 13:122–8.
35. Mashkova TD, Akopian TA, Romanova LY et al. (1994). Genomic organization, sequence and polymorphism of the human chromosome 4-specific alpha satellite DNA. Gene. 140:211–17.
36. Puechberty J, Laurent AM, Gimenez S, et al. (1999). Genetic and physical analyses of the centromeric and pericentromeric regions of human chromosome 5: recombination across 5cen. Genomics. 56:274–87.
37. Sugimoto K, Furukawa K, Kusumi K, Himeno M (1997). The distribution of binding sites for centromere protein B (CENP-B) is partly conserved among diverged higher order repeating units of human chromosome 6-specific alphoid DNA. Chromosome Res. 5:395–405.
38. Dela-Puente A, Velasco E, Perez-Jurado L et al. (1997). Analysis of the structural repetitive sequences adjacent to the centromeric alphoid DNA array of human chromosome 7 (unpublished).
39. Ge Y, Wagner MJ, Siciliano M, Wells DE (1992). Sequence, higher order repeat structure, and long-range organization of alpha satellite sequences specific to human chromosome 8. Genomics. 13:585–93.

40. Rocchi M, Archidacono N, Ward DC, Baldini A (1991). A human chromosome 9-specific alphoid DNA repeat spatially resolvable from satellite 3 DNA by fluorescent in situ hybridization. Genomics. 9:517–23.

41. Alexandrov IA, Mashkova TD, Romanova LY, Yurov YB, Kisselev LL (1993). Segment substitutions in alpha satellite DNA. Unusual structure of human chromosome 3-specific alpha satellite repeat unit. J Mol Biol. 231:516–20.

42. Joergensen AL, Bostock CJ, Bak AL (1987). Homologous subfamilies of human alphoid repetitive DNA on different nucleolus organizing chromosomes. Proc Natl Acad Sci USA. 84:1075–9.

43. Heilig R et al. (2001). Sequences of the Human Chromosome 14 (unpublished).

44. O'Keefe CL, Matera AG (2000). Alpha satellite DNA variant-specific oligoprobes differing by a single base can distinguish chromosome 15 homologs. Genome Res. 10:1342–50.

45. Greig GM, England SB, Bedford HM, Willard HF (1989). Chromosome-specific alpha satellite DNA from the centromere of human chromosome 16. Am J Hum Genet. 45:862–72.

48. Waburton PE, Waye JS, Willard HF (1993). Nonrandom localization of recombinant events in human alpha satellite repeats unit variants: implications for higher order structural characteristics within centromeric heterochromatin. Mol Cell Biol. 13:6520–9.

47. Bassi C, Magnani I, Sacchi N et al. (2000). Molecular structure and evolution of DNA sequences located at the alpha satellite boundary of chromosome 20. Gene. 256:43–50.

48. McDermid HE, Duncan AMV, Higgins MJ et al. (1986). Isolation and characterization of an alpha-satellite repeated sequence from human chromosome 22. Chromosoma. 94:228–34.

49. Laursen HB, Jorgensen AL, Jones C, Bak AL (1992). Higher rate of evolution of X chromosome alpha-repeat DNA in human than in the great apes. EMBO J. 11:2367–72.

50. Haaf T, Willard HF (1998). Orangutan alpha-satellite monomers are closely related to the human consensus sequence. Mamm Genome. 9:440–7.

51. Altschul SF, Madden TL, Schäffer AA et al. (1997). Gapped BLAST and PSI-BLAST: a new generation of protein database search programs. Nucl Acids Res. 25:3389–402.

52. Phylip. Free Package of programs for interfering phylogenies. Available free at http://evolution.genetics.washington.edu/phylip.

53. Modeltest version 3.06 by David Posada, April 2001. Department of Zoology, Brigham Young University, Provo UT 84602, USA.

54. Willard HF (1998). Centromeres: the missing link in the development of human artificial chromosomes. Curr Opin Genet Dev. 8:219–25.

55. Grimes BR, Rhoades AA, Willard HF (2002). Alpha-satellite DNA and vector composition influence rates of human artificial chromosome formation. Mol Ther. 5:798–805.

56. Wong LH, Saffery R, Choo KH (2002). Construction of neocentromere-based human minichromosomes for gene delivery and centromere studies. Gene Ther. 9:724–6.

57. Ando S, Yang H, Nozaki N, Okazaki T, Yoda K (2002). CENP-A, -B, and -C chromatin complex that contains the I-type alpha-satellite array constitutes the prekinetochore in HeLa cells. Mol Cell Biol. 22:2229–41.

58. Swofford DL (2000). PAUP*. Phylogenetic analysis using parsimony (*and other methods). Version 4. Sunderland, MA: Sinauer Associates.

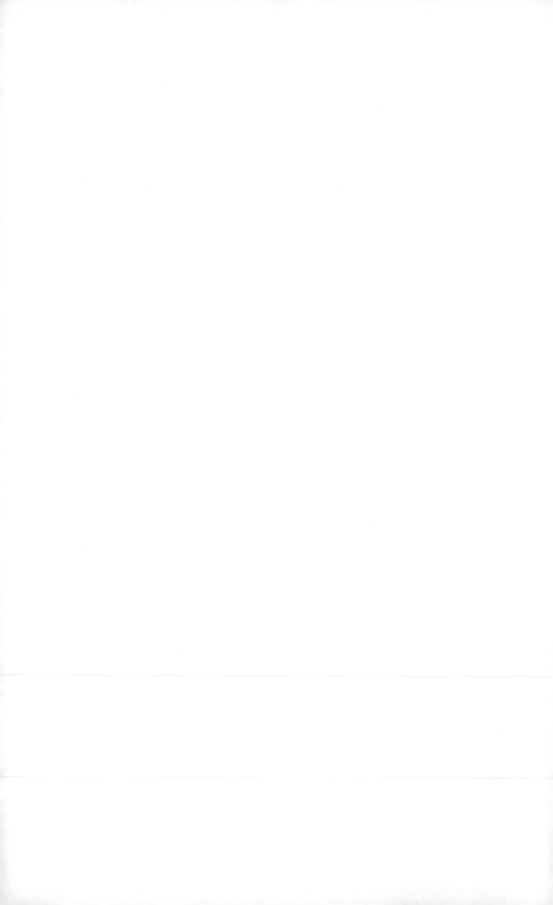

Part II
Plates

ORGANIZATION OF PART II

The following plates represent examples of human chromosome heteromorphisms that have been contributed by individual investigators specifically for this volume, by us or have been reprinted with permission from various published sources. Individual contributions have been identified by a numerical designation prefixed with the letter "c," after the name of the contributor, i.e. Lauren Jenkins (c2). A complete alphabetical listing of contributors, their titles, and affiliations is given in the List of Contributors at the front of Part I, followed by c2, c6, etc. to indicate the number(s) of their contribution(s).

All figures reprinted from published sources are acknowledged in the figure captions.

Numerical citations are used in the text throughout the book and are listed in the order cited at the end of each section, as is the usual case, in order to keep the text less cluttered and easier to read.

Each group of plates representing a chromosome is preceded by a set of ideograms representing the G-chromosome banding pattern of each chromosome at three different levels of resolution. The following description of the ideograms is reprinted with permission from ISCN 1995. "The left ideogram in each set represents the chromosome of a haploid karyotype of approximately 400 bands and the central ideogram, the 550 band level. These ideograms correspond to ISCN (1981) nomenclature. The location and width of bands are not based on any measurements. The dark G bands correspond to bright Q bands, with the exception of the variable regions. The numbering of R-banded chromosomes is exactly the same with a reversal of light and dark bands. The right ideogram represents the chromosome from a haploid karyotype of 850 bands and replaces the ISCN (1981) version. While the band numbers are exactly the same, the relative widths of euchromatic bands are based on measurements and the staining intensities reflect GTG bands (Francke, 1981, 1994). The ideogram of the Y chromosome has undergone a revision suggested by observations of Magenis and Barton (1987). While the number of bands on the euchromatic portion of the long arm has been expanded, the designations for the light versus dark bands have been maintained".

References

ISCN (1995). An International System for Human Cytogenetic Nomenclature (1995), Mittelman F, editor. Basel: S Karger.

Francke U (1981). High resolution ideograms of trypsin-Giemsa banded chromosomes. Cytogenet Cell Genet. 31:24–32.

Francke U (1994). Digitized and differentially shaded human chromosome ideograms for genomic applications. Cytogenet Cell Genet. 65:206–19.

Magenis E, Barton SJ (1987). Delineation of human prometaphase paracentromeric regions using sequential GTG- and C-banding. Cytogenet Cell Genet. 45:132–40.

CHROMOSOME 1

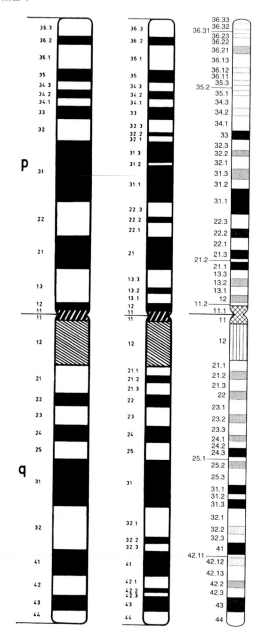

Plate 1. **A**: Normal no. 1's by G-banding showing increasing length of the secondary constriction, band 1q12. As the region increases in size, it appears to be divided into blocks, sometimes with a lighter proximal block (A2), a smaller dark-staining proximal block (A4), two clearly separated blocks of equal size and intensity (A5), or more rarely a small block and a very large block (A6). **B**: Giemsa-11 staining and C-banding variations from eight individuals. Top row, from left to right: chromosome 1 with Giemsa-11-positive staining; five chromosomes with single Giemsa-11-positive bands at varying distances from the centromere; two chromosomes with two Giemsa-11-positive bands. Bottom row: C-banding of chromosomes 1 from the same individuals. [Reprinted from Magenis RE, Donlon TA, Wyandt HE (1978). Giemsa-11 staining of chromosome 1: a newly described heteromorphism. Science. 202:64–5, Figure 1.] **C**: Further heterogeneity is revealed by lateral asymmetry in staining within the heterochromatin, due to interstrand compositional bias (i.e. T-rich strand vs. A-rich strand), revealed by substitution of T with 5-bromodeoxyuridine after 1 round of DNA synthesis. The longer chromosome on the left of each pair is a der(1)t(1;15) allowing it to be distinguished from the normal homolog (right member of each pair). Ideogram at the left depicts regions stained with the lateral asymmetry technique. Blocks B and C stain with Giemsa-11. Blocks A and D do not. [Reprinted from Magenis RE, Donlon TA, Wyandt HE (1978). Giemsa-11 staining of chromosome 1: a newly described heteromorphism. Science. 202: 64–5, Figure 3.]

Contributors
(A1–A3). Center for Human Genetics, Boston University (c1).
(A4–A6). Lauren Jenkins, Kaiser Permanente (c2).

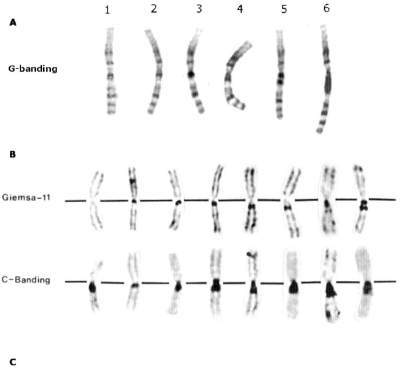

A

G-banding

1   2   3   4   5   6

B

Giemsa-11

C-Banding

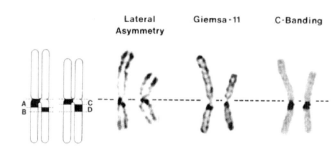

C

Lateral   Giemsa-11   C-Banding
Asymmetry

Plate 2. (**a**) Pair of 1's by G-banding showing duplication of bands q12 in right-hand homolog. (**b–g**) Pairs of 1's from five different individuals showing pericentric inversion of band q12 into the short arm.

Contributors
(a, c, f, g) Lauren Jenkins, Kaiser Permanente (c2).
(b,c) Center for Human Genetics, Boston University (c1).
(d) Patricia Miron, Brigham and Womens Hospital (c33).

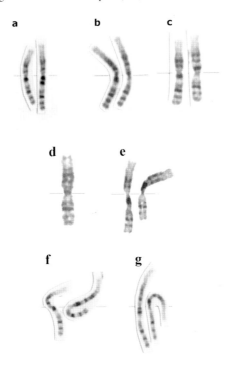

Plate 3. (a) Variations of 1qh region by C-banding. Numbers (top row) are scores arbitrarily assigned by the investigators to designate size (2–9) and (bottom row) complete (0) or (1) partial inversion. [Reprinted from Magenis RE, Palmer CG, Wang L *et al.* (1977). Heritability of chromosome banding variants. In: Hook EB, Porter IH, editors. Population Cytogenetics. Studies in Humans. New York: Academic Press, pp. 179–88.] (b, c) Sequential staining of same chromosomes 1 by Q-banding (left) and C-banding (right) with typical 1qh region (b) and homolog with complete 1qh inversion (c) [Reprinted from Magenis RE, Palmer CG, Wang L *et al.* (1977). Heritability of chromosome banding variants. In: Hook EB, Porter IH, editors. Population Cytogenetics. Studies in Humans. New York: Academic Press, pp. 179–88.]

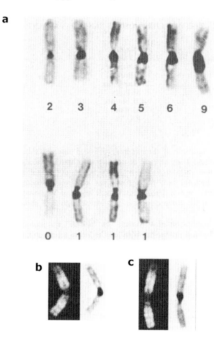

134

Plate 4. Apparently unremarkable paternal pericentric inversion in a family with a history of multiple miscarriages. (**a, b**). At lower resolution, by G- and C-banding, the inversion appears to be a typical complete inversion of the 1qh region. (**c**) At higher resolution, breakpoints were determined to be in euchromatic bands p13.3 and q21.3, respectively.

Contributor
Center for Human Genetics, Boston University (c1).

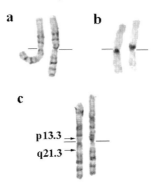

Plate 5. The chromosomes stained for C-bands (CBG), for regions resistant to the restriction endonucleases AluI and HaeIII and by the G-11 and DA/DAPI techniques. Rows **a** and **b** show the chromosomes from two normal subjects. Rows **c** and **d** are from [a balanced] translocation carrier [46,XY,t(1;7)(q11.1;q22)] showing the normal and derivative chromosomes 1 and 7, respectively. The derivative chromosomes are placed to the right [Reprinted from Babu A, Verma RS (1986). Cytochemical heterogeneity of the C-band in human chromosome 1. Histochem J. 18(6):329–33, Figure 2.]

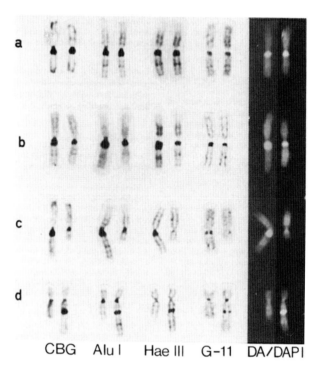

CBG   Alu I   Hae III   G-11   DA/DAPI

Plate 6. (a) Three fluorescent images of the same chromosome 1 after subsequent quinacrine (Q), DIPI* and mithramycin (MM) treatment. Note that most of the material in the secondary constriction is DIPI-positive; a small segment close to the centromere is brightly stained by mithramycin and remains unstained by DIPI. On the right, another chromosome 1, treated with chromomycin A3 (CMA) and subsequently digested by DNAse I is shown; a reverse pattern is obtained by staining the remaining DNA with Giemsa or Pinacyanol (for this preparation Pinacyanol was used). (b) Chromosomes 1 from four different individuals, showing different lengths of the secondary constriction. The polymorphic material is DIPI-positive [Reprinted from Schnedl W (1978). Structure and variability of human chromosomes analyzed by recent techniques. Hum Genet. 41:1–9].

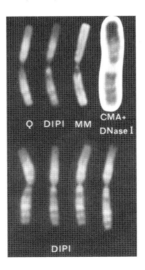

*DIPI = 6-imidazolino-2(imidazolinophenyl) indole is closely related to DAPI, with similar staining affinity.

Plate 7. Rosette formation of multiple copies of chromosome 1 attached at the 1qh region, associated with ICF syndrome [Reprinted from Swanson CM, Wheeler G, Cunniff C (1995). Chromosome instability in ICF syndrome: formation of micronuclei from multibranched chromosomes 1 demonstrated by fluorescence *in situ* hybridization. Am J Med Genet. 56:203–9.]

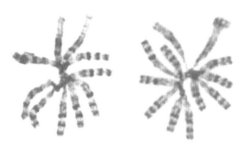

Plate 8. Ideogram of chromosome 1 and trypsin-Giemsa banded partial chromosome numbers 1 from [a] fetus (top) and mother (bottom) [Reprinted from Zaslav AL, Blumenthal D, Fox JE, Thomson KA, Segraves R, Weinstein ME (1993). A rare inherited euchromatic heteromorphism on chromosome 1. Prenat Diagn. 13(7):569–73, Figure 1.]

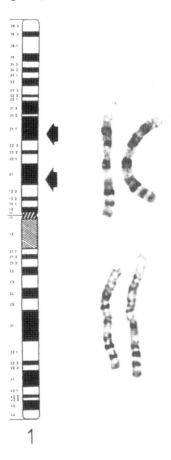

Chromosome 1: Summary

Variations in the size of band 1q12 (1qh region) of chromosome 1 were early noted to occur in 1/100 to 1/1000 newborns [1]. An elongated 1qh region referred to the "uncoiler" was used as a familial marker in the first successful effort to map an autosomal gene, the Duffy blood group, to chromosome 1 [2,3]. Linkage studies using variants of the 1qh region were subsequently used to establish the relative order of Duffy, Rh, phosphoglucomutase and amylase loci on 1q [4,5]. From a sample of 4000 7- and 8-year-olds [6], a subpopulation of 400 children was studied by C-banding. Variations in size of C-bands were compared with the length of the short arm of chromosome 16 (see Chapter 3). Variants that were smaller than 16p were graded as *levels 1 and 2*, equal to the length of the short arm, *level 3* and greater than the length of the short arm, *levels 4 and 5* [7,8]. Chromosome 1 showed 1qh-size variations in 7.5% of subjects, 80% of which were *level 5* variants, and 20% of which were *level 1* variants. There were no significant size differences between Black and White children. Partial inversions in chromosome 1 determined by G- and C-banding from the same study were less frequent, occurring with a frequency of 0.55% in White children and only 0.07% in Black children. Complete inversions of the 1qh region were not reported in the study [6]. Magenis *et al.* [9] reported on segregation of C-band variants of 1qh from 42 families used in gene mapping and classified them into 10 morphological categories, based on size and partial or complete inversion (**Plate 3**). One case with complete inversion was found by sequential Q- and C-banding. By C-banding alone the inversion might have been missed. Verma *et al.* [10] also provided a classification of inversions in chromosomes 1, 9 and 16 by CBG banding (see Chapter 3). Hsu *et al.* [11] reported a frequency of complete 1qh inversion of 0.04–0.06% in Black and Caucasian, and absence in Hispanic and Asian populations. The frequency of the inversion appeared to be correlated with size of the heterochromatin. For the most part, no increases in fetal loss have been associated with any of these common or rare 1qh heteromorphisms (**Plates 1–3**). Recently, a pericentric inversion was found that at first glance is not easily distinguishable from the inversions shown in the previous plates. However, at higher resolution breakpoints were determined to be in euchromatic bands on either side of the centromere (**Plate 4**). The patient in this instance has a history of multiple miscarriages (Center for Human Genetics, unpublished observation).

Heterogeneity is evident in 1qh heterochromatin not only by C-banding but also by Giemsa-11 staining (**Plate 1B**), and by lateral asymmetry (**Plate 1C**) [12]. Further heterogeneity is revealed by C-bands treated with restriction enzymes (Alu1 and HaeIII) and compared with DA/DAPI staining and G-11 bands. C-bands are Alu1-resistant, but bands remaining after HaeIII treatment are smaller and appear to correspond to DAPI staining. G-11 stained regions appear to be sub-bands of DA/DAPI-positive regions [13,14] (**Plate 5**). Heterogeneity in banding was also revealed by comparison of different fluorochromes such as DIPI, and mithramycin, which reportedly have different affinities for AT, or GC richness of different regions as demonstrated by Schnedl [15] (**Plate 6**).

Gardner *et al.* [16] raised the question of whether cases with 1qh+ are always innocuous, citing six cases with various anomalies, including two with severe anomalies resembling Patau and Meckel syndromes. In all six cases both parents, one of which carried the same heteromorphism, were normal. They also wrote of the variability in appearance of the 1qh region within the same individual and of possible epigenetic expression involving 1qh+ in some cases.

C-bands of chromosome 1 have been reported to be more variable in patients with malignant disease compared to normal controls [17,18]. Rearrangements in the vicinity of the centromere are over-represented in many types of human cancer [19], including the characteristic rosette formation (**Plate 7**) in a rare disease called ICF (immune deficiency, centromeric instability and facial anomalies) [20]. Hypomethylation of DNA has been implicated in some of these cancers and Ji *et al.* [21] have shown that inhibiting DNA methylation with 5-azadeoxycytidine and 5-azacytidine produced configurations similar to those in ICF disease. The alpha-satellite regions in chromosome 1 appear to be prone to breakage [22]. Surralles *et al.* [23] showed that breaks in 1q12 heterochromatin show a lower than normal rate of DNA excision repair.

Euchromatic variants. Euchromatic variants of chromosome 1 have been reported (see Chapter 6). Verma *et al.* [24] reported an unusual G-negative band with the heterochromatic qh region, and Zaslav *et al.* [25] reported a tandem duplication of bands 1p21–1p31 shared by a phenotypically normal mother and her fetus (**Plate 8**).

References

1. Lubs HA, Ruddle FH (1971). Chromosome polymorphism in American negro and white populations. Nature. 233:134–6.
2. Donahue RP, Bias WB, Renwick JH, McKusick VA (1968). Probable assignment of the Duffy blood group locus to chromosome **1** in man. Proc Natl Acad Sci (USA). 61:949–55.
3. Ying KL, Ives EJ (1968). Asymmetry of chromosome number 1 pair in three generations of a phenotypically normal family. Canad J Genet Cytol. 10:575–89.
4. Rivas ML, Conneally PM, Hecht F *et al.* (1975). Linkage relationships of 1qh to Amy, Fy, PGM1, and Rh. Cytogenet Cell Genet. 14:409–17.
5. Meyers DA, Conneally PM, Hecht F *et al.* (1975). Linkage group I: multipoint mapping. Cytogenet Cell Genet. 14:381–9.
6. Lubs HA, Kimberling WJ, Hecht F *et al.* (1977). Racial differences in the frequency of Q and C chromosomal heteromorphisms. Nature. 268:631–3.
7. Lubs HA, Patil SR, Kimberling WJ *et al.* (1977). Q and C-banding polymorphisms in 7 and 8 year old children: racial differences and clinical significance. In: Hook EB, Porter IH, editors. Population Cytogenetic Studies in Humans. New York: Academic Press, pp. 133–159.
8. Patil SR, Lubs HA (1977). Classification of qh regions in human chromosomes 1, 9 and 16 by C-banding. Hum Genet. 19:377–80.
9. Magenis RE, Palmer CG, Wang L *et al.* (1977). Heritability of chromosome banding variants. In: Hook EB, Porter IH, editors. Population Cytogenetics. Studies in Humans. New York: Academic Press, pp. 179–88.
10. Verma RS, Dosik H, Lubs HA (1978). Size and pericentric inversion heteromorphisms of secondary constriction regions (h) of chromosomes 1, 9 and 16 as detected by CBG technique in Caucasians: classification, frequencies and incidence. Am J Med Genet. 2:331–9.
11. Hsu LYF, Benn PA, Tannenbaum HL, Perlis TE, Carlson AD (1987). Chromosomal polymorphisms of 1, 9, 16 and Y in 4 major ethnic groups: a large prenatal study. Am J Med Genet. 26:95–101.
12. Magenis RE, Donlon TA, Wyandt HE (1978). Giemsa-11 staining of chromosome 1: a newly described heteromorphism. Science. 202:64–5.
13. Babu A, Verma RS (1986). Cytochemical heterogeneity of the C-band in human chromosome 1. Histochem J. 18:329–33.
14. Hedemann U, Schurmann M, Schwinger E (1988). The effect of restriction enzyme digestion of human metaphase chromosomes on C-band variants of chromosomes 1 and 9. Genome. 30:652–5.

15. Schnedl W (1978). Structure and variability of human chromosomes analyzed by recent techniques. Hum Genet. 41:1–9.
16. Gardner RJM, McCreanor HR, Paraslow MI, Veale AMO (1974). Are 1q+ chromosomes harmless? Clin Genet. 6:383–93.
17. Atkin NB, Baker MC (1977). Pericentric inversion in chromosome 1: frequency and possible association with cancer. Cytogenet Cell Genet. 19:180–4.
18. Tsezou A, Kitsiou-Tzeli S, Kosmidis H, Paidousi K, Katsouyanni K, Sinaniotis C (1993). Constitutive heterochromatin polymorphisms in children with acute lymphoblastic leukemia. Pediatr Hematol Oncol. 10:7–11.
19. Verma RS, Macera MJ, Babu A (1988). The role of heterochromatin in the origin of isochromosome 1 in neoplastic cells. Eur J Cancer Clin Oncol. 24:821–3.
20. Sawyer JR, Swanson CM, Wheeler G, Cunniff C (1995). Chromosome instability in ICF syndrome: formation of micronuclei from multibranched chromosomes 1 demonstrated by fluorescence in situ hybridization. Am J Med Genet. 56:203–9.
21. Ji W, Hernandez R, Zhang XY et al. (1997). DNA methylation and pericentromeric rearrangements of chromosome 1. Mut Res. 379:33–41.
22. Verma RS, Ramesh KH, Mathews T, Kleyman SM, Conte RA (1996). Centromeric alphoid sequences are breakage prone resulting in pericentromeric inversion heteromorphism of qh region of chromosome 1. Ann Genet. 39(4):205–8.
23. Surralles J, Darroudi F, Natarajan AT (1997). Low level DNA repair in human chromosome 1 heterochromatin. Genes Chromosomes Cancer. 20:173–84.
24. Verma RS, Kleyman SM, Conte RA (1997). An unusual G-negative band within 1qh region: a rare variant or an abnormality? Ann Genet. 40:229–31.
25. Zaslav AL, Blumenthal D, Fox JE, Thomson KA, Segraves R, Weinstein ME (1993). A rare inherited euchromatic heteromorphism on chromosome 1. Prenat Diagn. 13:569–73.

CHROMOSOME 2

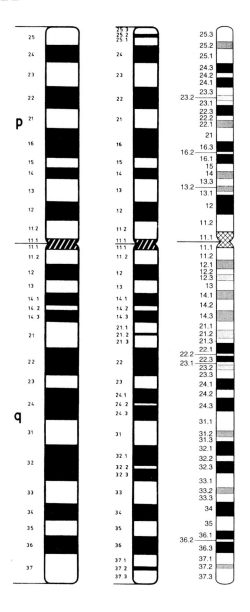

143

Plate 9. (**a–f**) Normal chromosomes 2 by G-banding. (**g–i**) Inversion in chromosome 2, inv(2)(p11.2q13).

Contributors
(**a–f, i**) Center for Human Genetics, Boston University School of Medicine (c1).
(**g, h**) Lauren Jenkins, Kaiser Permanente (c2).

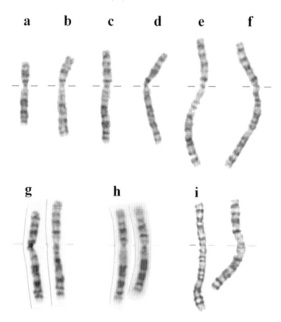

Plate 10. **A**: Normal chromosome 2 (left) and inversion 2 (p11q13) (right) with the ideogram with arrows to show the breakpoints [Reprinted from MacDonald IM, Cox DM (1985). Inversions of chromosome 2 (p11p13): frequency and implications for genetic counselling. Hum Genet. 69(3):281–3.] **B**: Six examples of inversion 2, two with pericentric inversions: Case 42, inv(2)(p13q21); Case 51, inv(2)(p11q13). Four other examples are paracentric inversions. G-banding (42,48), Q-banding (50–53), R-type replication pattern (50, 51). The inverted segments are indicated by brackets [Reprinted from Djalali M, Steinbach P, Bullerdiek J, Holmes-Siedel M, Verschraegen-Spae MR, Smith A (1986). The significance of pericentric inversions of chromosome 2. Hum Genet. 72(1):32–6.]

A

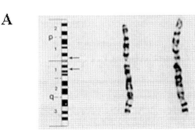

B

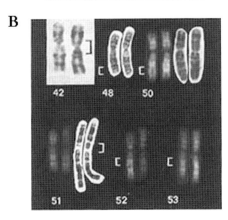

Chromosome 2: Summary

In the study of 400 subjects of 7 and 8 year old, by Lubs *et al.* [1], 0.8% of subjects had a distinguishable variation in the amount of C-band, centromeric heterochromatin in chromosome 2.

A more visible heteromorphism of chromosome 2, by conventional techniques, was a pericentric inversion. In initial unbanded studies of newborns the frequency in the population was between 0.0001 and 0.013 [2,3]. By banding, Vejerslev and Friedrich [4] found six cases in 5547 prenatal diagnoses, and Dejalali *et al.* [5] found seven cases of inversion 2 in 9500 prenatal diagnoses. Technically, because the band in the long arm of chromosome 2 that is inverted is non-heterochromatic, the inversion is regarded by some as a structural abnormality. Most inv(2) involve bands p11.2 in the short arm and q13 in the long arm (**Plate 9, Plate 10A**). Phillips [6] reported two families with inversions, one with inv(2)(p11q13) and one with inv(2)(p13q11). In the first family there reportedly was no effect on reproduction. In the second family some reproductive abnormalities were noted. Dejalali *et al.* [5] describe one case with breakpoints in p13 and q21 (**Plate 10B**) and review other cases with deviant breakpoints. Leonard *et al.* [7] and Baccichetti *et al.* [8] each describe four families with inv(2)(p11q13) and suggest there is some evidence of reproductive failure.

Although inv(2) is more often found in normal individuals, it was often ascertained through individuals with mental retardation [9–11] and/or a variety of congenital abnormalities. Anomalies included Pierre Robin anomaly [12], congenital heart defects [9–11], gonadal dysgenesis or hypogonadism (13,14), de Lange syndrome [5], adrenogenital syndrome [15], spina bifida [7], motor retardation [16] and psychiatric problems [17]. A number of cases of inv(2) have been associated with unrelated chromosome abnormalities, including Down syndrome [18] trisomy 13 [19], duplication in 7p [20], and Turner syndrome [14,21]. None of the phenotypic abnormalities associated with inv(2) is consistent and there has been no increased risk for congenital anomalies due to a chromosomal imbalance resulting from inv(2) in a liveborn child.

MacDonald and Cox [22] reviewed all banded cases from a 6-year period in a Canadian children's hospital and found two cases of inversion 2 among 3619 patients referred for chromosome studies. An additional three cases were found among 1820 prenatal chromosome studies. The first two cases were normal females referred for recurrent miscarriages; the last three cases were mothers referred for amniocentesis because of maternal age. All three carried the pericentric inversion and all three had previous normal pregnancies. Only one had a prior miscarriage.

Dejalali *et al.* [5] reviewed pedigrees of 41 published cases of inversion 2 and analyzed the data for 13 new cases obtained from 16,047 prenatal diagnoses [4,5]. From the pooled data, using Weinberg's proband method, they evaluated the risk for congenital anomalies and fetal wastage. In a corrected sample of 187 liveborn offspring, born to carriers of pericentric inversions, their review revealed 3.7% of cases with heterogeneous phenotypic anomalies. Excluding two that died after delivery, this frequency was reduced to 3%, interpreted to be the same as the basic risk for abnormal offspring for any couple. Of the 187 offspring, 11.2% were fetal wastage (stillbirths and spontaneous miscarriages) and 85% had a normal phenotype. The rate of stillborn and spontaneous abortions for carriers was determined to be about twice the rate for the general population. Carriers of inv(2) passed it on to about half of their children, and inv(2) occurred with equal frequency in male and female carriers. With a couple of exceptions [20,23], the breaks typically occurred in bands p11 and q13, both noted to be common fragile sites [24]. About 3% of cases were *de novo* [25,26].

Euchromatic variants

Euchromatic variants of chromosome 2 have been of two types (see Chapter 6). Interstitial deletion of 2q13–q14, detectable by G-banding, has been reported [27]. In addition, a number of cases of deletions of the subtelomeric region of 2q (not detectable cytogenetically) have been reported using FISH techniques (**Plate 66**) [28].

References

1. Lubs HA, Patil SR, Kimberling WJ *et al.* (1977). Q and C-banding polymorphisms in 7 and 8 year old children: racial differences and clinical significance: In: Hook EB, and Porter IH, editors. Population Cytogenetic Studies in Humans. New York: Academic Press, pp. 133–59.
2. Jacobs PA, Melville M, Ratcliffe S (1974). A cytogenetic survey of 11,680 newborn infants. Ann Hum Genet. 37:359–76.
3. Nielsen J, Sillesen I (1975). Incidence of chromosome aberrations in 11,148 newborn children. Hum Genet. 30:1–12.
4. Vejerslev LO, Friedrich U (1984). Experiences with unexpected structural chromosome aberrations in prenatal diagnosis in a Danish series. Prenat Diagn. 4:181–6.
5. Djalali M, Steinbach P, Bullerdiek J, Holmes-Siedel M, Verschraegen-Spae MR, Smith A (1986). The significance of pericentric inversions of chromosome 2. Hum Genet. 72(1):32–6.
6. Phillips RB (1978). Pericentric inversions inv(2)(p11q13) and inv(2)(p13q11) in two unrelated families. J Med Genet. 15:388–90.
7. Leonard C, Hazael-Massieux P, Bocquet L, Larget-Piet L, Boue J (1975). Inversion pericentrique inv(2)(p11q13) dans des familles no apparentees. Humangenetik. 28:121–8.
8. Baccichetti C, Lanzini E, Peserico A, Tenconi R (1980). Study on segregation and risk for abnormal offspring in carriers of pericentric inversion of the (p11->q31) segment of chromosome 2. Clin Genet. 18:402–7.
9. Fryns JP, Petit P, Heffinck R, and van den Berge H (1983). Mosaic pericentromeric inversion of chromosome 2. J Genet Hum. 31:157–61.
10. De Grouche J, Emerit I, Corone P, Vernant P, Lamy M, Soulie P (1963). Inversion pericentric probable du chromosome No. 2 et malformations congenitales chez un garcon. Ann Genet (Paris). 6:21–3.
11. De Grouche J, Aussuannaire M, Brissaud HE, Lamy M (1966). Aneusomie de recombinaison: three further examples. Am J Hum Genet. 18:21–3.
12. Singh RP, Jaco NT, Vigna MV (1970). Pierre Robin syndrome in siblings. Am J Dis Child. 120:560–1.
13. Podulgolnikova OA, Blymina MG (1972). Pericentric inversion of chromosome 2 in a girl with congenital mental deficiency and in her mother. Genetika (Moskva). 8:156–61.
14. Cohen MM, Rosenmann A, Hacham-Zadeh S, Dahan S (1975). Dicentric X-isochromosome (Xqidic) and pericentric inversion of No. 2 inv(2)(p15q12) in a patient with gonadal dysgenesis. Clin Genet. 8:11–17.
15. Weitkamp LR, Janzen MK, Guttormsen SA, Gershowitz H (1969). Inherited pericentric inversion of chromosome number two: a linkage study. Ann Hum Genet. 33:53.
16. Ayme S, Mattei MG, Mattei JF, Giraud F (1979). Abnormal childhood phenotypes associated with the same balanced chromosome rearrangements as in the parents. Hum Genet. 48:7–12.
17. Romain DR, Chapman CI, Columbano-Green C, Smythe RH, Gebbie O (1982). Two pericentric inversions, inv(2)(p11q13) and inv(5)(p13q13), in a patient referred for psychiatric problems. J Med Genet. 19:153–61.

18. Wikramanayake E, Renwick JH, Feguson-Smith MA (1971). Chromosomal heteromorphisms in the assignment of loci to particular autosomes: a study of four pedigrees. Ann Genet (Paris). 14:245–56.
19. Verma RS, Dosik H, Wexler IB (1977). Inherited pericentric inversion of chromosome no. 2 with Robertsonian translocation (13q14q) resulting in trisomy for chromosome 13q. J Genet Humaine. 25:295–301.
20. Subrt I, Kozak J, Hnikova O (1973). Microdensitometric identification of the pericentric inversion of chromosome No. 2 and of duplication of the short arm of chromosome No. 7 in a reexamined case. Hum Hered. 23:331–7.
21. Hooft C, Coetsier H, Orye E (1968). Syndrome de Turner et inversion pericentrique probable du chromosome No. 2. Ann Genet (Paris). 11:181–3 [French].
22. MacDonald IM, Cox DM (1985). Inversions of chromosome 2 (p11p13): frequency and implications for genetic counselling. Hum Genet. 69(3):281–3.
23. Mattevi MS, Pinheiro CEA, Erdtman B, Flores RZ, Salzano FM (1981). Familial pericentric inversion of chromosome 2. J Genet Hum. 29:161–9.
24. Hecht F, Hecht BK (1984). Fragile sites and chromosome breakpoints in constitutional rearrangements. II. Spontaneous abortions, stillbirths and newborns. Clin Genet. 26:174–7.
25. Hesselbjerg U, Friedrich U (1979). Pericentric inversion in chromosome No. 2 as a *de novo* mutation. Humangenetik. 53:117–19.
26. Kozma C, Subasinghe C, Meck J (1996). Prenatal detection of *de novo* inversion of chromosome (2)(p13q11.2) and postnatal follow-up. Prenat Diagn. 16(4):366–70.
27. Sumption ND, Barber JCK (2001). A transmitted deletion of 2q13 to 2q14.1 causes no phenotypic abnormalities. J Med Genet. 38:125–7.
28. Ballif BC, Kashork CD, Shaffer L (2000). The promise and pitfalls of telomere region-specific probes. Am J Hum Genet. 67:1356–9.

CHROMOSOME 3

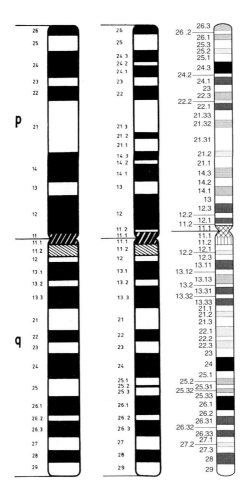

Plate 11. (**a–d**) Normal chromosomes 3 by G-banding. (**e–j**) Variation in intensity, size and location of 3cen variants by Q-banding, including apparent inversion of a Q-bright variant (**j**) into the short arm [Reprinted from Olson SB, Magenis RE, Lovrien EW (1986). Human chromosome variation: the discriminatory power of Q-band heteromorphism (variant) analysis in distinguishing between individuals, with specific application to cases of questionable paternity. Am J Hum Genet. 38(2):235–52, Figure 1.] (**k, l**) C-banding of 3cen (**k**) in normal pair of homologs; (**l**) C-banding of 3cen showing slightly larger C-band variant in one homolog than the other. [Reprinted from Craig-Holms AP, Moore FB, Shaw MW (1973). Polymorphism of human C-band heterochromatin I: frequency of variants. Am J Hum Genet. 25:181–92].

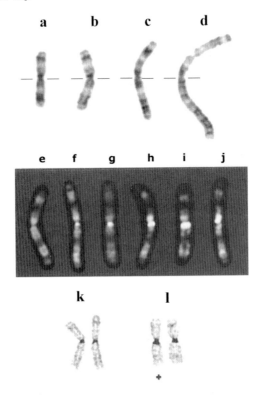

Chromosome 3: Summary

C- and/or Q-band variants were assessed by a number of investigators (see Chapter 3). Variation in size of the centromeric region of chromosome 3, 3cen, was described mainly by C-banding (**Plate 11k–l**). Lubs and colleagues [1–3], in their study of 7- and 8-year olds, found C-band polymorphisms of 3cen in approximately 10% of cases. Q-banding revealed variation in both size and intensity of the 3cen region. Q-bright centromeric regions (classified as levels 4 or 5) were found in 57% of cases studied. The slightly less intense variant (level 4 intensity) was found with a slightly higher frequency in White children compared to Black. Although numbers were small there was no significant difference in frequency between mentally retarded and intellectually normal children.

A second form of variant involving the Q-bright, C-positive 3cen region, normally in the long arm of chromosome 3, is an inversion into the short arm, i.e. inv(3) (**Plate 11j**). Inversion 3 in a number of studies [4–6] of mentally retarded and normal populations was reviewed by Soudek and Sroka [6]. Of 515 retarded individuals representing different populations, the frequency of inv(3) ranged from 1% to 11.1% with an overall frequency of 4.07% [6]. The frequency of inv(3) in over 3000 normal individuals ranged from 0% to 8.3% with an overall frequency of 1.26%. The highest frequency (8.3%) in the normal population was in a small selected Canadian population [5] and the highest frequency (11.1%) in the retarded population was in a small selected population from Estonia [6], leading both groups of investigators to conclude that differences between normal and retarded populations were not significant.

Q-band heteromorphisms were studied in 57 presumably normal subjects for use in paternity testing [7]. Six different variants of chromosome 3, including inv(3), were distinguishable by Q-banding (**Plate 11e–j**). Verma and Dosik [8] studied 100 Caucasians by sequential QFQ and RFA for heteromorphisms of centromere of 3 and 4, classified into five QFQ intensity levels; 62% of 3cen and 15% of 4 cen had intensities ≥ level 3. When the centromere was brilliant by QFQ it was deep red by RFA; when pale, it was light red by RFA. Color variants could not be distinguished in a blind study. In a study of 100 normal American Blacks [9,10], the frequency of QFQ-bright 3cen (levels 3 and 4) was 54.5%. Subtle differences in intensity of Q-bright, C-positive regions by RFA banding also could not be discerned in a blind study. QFQ was more useful. Heteromorphisms of bands p11 and q11 also did not show a consistent relationship between CBG and QFQ techniques [8].

Molecular characterization

Conte *et al.* [11,12] molecularly characterized the pericentromeric heterochromatin of chromosomes 3 in a child with an inv(3), referred for short stature, and subsequently found to be 48,XXYY. The inversion was present in the mother and there was no other eventful family history. The homolog lacked a Q-bright region and did not have an inversion. Both the inverted region, which was Q-bright, and band q11.2 in the normal homolog were resistant to treatment with the restriction enzymes, AluI and TaqI. Resistance to the latter suggested the q11.2 region to be composed of alpha satellite DNA. The probe P5095B hybridized to the entire inverted segment, suggesting that p11 and q11.2 shared similar alphoid sequences. However, overall, the various techniques revealed overlapping but non-identical patterns suggesting considerable heterogeneity within the alphoid region.

References

1. McKenzie WH, Lubs HA (1975). Human Q and C chromosomal variations: Distribution and incidence. Cytogenet Cell Genet. 14:97–115.
2. Lubs HA, Patil SR, Kimberling WJ *et al*. (1977). Q and C-banding polymorphisms in 7 and 8 year old children: racial differences and clinical significance. In: Hook EB, and Porter IH, editors. Population Cytogenetic Studies in Humans. New York: Academic Press, pp. 33–59.
3. Geraedts JPM, Pearson PL (1974). Fluorescent chromosome polymorphisms; frequencies and segregation in a Dutch population. Clin Genet. 6:247–57.
4. Mikelsaar AV, Ilus T, Kivi S (1978). Variant chromosome 3 (inv3) in normal newborns and their parents, and in children with mental retardation. Hum Genet. 41:109–13.
5. Fogle TA, McKenzie WH (1980). Cytogenetic study of a large Black kindred: inversions, heteromorphisms and segregation analysis. Hum Genet. 58:345–52.
6. Soudek D, Sroka H (1978). Inversion of "fluorescent" segment in chromosome 3: a polymorphic trait. Hum Genet. 44:109–15.
7. Olson SB, Magenis RE, Lovrien EW (1986). Human chromosome variation: the discriminatory power of Q-band heteromorphism (variant) analysis in distinguishing between individuals, with specific application to cases of questionable paternity. Am J Hum Genet. 38:235–52.
8. Verma RS, Dosik H (1979). Frequencies of centromeric heteromorphisms of human chromosomes 3 and 4 as detected by QFQ technique: can they be identified by RFA technique? Can J Genet Cytol. 21:109–13.
9. Verma RS, Dosik H (1980). Human chromosomal heteromorphisms in American Blacks. I. Structural variability of chromosome 3. J Hered. 71:441–2.
10. Verma RS, Dosik H (1981). Human chromosomal heteromorphisms in American Blacks. IV. Intensity variation in centromeric regions of chromosomes 3 and 4. Can J Cytol. 23:315–20.
11. Luke S, Verma RS (1991). Pericentromeric heterochromatin of chromosome 3. J Med Genet. 28:805–7.
12. Conte RA, Luke S, Verma RS (1992). Molecular characterization of "inverted" pericentromeric heterochromatin of chromosome 3. Histochemistry. 97: 509–10.

CHROMOSOME 4

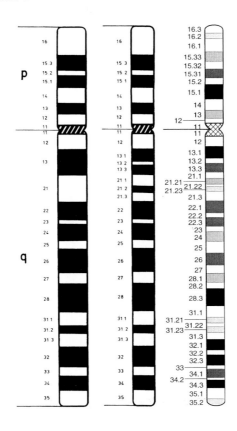

Plate 12. (**a**) Normal chromosomes 4 by G-banding. (**b**) Common Q-band heteromorphisms of 4cen [Reproduced from Olson SB, Magenis RE, Lovrien EW (1986). Human chromosome variation: the discriminatory power of Q-band heteromorphism (variant) analysis in distinguishing between individuals, with specific application to cases of questionable paternity. Am J Hum Genet. 38(2): 235–52, Figure 2.]

Contributor
(a) Center for Human Genetics, Boston University (c1).

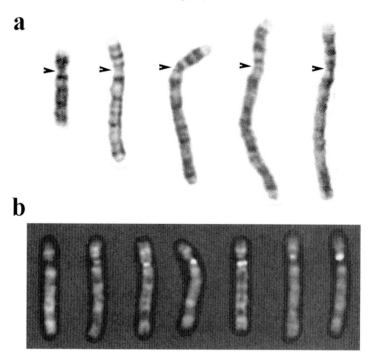

Plate 13. Partial karyotypes of antenatally screened fetus (**a, d**) and of the father (**b, c**) showing the variant chromosome 4 (arrows). (**a**) G-banding using trypsin after pretreatment with acetic saline. (**b**) G-banding using trypsin after treatment with hydrogen peroxide. (**c**) C banding. (**d**) Silver staining. [Reproduced from Docherty Z, Bowser-Riley SM (1984). A rare heterochromatic variant of chromosome 4. J Med Genet 21(6):470–2, Figure 1.]

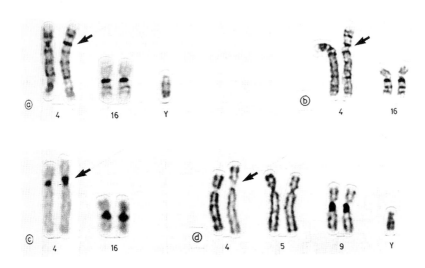

Plate 14. Euchromatic variants: (**a, b**) Rare variant in chromosome 4: inv(4)(p16.1p16.3). (**c, d**) Rare variant in chromosome 4: dup(4)(q35q35).

Contributors
(a,b) Center for Human Genetics, Boston University (c1).
(c,d) Steve Gerson, Dianon Systems, Inc (c18).

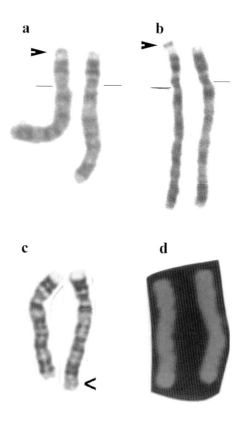

Chromosome 4: Summary

In the study of Q- and C-band heteromorphism in a subsample of 400 7- and 8-year olds from a collaborative study by Lubs *et al.* [1], Q-band heteromorphisms, consisting of level 4 and 5 intensities (> major 9q bands and distal Yq, respectively) were seen in about 20% of the Caucasian children and in 9% of the Black children. C-band variants of 4cen were seen in approximately 7:6% of children overall. In 100 normal American Blacks, Verma and Dosik [2] found bright QFQ variants (levels 3 and 4) in 7% of individuals. QFQ-band variants studied in 302 individuals [3] revealed two types of common heteromorphisms, one showing an intensely fluorescent band in 4cen and the other an intensely Q-bright band in the proximal 4p. A higher frequency of chromosome 4 Q-bright heteromorphism was reportedly found in patients with mental retardation, schizophrenia, hyperactivity, developmental delay and speech impediments. In a study of Q-band heteromorphisms for paternity testing [4], seven different variants were distinguishable in 57 subjects (**Plate 12f–l**).

In addition to the two common heteromorphisms described above, a rare variant involving an unusually large heterochromatic Q-, G- and C-band positive block of centromeric heterochromatin was described by Docherty and Bowser-Riley [5] (**Plate 13**). McKenzie and Lubs [6] also describe cases with a large C-positive region on 4 which may sometimes be missed if a Q-bright paracentromeric region and a striking non-fluorescent 4cen are present but C-banding is not done.

By molecular studies, two alpha satellites DNAs have been cloned and analyzed for chromosome 4 [7]. Under stringent hybridization conditions they hybridize only to the pericentromeric region of chromosome 4; under non-stringent conditions they hybridize to all chromosomes containing the suprachromosomal family 2 (chromosomes 2, 4, 8, 9, 13, 14, 15, 18, 20, 21 and 22). Southern blot yields a single 3.2 kb higher order MspI restriction fragment or a combination of a 2.6 kb and 0.6 kb MspI fragments. These two fragments together constitute about 60% of the length of the larger fragment.

Euchromatic variants

Two unusual cases involving euchromatic bands have come to our attention. Case 1 is an apparent paracentric inversion in 4p16 with breaks in 4p16.1 and 4p16.3 (**Plate 14a, b**). By FISH analysis a probe for Wolf-Hirschhorn syndrome is split by the inversion. The individual is phenotypically normal. The second case involves apparent additional material at 4q35 in a fetus and phenotypically normal father (**Plate 14c, d**) without other detectable chromosome abnormalities. It should be emphasized that such cases cannot be regarded as true variants, but may in fact represent subtle rearrangements that do presumably carry increased risks for pregnancy loss or liveborn offspring with anomalies due to recombinant products at meiosis that have a different genetic constitution than the carriers (see Chapter 6).

References

1. Lubs HA, Patil SR, Kimberling WJ *et al.* (1977). Q and C-banding polymorphisms in 7 and 8 year old children: racial differences and clinical significance: In: Hook EB, Porter IH, editors. Population Cytogenetic Studies in Humans. New York: Academic Press, pp. 133–59.

2. Verma RS, Dosik H (1981). Human chromosomal heteromorphisms in American Blacks. IV. Intensity variation in centromeric regions of chromosomes 3 and 4. Can J Cytol. 23:315–20.
3. Bardham S, Singh DN, Davis K (1981). Polymorphism in chromosome 4. Clin Genet. 20:44–7.
4. Olson SB, Magenis RE, Lovrien EW (1986). Human chromosome variation: the discriminatory power of Q-band heteromorphism (variant) analysis in distinguishing between individuals, with specific application to cases of questionable paternity. Am J Hum Genet. 38:235–52.
5. Docherty Z, Bowser-Riley SM (1984). A rare heterochromatic variant of chromosome 4. J Med Genet. 21:470–2.
6. McKenzie WH, Lubs HA (1975). Human Q and C chromosomal variations: Distribution and incidence. Cytogenet Cell Genet. 14:97–115.
7. Mashkova TD, Akopian TA, Romanova LY et al. (1994). Genomic organization, sequence and polymorphism of the human chromosome 4-specific alpha-satellite DNA. Gene. 140:211–17.

CHROMOSOME 5

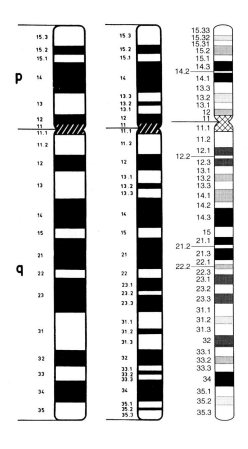

Plate 15. (**a**) Normal chromosomes 5 by G-banding. (**b–d**) Large 5cen by G-banding (arrow) compared with normal homolog (left) in each pair. (**e**) Chromosomes 5 from same patient by C-banding (arrow points to larger centromeric region).

Contributors
(a) Center for Human Genetics, Boston University (c1).
(b–e) Lauren Jenkins, Kaiser Permanente (c2).

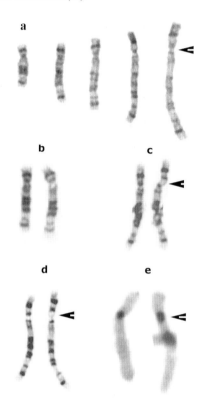

Plate 16. (a) Pairs of chromosomes 5 and 9 by G, C and G-11 banding. (b) Pedigree of family. [Figures 1 and 2 reproduced from Fineman RM, Issa B, Weinblatt V (1989). Prenatal diagnosis of a large heterochromatic region in a chromosome 5: implications for genetic counseling. Am J Med Genet. 32(4):498–9.]

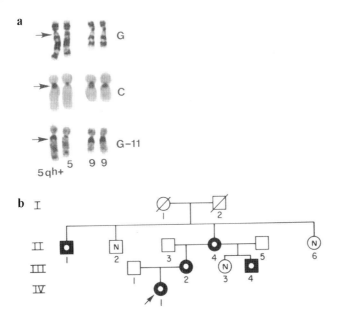

Plate 17. Euchromatic variant of chromosome 5 showing apparent deletion of 5p14 in child and mother. [Reprinted from Hand JL, Michels VV, Marinello MJ, Ketterling RP, Jalal SM (2000). Inherited interstitial deletion of chromosomes 5p and 16q without apparent phenotypic effect: further confirmation. Prenat Diagn. 20:144–8.]

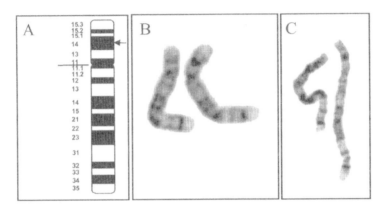

Chromosome 5: Summary

Two families with a rare variant of the centromeric region of chromosome 5 have been reported. The first by Fineman *et al.* [1] describes a C-band and G-11 band-positive large pericentromeric block of heterochromatin on chromosome 5 that was detected prenatally and subsequently found in several other family members, all of whom were phenotypically normal (**Plate 16**). A second case is described by Doneda *et al.* [2] in a three-generation family. Fluorescent in situ hybridization studies of the latter case showed the variant 5cen region to hybridize with satellite III sequences of chromosome 9. Beta-satellite sequences of chromosome 9 showed negative hybridization.

Euchromatic Variants

A euchromatic variant of chromosome 5 is reported by Hand *et al.* [3] (**Plate 17**) (see Chapter 6).

References

1. Fineman RM, Issa B, Weinblatt V (1989). Prenatal diagnosis of a large heterochromatic region in a chromosome 5: implications for genetic counseling. Am J Med Genet. 32:498–9.
2. Doneda L, Gandolfi P, Nocera G, Larizza L (1998). A rare chromosome 5 heterochromatic variant derived from insertion of 9qh satellite 3 sequences. Chromosome Res. 6:411–14.
3. Hand JL, Michels VV, Marinello MJ, Ketterling RP, Jalal SM (2000). Inherited interstitial deletion of chromosomes 5p and 16q without apparent phenotypic effect: further confirmation. Prenat Diagn. 20:144–8.

CHROMOSOME 6

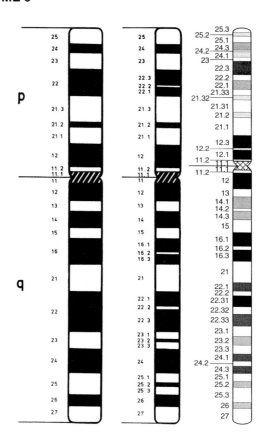

Plate 18. **(a–e)** Normal chromosomes 6 by G-banding. **(f, g)** Pairs of chromosome 6 showing large centromere (right chromosome of each pair). **(h)** Pair of chromosomes 6 by C-banding from same patient as **(g)** with large 6cen.

Contributors
(a–e) Center for Human Genetics, Boston University (c1).
(f–h) Lauren Jenkins, Kaiser Permanente (c2).

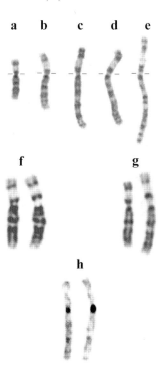

Plate 19. Pairs of chromosomes 6, from two different families (V2 and PB2) showing large 6cen (left chromosome of each pair) by C, G and Q-banding. Last row: hybridization shows amplification of the tritiated alpha-satellite sequence, ^{3}Hp308. [Reprinted from Jabs EW, Carpenter N (1988). Molecular cytogenetic evidence for amplification of chromosome-specific alphoid sequences at enlarged C-bands on chromosome 6. Am J Hum Genet. 43(1):69–74.]

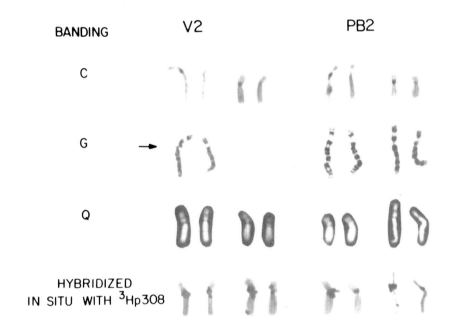

Chromosome 6: Summary

The frequency of heteromorphisms of the centromeric region of chromosome 6 was found by Lubs et al. [1] to be about 3% of their cohort of Black and White 7- and 8-year olds. About half had a small centromeric region and about half had a larger than average centromeric region (**Plate 18**). The frequency of the large 6cen was higher in the White children, although the numbers of cases were too small to be significant. Madan and Bruinsma [2] studied 92 consecutive individuals referred for cytogenetic testing and found 6p11 was enlarged in size in approximately 9% of their subjects. Polacek et al. [3] used C-band heteromorphism on chromosome 6 in seven families to establish linkage of the HLA region to chromosome 6.

Several investigators have isolated and characterized alpha satellite sequences in the centromeric region of chromosome 6 [4,5]. Jabs and Carpenter [6] characterized 6ph+ C-band region of chromosome 6 in two families which was 2–3 times the size of the region in the homolog. The region was not lengthened by 5-azacytidine. Alphoid repeat, D6Z1 (p308) localized to the 6ph+ region by in situ hybridization, was amplified 2–3-fold in the 6cen+ chromosome by tritium labeling (**Plate 19**) as well as by dot blot hybridization. Restriction enzyme studies showed no evidence of other amplified DNA sequences in this region. Lin et al. observed [7] a similar 6q11+ variant prenatally in a fetus and in the mother. The variant was G-negative, Q-negative and DA/DAPI-negative, but C-band-positive, and was approximately 3 times larger than the same region in the homolog. The region in neither chromosome decondensed when exposed to distamycin A or 5-azacytidine. It was late replicating and lateral asymmetry was observed after one cycle of 5-BrdU. The region hybridized with 6-specific alpha satellite D6Z1, indicating the variant was an amplification of the alpha repeat.

References

1. Lubs HA, Patil SR, Kimberling WJ et al. (1977). Q and C-banding polymorphisms in 7 and 8 year old children: Racial differences and clinical significance: In: Hook EB, Porter IH, editors. Population Cytogenetic Studies in Humans. New York: Academic Press, pp. 133–59.
2. Madan K, Bruinsman AH (1979). C-band polymorphism in human chromosome no. 6. Clin Genet. 15:193–7.
3. Polacek LA, Phillips RB, Hackbarth SA, Duquesnoy RJ (1983). A linkage study of the HLA region using C-band heteromorphisms. Clin Genet. 23:177–85.
4. Jabs EW, Wolf SF, Migeon BR (1984). Characterization of a cloned DNA sequence that is present at the centromeres of all human autosomes and the X chromosome and shows polymorphic variation. Proc Natl Acad Sci (USA). 81:4884–8.
5. Gar'kavtsev IV, Tsvetkova TG, Maksimova EV, Gonsales-Patine ME (1989). [Isolation and molecular cytogenetic characteristics of the alpha-satellite DNA of human chromosome 6] [Russian]. Biull Eksp Biol Med. 107:735–7.
6. Jabs EW, Carpenter N (1988). Molecular cytogenetic evidence for amplification of chromosome-specific alphoid sequences at enlarged C-bands on chromosome 6. Am J Hum Genet. 43:69–74.
7. Lin MS, Zhang A, Fujimoto A, Wilson MG (1994). A rare 6q11+ heteromorphism: cytogenetic analysis and in situ hybridization. Hum Hered. 44:31–6.

CHROMOSOME 7

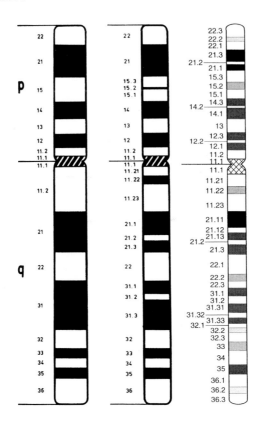

Plate 20. **(a)** Normal chromosomes 7 by G-banding. **(b)** Heteromorphism in a mother and in her son who is homozygous for 7cen+. Molecular studies indicated the son has uniparental disomy for the maternal chromosome 7. [Figure 3 reprinted from Voss R, Ben-Simon E, Avital *et al.* (1989). Isodisomy of choromosome 7 in a patient with cystic fibrosis: could uniparental disomy be common in human? Am J Hum Genet: 45(3):373–80.]

Contributors

(a) Center for Human Genetics, Boston University (c1)

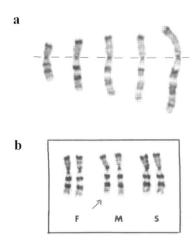

Chromosome 7: Summary

An enlarged centromeric region is reported in about 4% of individuals [1], generally of no known clinical significance. Of interest, however, is one case reported by Voss et al. [2] of uniparental disomy for a centromeric heteromorphism of chromosome 7cen+ that is maternal in origin. The cen+ was homozygous in a 4-year-old son with cystic fibrosis (CF) and very short stature. DNA polymorphisms of 11 paternal polymorphic loci spanning chromosome 7 were all negative in the child. Non-paternity was ruled out with a probability of 3.7×10^{-9}. The results indicated maternal uniparental disomy for the entire chromosome 7 (**Plate 20**). Uniparental disomy theoretically occurs in the population with a frequency of 1/30,000 [3,4]. However, the frequency in CF may be approximately 1/1000. Two cases of uniparental disomy in CF were maternal, suggesting a mechanism of nullisomic sperm and maternal isodisomic rescue [2].

The alpha satellite DNA on chromosome 7 reportedly consists of two distinct alphoid domains, arranged in higher order monomers [5,6]; on the short arm side, D7Z2 and long arm side, D7Z1. D7Z1 appears to be important for centromeric function. In a screen for centromeric sequences, four clones were observed that contained alpha satellite as well as L1 repeat units, an Alu element and a novel A-T rich repeated sequence [7,8].

References

1. Lubs HA, Patil SR, Kimberling WJ et al. (1977). Q and C-banding polymorphisms in 7 and 8 year old children: Racial differences and clinical significance. In Hook EB, Porter IH, editors. Population Cytogenetic Studies in Humans. New York: Academic Press, pp. 133–59.
2. Voss R, Ben-Simon E, Avital A et al. (1989). Isodisomy of chromosome 7 in a patient with cystic fibrosis: could uniparental disomy be common in humans? Am J Hum Genet. 45:373–80.
3. Warburton D (1988). Editorial: Uniparental disomy; a rare consequence of the high rate of aneuploidy in human gametes. Am J Hum Genet. 45:215–16.
4. Spence JE, Periaccante RG, Greig GM et al. (1988). Uniparental disomy as a mechanism for human genetic disease. Am J Hum Genet. 42:217–26.
5. Waye JS, England SB, Willard HF (1987). Genomic organization of alpha satellite DNA on human chromosome 7: evidence for two distinct alphoid domains on a single chromosome. Mol Cell Biol. 7:349–56.
6. Fetni R, Richer CL, Malfoy B, Dutrillaux B, Lemieux N (1997). Cytological characterization of two distinct alpha satellite DNA domains on human chromosome 7, using double-labeling hybridizations in fluorescence and electron microscopy on a melanoma cell line. Cancer Genet Cytogenet. 96:17–22.
7. Wevrick R, Willard HF (1991). Physical map of the centromeric region of human chromosome 7: relationship between two distinct alpha satellite arrays. Nucleic Acids. 19:2295–301.
8. Wevrick R, Willard VP, Willard HF (1992). Structure of DNA near long tandem arrays of alpha satellite DNA at the centromere of human chromosome 7. Genomics. 14:912–23.

CHROMOSOME 8

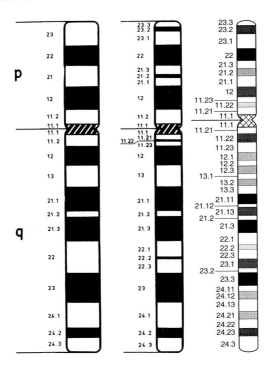

171

Plate 21. **(a)** Normal chromosomes 8 by G-banding. **(b)** Normal chromosomes 8 by C-banding (enlarged C-band in left-hand chromosome of each pair) [Modified from Figure 6 from McKenzie WH, Lubs HA (1975). Human Q and C chromosomal variations: distribution and incidence. Cytogenet Cell Genet. 14: 97–115]. **(c)** Normal chromosome 8 and ideogram (left), and chromosome 8 and ideogram (right) with duplication of 8p23.2 (arrowhead) and parts of bands 8p23.1 and 8p23.3. FISH studies confirm the extra band to be from chromosome 8 (see Summary).

Contributors
(a) Center for Human Genetics (c1).
(c) JJM Engelen, Universiteit Maastricht, The Netherlands (c40).

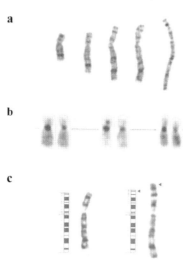

Chromosome 8: Summary

Only one case had a large chromosome 8 centromere among 192 White and Black 7- and 8-year olds studied by Lubs *et al.* [1] Earlier studies by McKenzie and Lubs [2], however, also revealed one case among 77 with a C-band-positive 8cen+, which they reported was not detected by Q-banding alone (**Plate 21b**).

Euchromatic variants

Euchromatic variants involving the distal band of 8p, transmitted from parents to children, have been reported in more than a dozen cases [3–5]. By molecular and cytogenetic studies and review of 12 families, Barber *et al.* [6] conclude these duplications do not have clinical significance. O'Malley and Storto [5] report an apparent duplication in 8p23.1 in a fetus and the phenotypically normal father. Chromosome painting showed no evidence of a translocation with any other chromosome. A previous normal pregnancy by the same couple did not have the paternal variant 8, suggesting there was not a translocation between the father's two homologs, which, if the case, might have resulted in the first child having a deleted 8. An unusual euchromatic variant of 8p is also reported by Engelen *et al.* [7], in which the most distal band of 8p at the 850 band resolution level is duplicated (**Plate 21c**) in a 34-year-old male with oligoasthenozoospermia and in his 57-year-old mother and 27-year-old brother, both of whom are phenotypically normal. There is no history of miscarriages. FISH confirmed duplication of probes specific to bands 8p23.3 and 8p23.2, distal to the telomeric region, but not in the telomeric region itself.

Reported deletions in 8q24 have variable phenotypes ranging from lethal to normal [8,9]. Deletions in the region 8q24.11–8q24.13 have been associated with Langer-Giedion (LGS) or trichorhinophalangeal syndromes [9,10]. Batanian *et al.* [8] also report an interstitial deletion of chromosome 8q24.13–8q24.22 in a phenotypically normal mother and in her stillborn fetus that showed no abnormalities by prenatal ultrasound. There was a family history of pregnancy losses by the maternal grandmother and by two maternal aunts, both of whom also had normal children. FISH showed no evidence of rearrangement with another chromosome, but revealed deletion of c-myc with a commercial probe from Vysis (Downers Grove, IL). There was no history of hematological disorder in the family. Two *de-novo* cases of interstitial deletions in distal 8q24.1 reportedly had mild anomalies, but not LGS [11]. One case with LGS features, but normal intelligence, had an interstitial deletion of 8q24.11–8q24.12 [9].

References

1. Lubs HA, Patil SR, Kimberling WJ *et al.* (1977). Q and C-banding polymorphisms in 7 and 8 year old children: Racial differences and clinical significance. In: Hook EB, Porter IH, editors. Population Cytogenetic Studies in Humans. New York: Academic Press, pp. 133–59.
2. McKenzie WH, Lubs HA (1975). Human Q and C chromosomal variations: distribution and incidence. Cytogenet Cell Genet. 14:97–115.
3. Williams L, Larkins S, Roberts E, Davidson EV (1996). Two further cases of variation in band 8p23.1. Not always a benign variant? J Med Genet. 33:A3.020.
4. Joyce C, Collinson M, Barber J (1996). Validation of a subtelomeric probe and its amplification in cytogenetic duplications of 8p with no detectable phenotypic effect. J Med Genet. 33:A3.014.

5. O'Malley DP, Sorto PD (1999). Confirmation of the chromosome 8p23.1 euchromatic duplication as a variant with no clinical manifestations. Prenat Diagn. 19:183–4.
6. Barber JCK, Joyce CA, Collinson MN *et al.* (1998). Duplication of 8p32.1: a cytogenetic anomaly with no established clinical significance. J Med Genet. 35:491–6.
7. Engelen JJM, Moog U, Evers JLH, Dassen H, Albrechts JCM, Hamers AJH (2000). Duplication of chromosome region 8p23.1→p23.3. Am J Med Genet. 91:18–21.
8. Batanian JR, Morris K, Ma E, Huang Y, McComb J (2001). Familial deletion of (8)(q24.1q24.22) associated with a normal phenotype. Clin Genet. 60:371–3.
9. Ludecke H, Johnson C, Wagner M *et al.* (1991). Molecular definition of the shortest region of deletion overlap in the Langer-Giedion syndrome. Am J Hum Genet. 49:1197–206.
10. Bowen P, Biederman B, Hoo JJ (1985). The critical segment of the Langer–Giedion syndrome: 8q24.11–q24.12. Ann Genet (Paris). 4:224–7.
11. Fennel SJ, Benson JW, Kindley AD, Schwarz MJ, Czepulkowski B (1989). Partial deletion 8q without Langer-Giedion syndrome: a recognizable syndrome. J Med Genet. 26(3):167–71.

CHROMOSOME 9

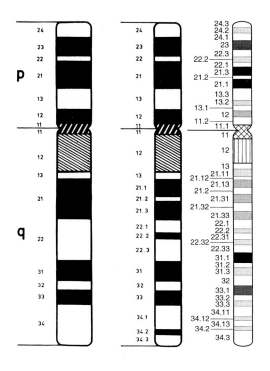

Plate 22. (**a–f**) Chromosomes 9 showing variations in length by G-banding of the heterochromatic secondary constriction (9qh region). (**g–i**) Pairs of chromosomes 9 from the same subject at three different resolutions of G-banding. Note difference in size between the homologs in all three pairs. (**j–l**) Pairs of chromosomes 9 from the same subject showing a G-positive band in the right-hand homolog (**j**) and two blocks of heterochromatin by C-banding (**k**) and by DA/DAPI staining (**l**). (**m, n**) Pairs of 9's from normal male showing large 9qh region by G-banding (**m**) and C-banding (**n**).

Contributors
(a–e) Center for Human Genetics, Boston University (c1).
(f) Jacqueline Schouman, Haukeland University Hospital (c25).
(g–l) Lauren Jenkins, Kaiser Permanente (c2).
(m,n) Jim Malone, Akron Childrens Hospital (c39).

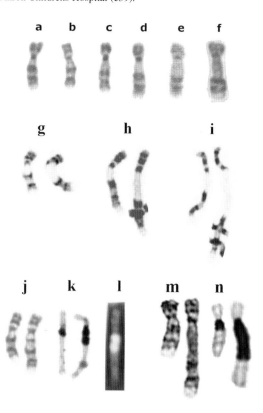

Plate 23. (**a–m**) Pairs of chromosomes 9 (except for c and d) showing various pericentric inversions in one of the homologs. An example of a partial inversion is shown (**b**, left). All remaining pairs appear to be complete inversions. (**i–k**) G-, Q- and C-banding of pairs of homologs from the same subject. (**l, m**) Q- and C- banding of chromosomes 9 from a different subject. Inversions are on the left in each pair of homologs.

Contributors
(a) Center for Human Genetics, Boston University (c1).
(b) Sharon Wenger, West Virginia University (c41).
(c) Jacqueline Schoumans, Haukeland University Hospital (c22).
(d,e) Center for Human Genetics, Boston University (c1).
(f–m) Lauren Jenkins, Kaiser Permanente (c2).

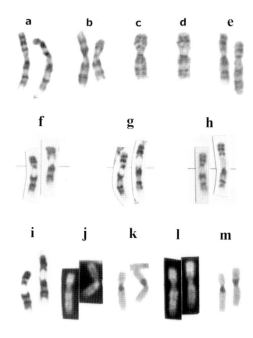

Plate 24.   Three different types of pericentric inversions involving shuffling of satellite DNAs within the 9qh region. [Figure 1, reprinted from Ramesh KH, Verma RS (1996). Breakpoint in alpha, beta and satellite III DNA sequences of chromosome 9 result in a variety of pericentric inversion. J Med Genet. 33(5):395–8.]. Characterization of pericentric inversion by FISH. **A:** Arrows indicate the two alphoid (top), one β (middle), and one satellite III (bottom) hybridization signal(s); inversion type A (five cases). **B:** Arrows indicate one alphoid (top), two β (middle), and one satellite III (bottom) hybridization signal(s); inversion type B (two cases). **C:** Arrows indicate two alphoid (top), two β (middle), and two satellite III (bottom) hybridization signal(s); inversion type C (one case). The normal non-rearranged chromosome 9 is shown on the left for the chromosomes hybridized with β and satellite III DNA probes.

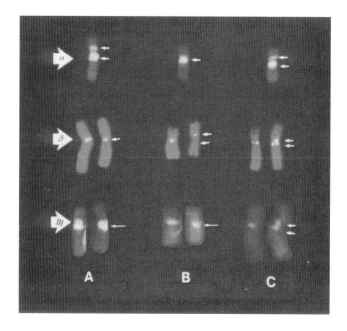

Plate 25. Mechanisms of formation of three different types of pericentric inversions involving different satellite DNAs within the 9qh region [Figure 3 reprinted from Ramesh KH, Verma RS (1996). Breakpoint in alpha, beta and satellite III DNA sequences of chromosome 9 result in a variety of pericentric inversion. J Med Genet. 33(5):395–8]. Schematic representation of the three different types of pericentric inversions involving the qh region of chromosome 9. **A:** Inversion type A showing the two separated alphoid regions, the normal chromosome 9 on the left shows the position of α, β, and satellite III DNA regions, with long arrows (on the left) indicating the breakpoints. **B:** Inversion type B showing two separated β satellite DNA regions; on the left is the normal chromosome 9 with long arrows indicating the breakpoints. **C:** Inversion type C showing two alphoid, β, and satellite III DNA regions; breakpoints involved in the first and second inversions are shown by the long arrows.

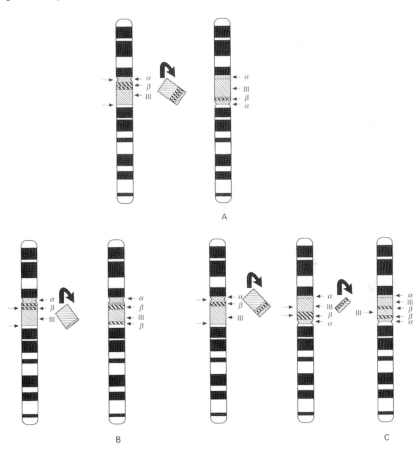

Plate 26. (**a–e**) Pairs of chromosomes 9 showing extra euchromatic (G-positive) band (**a, d**) that is C-band negative (Arrowhead, b and e) and Q-band positive (Arrowhead, **c**). The extra band was found segregating as a normal variant in this family. A similar extra band was segregating in a second family. (**f**) Duplication of 9q13->9q21 in a phenotypically normal mother and a fetus with fetal hydrops [Reported by Jalal SM, Kukolich MK, Garcia M, Day DW (1990). Euchromatic 9q+ hetromorphism in a family. Am J Hum Genet. 37(1):155–6.]

Contributor
(a–e) Birgitte Roland, University of Calgary (c30).

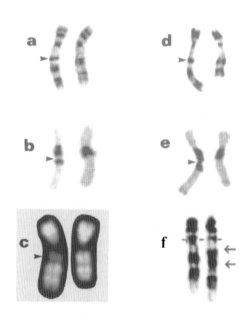

Plate 27. Extra euchromatic band in chromosome 9 in a 16.5-year-old female with mental retardation and multiple congenital abnormalities. Mother's chromosomes were normal; father was unavailable for study. [(**a, b**). Figures 1 and 3, reprinted from Luke S, Verma RS, PeBenito R, Macera MJ (1991). Inversion-duplication of bands q13–q21 of human chromosome 9. Am J Med Genet. 40(1):57–60.]

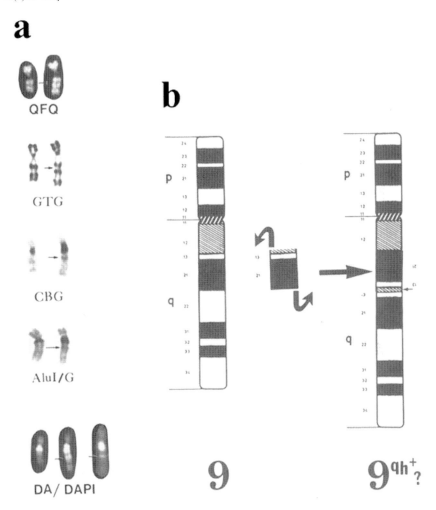

Plate 28. Inversion in chromosome 9 (**A**) and extra euchromatic band (**B**) in two patients studied by multiple staining techniques (**a**) and by FISH (**b**). [Figures 1 and 2 reprinted from Verma RS, Luke S, Brennan JP, Mathews T, Conte RA, Macera MJ (1993). Molecular topography of the secondary construction region (qh) of the human chromosome 9 with an unusual euchromatic band. Am J Genet. 52(5):981–6.]

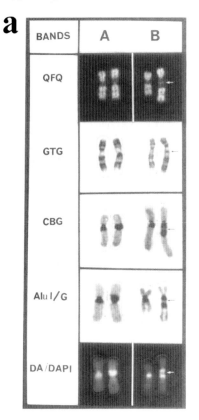

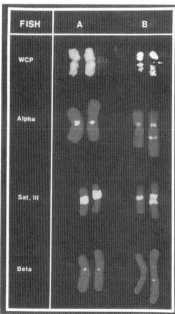

Plate 29. Extra euchromatic bands in the short arm of chromosome 9 (**a, b**). Partial pericentric inversions of C-band-positive material in two normal amniotic prenatal cases. Right-hand pair of chromosome in (**a**) is C-banded. (**c**) Pair of 9's representing a familial extra euchromatic band in the short arm of a mildly retarded 9-year-old girl and her father who also had learning disability and poor school performance. Mild dysmophic features were also present in both. [Reprinted from Haddad BR, Lin AE, Wyandt H, Milunsky A (1996). Molecular cytogenetic characterization of the first familial case of partial 9p duplication (p22p24). J Med Genet. 33(12):1045–7.]

Contributor
(a,b) Center for Human Genetics, Boston University (c1).

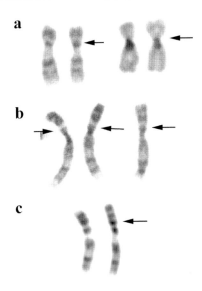

Chromosome 9: Summary

The lightly stained secondary constriction of chromosome 9 by plain Giemsa distinguishes it from other C-group chromosomes [1–3]. By G-banding (**Plate 22a–f**), the secondary constriction itself stains lightly, but bands on either side of the centromere typically stain as intensely as the pericentromeric regions of other chromosomes. By C-banding or DA/DAPI staining (**Plate 22k, l, n**), the entire region, including the pericentromeric bands, usually consists of a uniform block of dark staining heterochromatin but, when larger, is often separable into two or more blocks of heterochromatin separated by one or more G-positive (**Plate 22f, j**), C-negative bands (**Plate 22k**). The 9qh region is also the region most strikingly stained by Giemsa-11 (G-11) staining [4–6].

While variations in the length of the 9qh region have been frequently noted, it is not always clear whether or not such variations are innocuous [7–9]. Palmer and Schroder [10] and Fitzgerald [11] studied segregation of variant 9's in families with abnormal probands and concluded that the 9's with elongated qh regions probably represented duplications of the heterochromatin and that they were normal variants. Early banding studies of 9qh by Lubs *et al.* [12,13] of 7- and 8-year-olds, reported a frequency of 20–25% with variants of chromosome 9. As with other heterochromatic regions, in these studies the frequency of elongated 9qh (9qh+) was higher in Black children with mental retardation (17%). However, the frequency of 9qh+ in intellectually normal White children (9%) was higher than in White children with mental retardation (2%).

9qh inversions

A frequent variant of the 9qh region, besides length, is the apparent presence of a partial or complete inversion (**Plates 23–25, 27 and 28a**). The reported frequency range is 1–2.8% [15,16]. The frequency of partial 9qh inversions is 0.45–0.55% and of complete 9qh inversions, 0.13–1.07%. The latter are higher in the African-American than in the Caucasian population. Hansmann [14] studied the variability of 9qh inversions and classified them into three structural types: Type I showing total heterochromatin in the short arm, Type II showing part of the heterochromatin in the short arm, and Type III showing most of the heterochromatin in the long arm. At least one group of investigators [17] questioned whether partial inversions actually exist. Homozygous carriers of inversion 9 have been reported in at least four cases without apparent phenotypic effects [18–21].

Adverse effects

Metaxotou *et al.* [22] studied polymorphism of chromosome 9 in 600 Greek subjects, including individuals with sex problems, congenital abnormalities and mental retardation, couples with multiple abortions and stillbirths, parents of children with Down syndrome or other malformations and relatives of affected individuals. Four percent of individuals carried a partial inversion of chromosome 9, 4% had a complete inversion and 7.5% had an elongated 9qh region. Howard-Peebles and Stoddard [23] reviewed literature on inversions of the 9qh region. They outlined five possible effects of 9qh inversion: (1) no effect; (2) reduced fertility or reproductive failure [18,19,25]; (3) duplication/deletion in meiosis [16];

184

(4) chromosome interactions [24]; (5) disturbances of RNA synthesis during meiosis [19]. Of the five, most data support the first possibility. Of cases with reduced fertility [25], most were reported to be males [19]. However, studies of testicular morphology and of diakinesis in meiosis in two male carriers [18] showed no abnormalities. More recently Teo *et al.* [26] retrospectively studied the significance of inv(9qh) in 2448 antenatal patients and 1058 peripheral blood karyotypes collected over 3 years. Thirty cases of inv(9qh) from 29 families were found in the antenatal group and six cases were found in the peripheral blood group. Parents of the antenatal group contributed equally and inv(9qh) was not preferentially found in either fetal sex. None of the babies born with inv(9) was phenotypically abnormal. Of the six cases studied from peripheral blood, one had tri(21) and one had del(13q). Four adult patients had obstetrical and fertility problems. Subfertility appeared to be high among patients with inv(9) (36%) but was interpreted to represent a bias of older subfertile women seeking antenatal diagnosis. Occurrence of duplication/deletion, although possible for inversion carriers, was low.

A variety of case reports with chromosome abnormalities in addition to inversion 9 suggest some possible interchromosomal or meiotic effects [27–30]; however, the high frequency of 9qh inversions in the population does not preclude the possibility that such occurrences are coincidental. Luke *et al.* [31] describe an inv dup(9)(q13q21) associated with psychomotor retardation, microcephaly, narrow palpebral fissures, renal and genital abnormalities, vertebral anomalies, protruding tongue, and learning and behavioral abnormalities. Inversions in which at least one breakpoint has occurred in euchromatin have also been reported [32].

Structure of repeated sequences in 9qh

The structural organization of heterochromatin within the 9qh region has been studied by numerous investigators. Satellite DNAs were early localized to the centromeric and secondary constriction regions in human chromosomes [33–37]. Jones *et al.* [38–40] and others [41] isolated various subfractions of satellite DNA based on buoyant densities in a cesium chloride gradient and ultracentrifugation in cesium chloride or cesium sulfate in the presence of Ag+ or Hg+ ions. Satellite I [40,41] hybridized mainly to distal Yq with minor concentrations in centromeres of other chromosomes, including chromosome 9 [41]. Satellite II [41] hybridized mainly to chromosomes 1 and in low amounts to chromosome 16, but not to chromosome 9; satellite III [39] hybridized mainly to chromosomes 9 with smaller amounts to the D- and G-group chromosomes; satellite IV hybridized to chromosomes 9 and the Y [35,41] with smaller amounts on the D- and G-group chromosomes. These fractions of satellite DNA originally isolated by buoyant density in $CsSO_4$ have since come to be referred to as "classical satellite" DNA. Additional satellite fractions were isolated by Manuelidis [42,43] using Hoechst 33258 and EcoR1 restriction enzyme fractionation. The EcoR1 fraction, referred to as alpha (α) satellite DNA, hybridizes to the centromeric regions of every chromosome [44]. An additional fraction of satellite DNA, referred to as beta (β) satellite, hybridizes mainly to the centromere and short arm regions of the acrocentric chromosomes [45], but a specific fraction also hybridizes to the centromeric region of chromosome 9 (see Chapters 8 and 9).

The molecular characterization of the 9qh region represents a challenging example of attempts to understand the organization and significance of heterochromatic regions. Because of the variability in size and frequency of structural rearrangements involving the 9qh region and the location of various satellite DNA fractions within it, there has been much interest in its molecular dissection. Molecular characterization of inv(9qh) in normal individuals was studied by combined application of in situ hybridization, and classical staining and restriction enzyme techniques [46–9]. Luke *et al.* [46] studied five individuals using: (1) a 171 bp α-satellite sequence that hybridized to all human centromeres, (2) a classical (satellite III) probe [D9Z1, pentameric repeat (5′ATTCC 3′)] specific to chromosome 9qh, and (3) a β-satellite probe (D9Z5, 68 bp tandem repeat) specific to the centromeric region of chromosome 9. Four individuals had inverted alphoid sequences while one had a single intact alphoid site. Ramesh and Verma [48] studied breakpoints in α-, β- and satellite III sequences of inv(9qh) in eight individuals (**Plate 24**). Three similar-appearing inversions by CBG banding were classified by hybridization pattern: Type A (the most frequent) with two α-, one β- and one sat III; Type B with two β-, one α- and one sat III; Type C, more complex, appeared to involve two inversions. Samonte *et al.* [49] describe eight more 9qh inversions with four additional types of patterns with α-, β- and sat III probes: Type A: breaks within the α- and β-satellite sequences; Type B: breaks within the β-region; Type C: breaks within the β- and sat III regions and; Type D: breaks within the α- and sat III. Some of the latter cases were not as evident as having pericentric inversions at the microscope level. The outcome of these studies is that considerable reshuffling occurs with the alpha, beta and satellite III repeated sequences of the 9qh region. One question raised from these studies is "Is there formation of any functional dicentric in these reshufflings?" More recent work suggests that alphoid sequences themselves are not the requirement for a functional centromere. Vance *et al.* [50], for example, have reported an apparently acentric stable chromosome derived from chromosome 9 without detectable alpha or beta satellite regions.

Extra euchromatic band in 9qh

Extra euchromatic bands as normal variants in human chromosomes and their mechanisms of origin have been covered as a special topic in Chapter 6. Euchromatic variants in chromosome 9 consist of G-positive bands that are C-band negative and apparently have no phenotypic effect. Such euchromatic bands have been described both in the long arm of chromosome 9 [46–54] (**Plates 26–28**), and in the short arm [55–7] (**Plate 29**). Two types of euchromatic variants of chromosome 9 were characterized by Wang and Miller [47]; one with a G-band in the short arm near the centromere and one with heterochromatin above and below the centromere and a G-positive band in the short arm immediately distal to the heterochromatin. Both types were speculated to possibly represent stable dicentrics. It was determined that some G-positive, C-negative bands were extra alpha satellite bands [47,49,54]. It was also speculated that some euchromatic bands inserted into 9qh heterochromatin that were satellite negative could represent gene sequences that were inactivated by position effect [46,48,49,54]. Still other extra G-positive bands are reported that were C-positive (**Plate 27**)

[46,56]. At least one reported G-positive band was C-negative, but Q-bright (**Plate 26**) [58] and was confirmed to be euchromatin by FISH [62].

Some cases with extra G-positive or Q-positive bands have had associated phenotypic abnormalities. Silengo *et al.* [59] reported a normal father and a 7-month-old child with multiple congenital anomalies, both with an extra Q-positive band in the 9qh region. Luke *et al.* [46] report a paracentric inversion and duplication (**Plate 27**) in a 16.5-year-old female who has mental retardation and behavioral problems. They regarded this case to be a structural abnormality. However, Docherty and Hulten [60], responding to this case, refer to a similar-appearing chromosome 9 that they had reported earlier [61] with a large euchromatic region inserted into the qh-region in a child with trisomy 21 and Down syndrome. The same chromosome was present in a phenotypically normal mother and brother of the patient. Finally (**Plate 29c**) shows an extra widely separated G-band-positive, satellite III-negative band in the short arm of a chromosome 9 in a father and his 9-year-old daughter, both with mild learning disabilities and dysmorphic features, including clinodactyly [57].

References

1. Patau K, Smith DW, Therman E, Inhorn SL (1960). Multiple congenital anomalies caused by an extra chromosome. Lancet. 1:790–3.
2. Ferguson-Smith MA, Ferguson-Smith ME, Ellis OM, Dickson M (1962). The site and relative frequencies of secondary constrictions in human somatic chromosomes. Cytogenetics. 1:325–43.
3. Palmer CG, Funderburk S (1965). Secondary constrictions in human chromosomes. Cytogenetics. 4:261–76.
4. Bobrow M, Madan K, Pearson PL (1972). Staining of specific regions of human chromosomes, particularly the secondary constriction of No. 9. Nature New Biol. 238:122–4.
5. Gagne R, Laberge C (1972). Specific cytological recognition of the heterochromatic segment of chromosome number 9 in man. Exp Cell Res. 73:239–42.
6. Wyandt HE, Wysham DG, Minden SK, Anderson RS, Hecht F (1976). Mechanisms of Giemsa banding of chromosomes. Exp Cell Res. 102:85–94.
7. Hakansson L (1966). A case of Werdnig-Hoffman muscular dystrophy with an unusual chromosome complement. Hereditas Genetiskt Archiv. 55:358–61.
8. Moores EC, Anders JM, Emanuel R (1966). Inheritance of marker chromosomes from cytogenetic survey of congenital heart disease. Ann Hum Genet. 30:77–84.
9. Schmid W, Vischer D (1969). Spontaneous fragility of an abnormally wide secondary constriction region in a human chromosome No. 9. Humangenetik. 7:22–7.
10. Palmer CG, Schroder J (1971). A familial variant of chromosome 9. J Med Genet. 8:202–8.
11. Fitzgerald PH (1973). The nature and inheritance of an elongated secondary constriction on chromosome 9 of man. Cytogenet Cell Genet. 12:404–13.
12. Lubs HA, Patil SR, Kimberling WJ *et al.* (1977). Q and C-banding polymorphisms in 7 and 8 year old children: racial differences and clinical significance: In: Hook EB, Porter JH, editors. Population Cytogenetic Studies in Humans. New York: Academic Press, pp. 133–59.
13. Lubs HA, Kimberling WJ, Hecht F *et al.* (1977). Racial differences in the frequency of Q and C chromosomal heteromorphisms. Nature. 268:631–3.
14. Hansmann I (1976). Structural variability of human chromosome 9 in relation to its evolution. Hum Genet. 31:247–62.
15. Boue J, Taillemite JC, Hazael-Massieux P, Leonard C, Boue A (1975). Association of pericentric inversion of chromosome 9 and reproductive failure in ten unrelated families. Humangenetik. 30:217–24.
16. Madan K, Bobrow M (1974). Structural variation in chromosome no. 9. Ann Genet. 17:81–6.
17. Mattei MG, Mattei JF, Guichaoua M, Giraud F (1981). Partial inversion of the secondary constriction of chromosome 9. Does it exist? Hum Genet. 59:310–16.
18. Vine DT, Yarkoni S, Cohen MM (1976). Inversion homozygosity of chromosome no. 9 in a highly inbred kindred. Am J Hum Genet. 28:203–7.

19. Wahrman J, Atidia J, Goitein R, Cohen T (1972). Pericentric inversions of chromosome 9 in two families. Cytogenetics. 11:132–44.
20. De la Chapelle A, Schroder J, Stenstrand K et al. (1974). Pericentric inversions of human chromosomes 9 and 10. Am J Hum Genet. 26:746–66.
21. Zabel B, Hansen S, Hillig U, Groting-Imhof H (1977). A girl with partial long-arm deletion of chromosome 11 and familial pericentric inversion of chromosome 9. Hum Genet. 36:117–22.
22. Metaxotou C, Kalpini-Mavrou A, Panagou M, Tsengi C (1978). Polymorphism of chromosome 9 in 600 Greek subjects. Am J Hum Genet. 30:85–9.
23. Howard-Peebles PN, Stoddard GR (1976). A satellited Yq chromosome associated with trisomy 21 and an inversion of chromosome 9. Hum Genet. 34:223–5.
24. Lejeune J (1963). Autosomal disorders. Pediatrics. 32:326–37.
25. Kahn F, Verma RS, Dosik H, Warman J (1978). Primary amenorrhea in a black family with duplication and inversion of the secondary constriction regions of chromosome 9. J Clin Endocrinol Metab. 47:280–3.
26. Teo SH, Tan M, Knight L, Yeo SH, Ng I (1995). Pericentric inversion 9 – incidence and clinical significance. Ann Acad Med Singapore. 24:302–4.
27. Schinzel A, Hayashi K, Schmid W (1974). Mosaic trisomy and pericentric inversion of chromosome 9 in a malformed boy. Humangenetik. 25:171–7.
28. Bowen P, Ying KL, Chung GSH (1974). Trisomy 9 mosaicism in a newborn infant with multiple malformations. J Pediatr. 85:95–7.
29. Seabright M, Gregson M, Mould S (1976). Trisomy 9 associated with an enlarged 9qh segment in a liveborn. Hum Genet 34:323–5.
30. Sutherland GR, Gardiner AJ, Carter RF (1976). Familial pericentric inversion of chromosome 19, inv(19)(p13q13) with a note on genetic counseling of pericentric inversion carriers. Clin Genet. 10:54–9.
31. Luke S, Verma RS, PeBenito R, Macera MJ (1991). Inversion-duplication bands q13–q21 of human chromosome 9. Am J Med Genet. 40:57–60.
32. Hansmann I, Keutel J (1975). A subtelomeric chromosome 9 in a dysplastic 18-year-old boy with dissociated mental development. Humangenetik. 30:287–90.
33. Corneo G, Ginelli E, Polli EJ (1968). Isolation of complementary strands of a human satellite DNA. J Mol Biol. 33:331.
34. Corneo G, Ginelli E, Polli EJ (1970). Repeated sequences in human DNA. J mol Biol. 48:319.
35. Saunders GF, Hsu TC, Getz MJ, Simes EL, Arrighi FE (1972). Locations of human satellite DNA in human chromosomes. Nature New Biol. 236:244–6.
36. Ginelli E, Corneo G (1976). The organization of repeated DNA sequences in the human genome. Chromosoma. 56:55–68.
37. Miklos GLG, John B (1979). Heterochromatin and satellite DNA in man: Properties and prospects. Am J Hum Genet. 31:264–80.
38. Jones KW, Corneo G (1971). Location of satellite and homogenous DNA sequences on human chromosomes. Nature New Biol. 233:268–71.
39. Jones KW, Prosser J, Corneo G, Ginelli E (1973). The chromosomal localisation of human satellite DNA III. Chromosoma. 42:445–51.
40. Jones KW, Purdom IF, Prosser J, Corneo G (1974). The chromosomal localisation of human satellite DNA I. Chromosoma. 49:161–71.
41. Gosden JR, Mitchell AR, Buckland RA, Clayton RP, Evans HJ (1975). The location of four human satellite DNAs on human chromosomes. Exp Cell Res. 92:148–58.
42. Manuelidis L, Wu JC (1978). Homology between human and simian repeated DNA. Nature. 276:92–4.
43. Manuelidis L (1978). Complex and simple sequences in human repeated DNAs. Chromosoma. 66:1–22.
44. Willard HF (1985). Chromosome-specific organization of human alpha satellite DNA. Am J Hum Genet. 37:524–32.
45. Waye JS, Willard HF (1989). Human β satellite DNA: Genomic organization and sequence definition of a class of highly repetitive tandem DNA. Proc Natl Acad Sci USA. 86:6250–4.
46. Luke S, Verma RS, Conte RA, Mathews T (1992). Molecular characterization of the secondary constriction region (qh) of human chromosome 9 with pericentric inversion. J Cell Sci. 103:919–23.
47. Wang JC, Miller WA (1994). Molecular cytogenetic characterization of two types of chromosome 9 variants. Cytogenet Cell Genet. 67:190–2.

48. Ramesh KH, Verma RS (1996). Breakpoints in alpha, beta and satellite III DNA sequences of chromosome 9 result in a variety of pericentric inversions. J Med Genet. 33:395–8.
49. Samonte RV, Conte RA, Ramesh KH, Verma RS (1996). Molecular cytogenetic characterization of breakpoints involving pericentric inversions of human chromosome 9. Hum Genet. 98:576–80.
50. Vance GH, Curtis CA, Heerema NA, Schwartz S, Palmer CG (1997). An apparently acrocentric marker chromosome originating from 9p with a functional centromere without detectable alpha and beta satellite sequences. Am J Hum Genet. 71:436–42.
51. Jalal SM, Kukolich MK, Garcia M, Day DW (1990). Euchromatic 9q+ heteromorphism in a family. Am J Hum Genet. 37:155–6.
52. Knight LA, Soon GM, Tan M (1993). Extra G positive band on the long arm of chromosome 9. J Med Genet. 30:613.
53. Verma RS, Luke S, Brennan JP, Mathews T, Conte RA, Macera MJ (1993). Molecular topography of the secondary constriction region (qh) of the human chromosome 9 with an unusual euchromatic band. Am J Hum Genet. 52:981–6.
54. Macera MJ, Verma RS, Conte RA, Bialer MG, Klein VR (1995). Mechanisms of the origin of a G-positive band within the secondary constriction region of human chromosome 9. Cytogenet Cell Genet. 69:235–9.
55. Buckton KE, O'Riordan ML, Ratcliffe S et al. (1980). A G-band study of chromosomes in live-born infants. Ann Hum Genet. 43:227–39.
56. Sutherland GR, Eyre H (1981). Two unusual G-band variants of the short arm of chromosome 9. Clin Genet. 19:331–4.
57. Haddad BR, Lin AE, Wyandt H, Milunsky A (1996). Molecular cytogenetic characterization of the first familial case of partial 9p duplication (p22p24). J Med Genet. 33:1045–7.
58. Roland B, Chernos JE, Cox DM (1992). 9qh+ variant band in two families. Am J Med Genet. 42:137–8.
59. Silengo MC, Davi GF, Franeschini P (1982). Extra band in the 9qh+ chromosome in a normal father and in his child with multiple congenital anomalies. Hum Genet. 60:294.
60. Docherty Z, Hulten MA (1993). Rare variant of chromosome 9 (letter). Am J Med Genet. 45:105–6.
61. Docherty Z, Hulten MA (1985). Extra euchromatic band in the qh region of chromosome 9. J Med Genet. 22:156–7.
62. Hoo JJ, Szego K, Wong P, Roland B (1993). Evidence of chromosome 9 origin of the euchromatic variant band within 9qh. Clin Genet. 43: 309–11.

CHROMOSOME 10

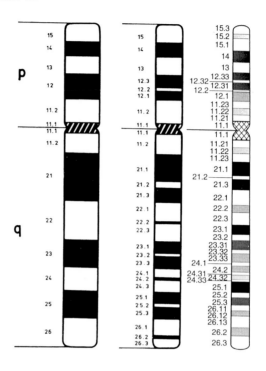

Plate 30. (a) Normal chromosomes 10 at increasing band resolution. (b) Pericentric inversion of chromosome 10 from prenatal sample. Inversion is maternal in origin. (c) Pair of chromosomes 10 from prenatal sample with pericentric inversion in chromosome at left. Parental studies were not done.

Contributors
(a) Center for Human Genetics, Boston University (c1).
(b) K. Yelavarthi and J. Nunich, Northwest Center for Medical Research (c13).
(c) Emilie Ongcapin, St. Barnabas Medical Center (c12).

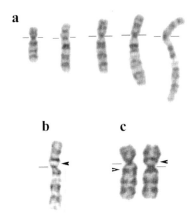

Chromosome 10: Summary

The only common variant that has been reported for chromosome 10 is a pericentric inversion, i.e. inv(10)(p11.2q21.2) (**Plate 30**). Collinson *et al.* [1] studied 33 families in which a pericentric inversion of chromosome 10 was segregating, and reviewed another 32 families in the literature. Twenty-one of their 33 families were ascertained through prenatal diagnosis. Twelve other families were ascertained for a wide variety of reasons as were data obtained from reported cases. They conclude from the compiled data that reasons for referral are unrelated to the chromosome abnormality. Of the 65 families there was no recorded instance of a recombinant 10 arising from inv(10). The rate of abortion from 94 pregnancies in their own cases was 7.4% (less than 15% for the general population). Stillbirth and neonatal death, corrected for ascertainment bias, was 1.3% (compared to 0.57% for the general population). Fertility also appeared not to be reduced in either male or female carriers. Overall, they conclude that inv(10) can be regarded as a variant analogous to the pericentric inversion in chromosome 2 and that investigation of carrier status in families with the inversion is unwarranted since there are no known consequences.

Isolation of a specific alpha satellite for chromosome 10 [2], consisted of eight tandem repeats of a 171-bp monomer unit. A cloned 8mer representative probe detected a polymorphic restriction enzyme pattern. Jackson *et al.* [3] studied a cosmid containing the junction between alphoid and satellite III sequences mapping to chromosome 10. They showed the alphoid sequences to consist of tandemly arranged dimers that were distinct from the known chromosome 10-specific alphoid family. PCR data confirmed the integrity of the sequence data. The results along with pulse field gel electrophoresis placed the boundary between alphoid and satellite III in the 10cen–10q11.2 interval. Sequence data showed the repetitive sequences to be separated by a partial L1 interspersed repeat sequence less than 500 bp in length.

References

1. Collinson MN, Fisher AM, Walker J, Currie J, Williams L, Roberts P (1997). Inv(10)(p11.2q21.2), a variant chromosome. Hum Genet. 101:175–80.
2. Devilee P, Kievits T, Waye JS, Pearson PL, Willard HF (1988). Chromosome-specific alpha satellite DNA: isolation and mapping of a polymorphic alphoid repeat from chromosome 10. Genomics. 3:1–7.
3. Jackson MS, Mole SE, Ponder BA (1992). Characterization of the boundary between satellite III and alphoid sequences on human chromosome 10. Nucleic Acids Res. 20:4781–7.

CHROMOSOME 11

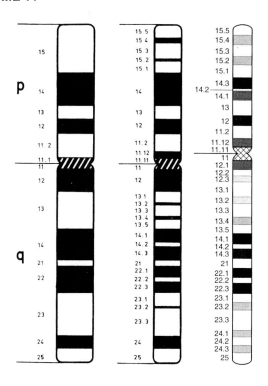

Plate 31. (**a**) Normal chromosomes 11 at increasing band resolution. (**b**) Chromosome 11 pairs showing prominent G-positive (GTG) and C-positive band in the short arm. Region is also R-positive (RBA) and Q-negative (QFQ). Arrows point to variant chromosome (right) in each pair. [Figure 1 modified from Aiello V, Ricci N, Palazzi P, D'Agostino G, Calzolari E (1994). New variant of chromosome 11. Am J Med Genet. 50:294–95.]

Contributors
(a) Center for Human Genetics. Boston University (c1).

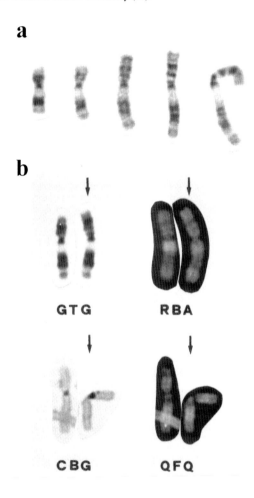

Plate 32. Chromosome 11 pairs from a prenatal chromosome study. (**a**) Two pairs showing large alpha satellite signal (arrows) with D11Z1 probe (green). Variant chromosome was paternal in origin. Red signals are for cyclin D1 at 11q13. (**b, c**) Two pairs of chromosome 11 from the same case by G-banding. Arrows point to a large heterochromatic region (right) in each pair. Heterochromatin is less condensed in the left-hand pair (**b**).

Contributor
(a–c) Patricia Miron, Brigham and Women's Hospital (c9).

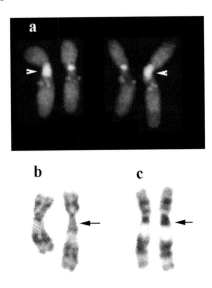

Chromosome 11: Summary

A rare variant involving the centromeric region of chromosome 11 has been observed in at least three cases. Till *et al.* [1] describe a new variant involving duplication of the centromere in a fetus and a 39-year-old mother. The fetus had no obvious anomalies when delivered. C- and G-banding suggest the variant chromosome is a pseudodicentric with inactivation of one centromere. Another case with an additional C-band positive, Q-band negative region in the centromeric region of chromosome 11 was observed in a man who was identified through fetal loss in his wife [2] (**Plate 31**). No additional details of family history are given. The authors report this as a familial variant whose clinical significance is unknown. Finally, a third case of a similarly large centromeric variant, ascertained prenatally, has come to our attention (contributed by Patricia Minor). The variant chromosome is paternal in origin. In this case fluorescent *in situ* hybridization with the alpha satellite centromeric probe, D11Z1, shows the extra material to be D11Z1-positive (**Plate 32**).

References

1. Till M, Rafat A, Charrin C, Planchu H, Germain D (1991). Duplication of chromosome 11 centromere in fetal and maternal karyotypes: a new variant? Prenat Diagn. 11:481–2.
2. Aiello V, Ricci N, Palazzi P, D'Agostino G, Calzolari E (1994). New variant of chromosome 11. Am J Med Genet. 50:294–5.

CHROMOSOME 12

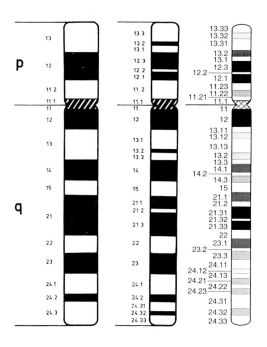

Plate 33. Normal chromosomes 12 at increasing levels of band resolution.

Contributor
Center for Human Genetics, Boston University (c1)

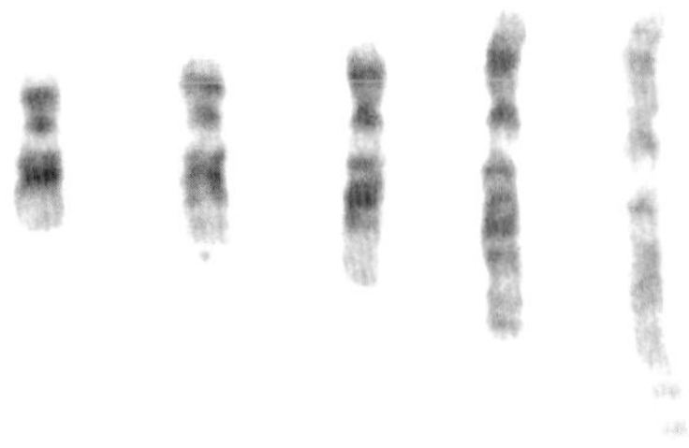

Chromosome 12: Summary

Mayer *et al.* [1] reported an enlarged centromere on a chromosome 12 in one patient with mental retardation that was also present in many normal relatives. The only similar heteromorphism was reported in three of 212 Japanese A-bomb survivors [2].

References

1. Mayer M, Matsuura J, Jacobs, P (1978). Inversions and other unusual heteromorphisms detected by C-banding. Hum Genet. 45:43–50.
2. Sofuni T, Tanabe K, Ohtaki K, Shimba H, Awa AA (1974). Two new types of C-band variants in human chromosome (6ph+ and 12ph+). Jpn J Hum Genet. 19:251–6.

CHROMOSOME 13

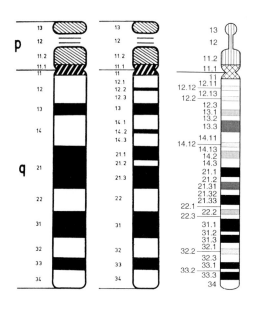

Plate 34. (**a**) Normal chromosomes 13 from seven different individuals showing increasing band resolution and variations in size and staining of short arms, stalks and satellites by G-banding (**Plate 35**). Note the range from an almost undetectable short arm and apparent lack of a satellite (extreme left) to a more prominent dark staining short arm and very prominent satellite (extreme right). (**b**) Pairs of homologs (different cells from same subject) showing almost no evidence of satellites by G-banding, but clearly showing the presence of satellites by Q-banding. (**c**) Pairs of homologs from a different subject showing similarly staining short arms by G-banding, but with a striking difference in size and intensity by Q-banding. (**d**) Chromosome 13 with prominent light and dark staining regions in the short arm, with the prominent dark band being intensely bright by Q-banding (note a less intensely fluorescent satellite is also evident by Q-banding). (**e**) G-banding variations in the size of stalk regions (regions separating short arm and satellite) in pairs of homologs from three different individuals. (**f**) Pair of 13's from a normal individual showing striking stalk region by G-banding (middle) with an unusual pattern of alternating light (constrictions) and darker bands and a terminal satellite. NOR (silver)-staining (left) reveals two prominent nucleolar organizing regions (NORs) more or less corresponding to the two constricted regions. (**g**) G-banding (left) showing a chromosome 13 with three tandem dark staining satellites. NOR-staining (middle and right) of the same chromosome from two different cells showing at least three NOR regions. In such tandemly repeated NOR regions the number of active NORs may vary in size and number in different cells.

Contributors
(a–e) Center for Human Genetics, Boston University (c1).
(f) Arturo Anguiano, Quest Diagnostics (c17).
(g) Lauren Jenkins, Kaiser Permanente (c2).

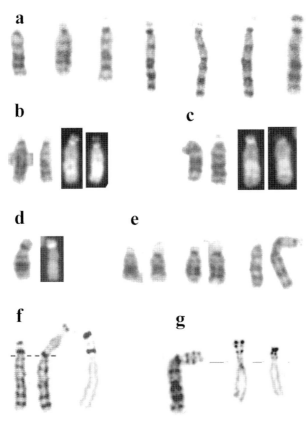

Plate 35. (**a**) Ideogram and photograph of chromosome 13 illustrating independently varying regions of acrocentric chromosomes. [Figure 1, reprinted with permission from Olson SB, Magenis RE, Lovrien EW (1986). Human chromosome variation: the discirminatory of Q-band heteromorphism (variant) analysis in distinguishing between individuals, with specific application to cases of questionable paternity. Am J Hum Genet. 38(2):235–52.] (**b**) Sequential banding of chromosome 13 homologs by G-, Q- and R-banding by acridine orange (AO)* followed by densitometry (graph at right) of the variable regions stained by AO. Note differences in intensity of Giemsa staining of Q-negative regions for the two homologs and additional variability in staining of both Q-positive and Q-negative regions by AO staining (HE Wyandt, unpublished).

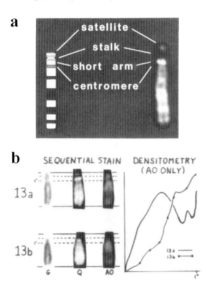

Acridine orange staining was performed following treatment of chromosomes with dilute alkali (0.07 M NaOH) to give RFA banding pattern [Wyandt et al, (1974). Humangenetik. 23:119–130].

Plate 36. Twenty-six variants of chromosome 13 from a population of 39 unrelated people. Each chromosome is serially printed to reveal heteromorphisms not visible at an exposure generally chosen to define the overall banding pattern. A1–A7 have satellites that would not have been observed at a routine exposure. Scores are determined by comparisons of serial prints against standards, including an internal standard. Very short, medium to intense short arms (scored 13, 14 and 15) as in C1 or D3 are relatively common on chromosomes 13, whereas bright short arms on chromosomes 14 and 15 are less frequent. [Figure 3, reprinted from Olson SB, Magenis RE, Lovrien EW (1986). Human chromosome variation: the discriminatory power of Q-band heteromorphism (variant) analysis in distinguishing between individuals, with specific application to cases of questionable paternity. Am J Hum Genet. 38(2):235–52.]

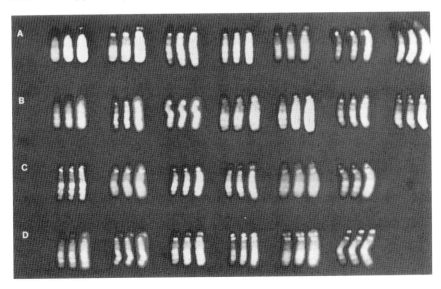

Chromosome 13: Summary

The most variable chromosomes in the human karyotype are the acrocentric chromosomes, 13, 14, 15, 21 and 22. Because of their similarities it seems reasonable to first summarize the features they hold in common, and then proceed to the features of each that appear to be characteristic. The features in common are: (1) they all carry nucleolar organizing regions (NORs) revealed by silver staining. (2) They all have four distinct regions that can be heteromorphic (**Plate 35a**) and/or may have different staining properties (**Plate 35b**). (3) All are involved in a particular type of translocation called a Robertsonian translocation in which there is typically loss of satellites, NORs and part or all of the short arms. It has long been known that the involvement of acrocentrics in Robertsonian translocations is non-random [1–3]. Chromosome 13 is the second most commonly involved acrocentric after chromosome 14. Translocation between chromosomes 13 and 14 is the most common Robertsonian rearrangement, followed by translocation between 14 and 21, followed by translocation between 13 and 21 [3]. Such non-random involvement appears to be correlated with the frequency that the acrocentrics share repeated sequences [4,5]. In situ hybridization studies have shown that the majority of Robertsonian translocations involving non-homologs are dicentric, whereas the majority involving homologs are monocentric [6,7]. Recent molecular studies reveal varying degrees of homology of repeated sequences, with breakpoints most frequently occurring in repeated sequences that are in common, typically in the short arm, less frequently in the NOR or satellite regions [8–11]. This, together with their common nucleolar organizing function, may bring these regions in proximity more often so that they are more frequently involved in this particular type of rearrangement.

There is also considerable shuffling of various repetitive DNA sequences comprising the centromeric, short-arm and satellites of these chromosomes. (See Chapters 8 and 9 for a detailed discussion of the dissection, evolution and possible function of satellite sequences in these regions that are the most highly heteromorphic in the human genome). Variations involve staining and/or size of the pericentromeric regions, short arms, and satellites as well as variation in the number and/or size of NORs. None of these variations appear to have any direct clinical consequences (**Plates 34–36**).

Occasionally, an acrocentric without any detectable satellite or NOR region and a very small or absent short arm is seen (**Plate 34a**). This may be a normal variant, without any direct clinical consequences, or may be symptomatic of a chromosome which is unstable [12].

Whether or not variations in size and composition correlate with any predisposition to nondisjunction or certain types of structural abnormalities such as deletion or formation of marker chromosomes have been topics of much speculation, with certain biases or inconsistencies making interpretation of the data difficult or inconclusive (see Chapter 4). Molecular dissection of these areas will eventually give more definitive answers.

Because of the high degree of heteromorphism, variants of the acrocentric chromosomes have been used in a variety of ways: (1) to determine parental and meiotic origin of chromosomal aneuploidy, (2) in the determination of origins of triploidy, (3) in ruling out maternal contamination and (4) as markers in determining paternity. Olson *et al.* (see Chapter 5), in particular, used Q-banding heteromorphisms of the most variable chromosome regions in determining paternity. Twenty-six different variants of chromosome 13 were discernible in a population of 39 unrelated people (**Plate 36**) [13]. Very short, intensely bright short arms were more frequent on chromosome 13 than on chromosomes 14 or 15. Such Q-band variants frequently correspond to intensely Giemsa-positive regions by G-banding, but the correlation is not definite. Dark G-bands also are not necessarily C-band positive or R-band negative (**Plates 34, 35b**). The correlation between G-, C- and Q-banding is shown in a few individual examples contributed for this volume (**Plate 34**). Although the cases presented here are presumably from normal individuals, they are not necessarily representative of what is normal. In all cases of striking or unusual heteromorphisms, multiple banding techniques and parental chromosome studies are recommended, even if the variant appears similar to one that has been seen before.

References

1. Hecht F, Case MP, Lovrien EW, Higgins JV, Thuiline HC, Melnyk J (1968). Non-randomness of translocations in man: preferential entry of chromosomes into 13-15-21 translocations. Science. 161:371–2.
2. Nagel M, Hoehn H (1971). On the non-random involvement of D-group chromosomes in centric fusion translocations in man. Humangenetik. 11:351–4.
3. Hecht F, Kimberling WJ (1972). Registry of data on Robertsonian (centric fusion) translocations. Lancet. 1:1342.
4. Jorgensen AL, Bostock CJ, Bak AL (1987). Homologous subfamilies of human alphoid repetitive DNA on different nucleolus organizing chromosomes. Proc Natl Acad Sci USA. 84:1075–9.
5. Choo KH, Vissel B, Brown R, Filby RG, Earle E (1988). Homologous alpha satellite sequences on human acrocentric chromosomes with selectivity for chromosome 13, 14 and 21: Implications for recombination between nonhomologs and Robertsonian translocations. Nucleic Acids Res. 16:1273–84.
6. Wolff DJ, Schwartz S (1992). Characterization of Robertsonian translocations by using fluorescence in situ hybridization. Am J Hum Genet. 50:174–81.
7. Gravholt CH, Friedrich U, Caprani M, Jorgensen AL (1992). Breakpoints in Robertsonian translocations are localized to satellite III DNA by fluorescence in situ hybridization. Genomics. 14:924–30.
8. Page SL, Shin JC, Han JY, Choo KH, Shaffer LG (1996). Breakpoint diversity illustrates distinct mechanisms for Robertsonian translocation mechanisms. Hum Mol Genet. 5:1279–88.
9. Sullivan BA, Jenkins LS, Karson FM, Leana-Cox J, Schwartz S (1996). Evidence for structural heterogeneity from molecular cytogentic analysis of dicentric Robertsonian translocations. Am J Hum Genet. 59:167–75.
10. Bandyopadhyay R, McQuillan C, Page SL, Choo KH, Shaffer LG (2001). Identification and characterization of satellite III subfamilies to the acrocentric chromosomes. Chromosome Res. 9:233–14.
11. Bandyopadhyay R, Berend SA, Page SL, Choo KH, Shaffer LT (2001). Satellite III sequences on 14p and their relevance to Robertsonian translocation formation. Chromosome Res. 9:235–42.
12. Lebo RV, Wyandt HE, Warburton P, Li S, Milunsky JM (2002). An unstable dicentric Robertsonian translocation in a markedly discordant twin. Clin Genet. 65:383–9.
13. Olson SB, Magenis RE, Lovrien EW (1986). Human chromosome variation: the discriminatory power of Q-band heteromorphism (variant) analysis in distinguishing between individuals, with specific application to cases of questionable paternity. Am J Hum Genet. 38:235–52.

CHROMOSOME 14

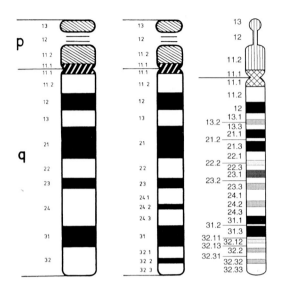

Plate 37. (**a**) Normal chromosomes 14 from six different subjects by G-banding showing increasing band resolution. (**b,c**) Pairs of homologs at standard band resolution from two different subjects. (**d**) Chromosome 14 with moderate-size satellite. (**e**) Chromosomes 14 from two different people showing large satellite (left) and lacking a visible short arm (right). (**f–h**) Pairs of chromosomes by G-banding (top) and Q-banding (bottom). (**h–j**) Pairs of chromosomes by G-banding (left) with chromosomes from same subjects stained for NOR regions by silver staining (right). A double NOR is shown in one of the chromosomes (**i**). A particularly striking variant of 14p by G-banding (**j**, middle) has a terminal constriction, corresponding to the large NOR by silver staining (**j**, right).

Contributors
(a–d, f–j) Center for Human Genetics, Boston University (c1).
(e) Jacqueline Schoumans, University Hospital Haukeland (c27, c28).

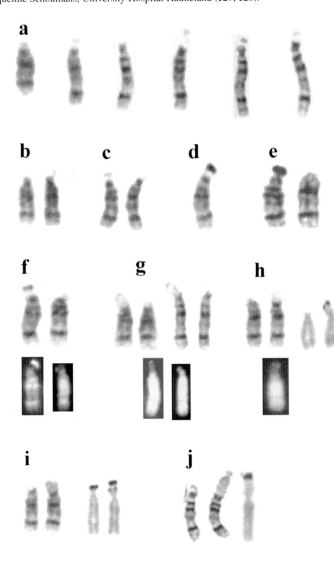

Plate 38. Sixteen different variants of chromosome 14 from a population of 39 unrelated people. Each chromosome is serially printed to reveal heteromorphisms not visible at an exposure generally chosen to define the overall banding pattern. [Figure 4, reprinted from Olson SB, Magenis RE, Lovrien EW (1986). Human chromosome variation: the discriminatory power of Q-band heteromorphism (variant) analysis in distinguishing between individuals, with specific application to cases of questionable paternity. Am J Hum Genet. 38(2):235–52.]

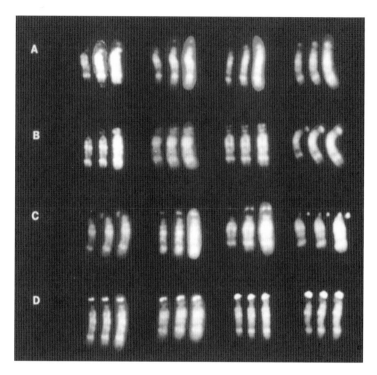

Plate 39. (a) Chromosome 14pss by different banding techniques (G, C, Q, R) and after treatment with 5-azacytidine (5-azacytidine, 5×10^{-6} M, last 7 h of culture). Silver staining at far right (Ag) shows two NOR regions. Unbanded (normal) 14pss (arrow, third from right) points to untreated chromosome. (**b**) The same unbanded 14pss chromosome from several mitoses treated with 5-azacytidine, stained with Giemsa. (**c**) Several chromosomes by RHG-banding. (**d**) Several chromosomes from same sample by silver staining showing variability in number, size and location of active NOR regions. See **Plate 40** and summary for more details.

Contributor
Petr Balicek, Division of Medical Genetics, University Hospital, Hradec Kralove (c16).

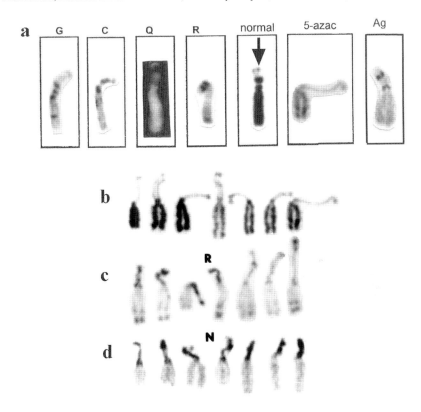

Plate 40. (a) Schematic representation of variability in the amount of GC-rich (RGH-positive) material. Any larger accumulation of such material tends to dissociate from the basal segment of short arms by a proximal secondary constriction. (b) Conventionally stained acrocentric chromosomes with different short arms derived from various individuals. The last chromosomes display double and triple satellites. (c) Chromosome with 14pss from several mitoses in prophase. The intercalar segment of double satellites can be dissociated by secondary constrictions (active NORs) in practically any site of the segment. See summary for more details.

Contributor
Petr Balicek, Division of Medical Genetics, University Hospital, Hradec Kralove (c16).

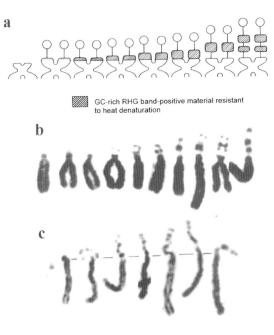

a

GC-rich RHG band-positive material resistant to heat denaturation

b

c

Chromosome 14: Summary

Chromosome 14 is the acrocentric most frequently involved in Robertsonian translocations. As with chromosome 13, variation in the number of satellites and NORs are observed (**Plate 37**). Q-band variants of the chromosome 14 include bright satellites, bright short arms, lack of satellites or NORs, and variable size short arms. A bright short arm region seems to be less frequent than for chromosome 13. In a study of 39 unrelated people, Olson *et al.* [1] found 14 different variants that were distinguishable by Q-banding (**Plate 38**).

Of particular interest with regard to NOR regions is a study of Balicek *et al.* [2,3] in which they found that multi-satellited, multi-NOR-positive chromosomes 14 showed correspondingly large blocks of R-banded (RGH-positive) material that were heat resistant (**Plates 39,40**). Intercallary NOR-positive regions corresponding to secondary constrictions were shown to punctuate these blocks anywhere along their length. From these observations they concluded that R-banded material represents genetically inactive blocks of rRNA genes. Treatment of lymphocytes with azacytidine in low doses (5×10^{-6} M) led to extreme undercondensation of RGH-positive regions.

FISH Variants of Chromosome 14

Fluorescent in situ hybridization has revealed at least one common variant on chromosome 14 that shows up when using the a chromosome 15-specific satellite sequence, D15Z1 (also referred to as satellite III). Cross-hybridization between chromosomes 14 and 15 occurs approximately 12% of the time (see Summary on chromosome 15). A case in which both chromosomes 14 homologs show a signal with D15Z1 has recently come to our attention. If the chance of both parents carrying the variant 14 is 1 per 100 couples, the chance of a child being homozygous for the variant is 1 in 300 (**Plate 69**). Although this is presumably a normal variant, the possibility of uniparental disomy for chromosome 14 should be ruled out, particularly if the proband (as in this case) has clinical abnormalities.

Complete loss of satellite III sequences from 14p and the centromeric region in a case of 14p- has been reported by Earle *et al.* [4]. This presumably normal variant showed absence of the short arm, NOR and possibly part of the centromeric region. A normal alpha satellite signal was obtained.

References

1. Olson SB, Magenis RE and Lovrien EW (1986). Human chromosome variation: the discriminatory power of Q-band heteromorphism (variant) analysis in distinguishing between individuals, with specific application to cases of questionable paternity. Am J Hum Genet. 38:235–52.
2. Balicek P, Zizka J (1980). Intercalar satellites of human acrocentric chromosomes as a cytological manifestation of polymorphisms in GC-rich material. Hum Genet. 54:343–7.
3. Balicek P, Zizka J, Skalska H (1982). RGH-band polymorphism of the short arms of human acrocentric chromosomes and relationship of variants to satellite association. Hum Genet. 62:237–9.
4. Earle E, Voullaire LE, Hills L, Slater H, Choo KH (1992). Absence of satellite III DNA in the centromere and the proximal long-arm region of human chromosome 14: analysis of a 14p-variant. Cytogenet Cell Genet. 61:78–80.

CHROMOSOME 15

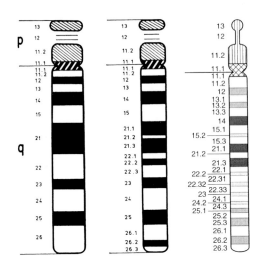

Plate 41. (**a**) Normal chromosomes 15 from five different subjects by G-banding showing increasing band resolution. (**b**) Normal chromosomes from five subjects showing gradations in size of short arms. (**c**) Normal chromosomes from five different subjects showing variations in size of satellites.

Contributors
(a–c) Center for Human Genetics, Boston University (c1).
(b) (second from right). Jacqueline Schoumans, Haukeland University Hospital (c19).

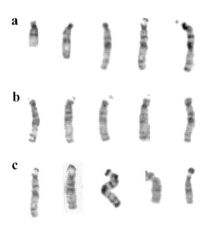

Plate 42. Twenty different variants of chromosome 15 from a population of 39 unrelated people. Each chromosome is serially printed to reveal heteromorphisms not visible at an exposure generally chosen to define the overall banding pattern. The large bright satellites in D5 are relatively uncommon and were present in only one person in the population studied. [Figure 5, reprinted from Olson SB, Magenis RE, Lovrien EW (1986). Human chromosome variation: the discriminatory power of Q-band heteromorphism (variant) analysis in distinguishing between individuals, with specific application to cases of questionable paternity. Am J Hum Genet. 38(2):235–52.]

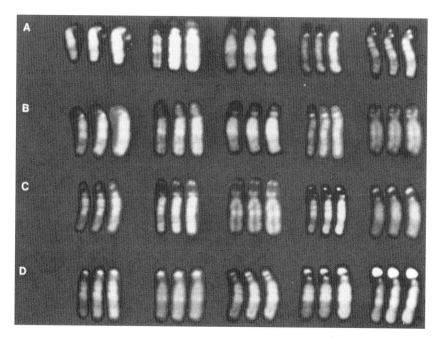

Plate 43. Variant short arm regions by different banding and FISH techniques. (**a**). Pair of homologs by G- and Q-banding showing dark short arm and Q-positive satellite in one homolog (left) and narrow Q-positive band in the other (right). (**b**) Similar comparison in a different subject with a 15p+ (left). Note that the chromosome does not have a Q-bright region, despite size and dark staining of the 15p+. (**c, d**) Pairs of homologs from a third subject by G-banding (c) and by Q-banding (**d**). Note large short arm (**c**, left) and bright satellites on both homologs. (**e–i**) Note large short arm (**e**, left) has similar G-banding to the 15p+ in (**b**), but has an intensely Q-positive terminal band (**f**). C-banding of same region (**g**, left) is negative and a rather large NOR region is evident by silver staining (**h**, left). Centromeric regions are similar in size in both homologs with the alpha satellite probe, D15Z4 (**i**). (**j**) Two chromosomes 15 from different mitoses with large pale staining short arm by G-banding (left) showing at least two NOR regions by silver staining (two chromosomes at right from different mitoses from same subject).

Contributor
(a–j) Center for Human Genetics, Boston University (c1).

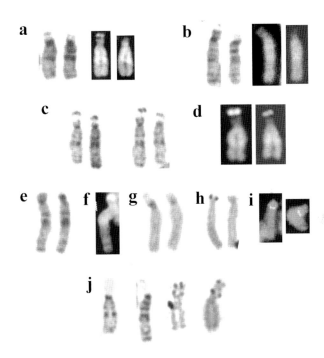

Plate 44. Variants of chromosome 15 studied by FISH. (**a–c**) Pairs of homologs showing diminutive short arm (arrow). (**a**) G banding. (**b**) FISH, using probe mixture of classical satellite (D15Z1, green) and D15S11 (red) in band q11.2 showing absence of D15Z1 from one homolog (right). (**c**) Homologs from same subject showing presence of alpha satellite (D15Z4) in centromeric region of both homologs. (**d–g**) Striking 15p+ from apparently normal subject by G-banding (**d–e**) showing two C-band positive regions (**f**, right) and two blocks of classical satellite (D15Z1) by FISH (**g**, right). Red signs are for SNRPN (proximal) and PML (distal).

Contributors
(a–c) Center for Human Genetics, Boston University (c1).
(d–g) KF Choeng, KK Womens and Childrens Hospital (c31).

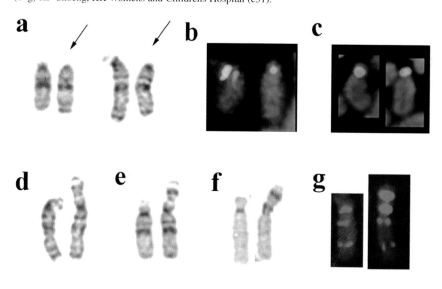

Plate 45. Variants of 15p due to translocations with distal Yq. (**a–d**) 15p+ by G-banding (**a, b**, right), by C-banding (**c**) and by Q-banding (**d**, right). (**e**) Metaphase treated with distamycin A produces under-condensation of 15p+ (large arrow) compared to normal homolog (small arrow). (**f**) FISH with painting library for 15 (wcp15, green) and distal Yq (DYZ1, red). Note absence of red signal from normal homolog (left). (**g–i**). Different normal male subject with 15p+ by G-banding (**g**), C-banding (**h**) and by FISH with DYZ1 (**i**). Note two green signals in interphase in the same metaphase (upper right).

Contributors
(a–f) KF Choeng, KK Womens and Childrens Hospital (c32).
(g–i) J M Fink, Hennepin County Medical Center (c37).

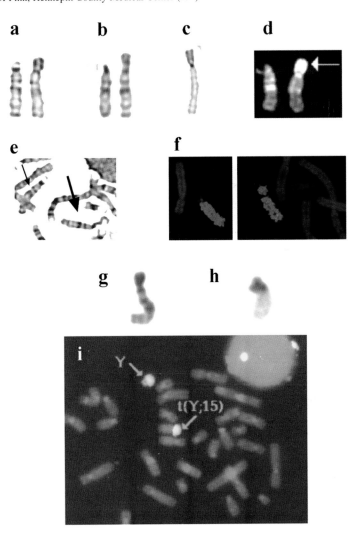

Plate 46. Apparently large satellite on 15p due to translocation from distal Yq. (**a**) G-banding of 15ps+ from two different cells and of Y from one cell. (**b**) Q-banding of 15s and Y from two different cells. (**c**) Silver staining showing large NOR corresponding to constriction in 15p+. Note small NOR in normal homolog (left). (**d**) Chromosomes 15 and Y by FISH with probe mixture of D15Z1 and D15Z4 showing classical and alpha satellites on both homologs. (**e**) Chromosome painting library (wcpY, including DYZ1) showing signals over both 15 ps+ and the Y chromosome.

Contributor
(a–e) Center for Human Genetics, Boston University (c1).

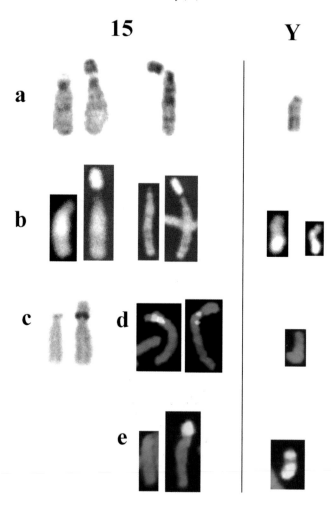

Plate 47. (**A**) An unstained area at 15q11.2 (G-banded, top left) was positive with Ag-NOR (bottom left) indicating an unusual insertional translocation of the nucleolar organizing region from an acrocentric short arm (Jalal and Ketterling, unreported case; see Chapter 6). (**B**) Pairs of 15 from a normal subject showing euchromatic variant of band 15q11.2. (**C, D**) Duplication variant of 15q11.2–q13.1 in a sequential G-banded partial metaphase (**D**), followed by wcp15 probe analysis (**C**) has been reported by Jalal *et al.* (1994) from 15 cases in seven unrelated families (see Chapter 6).

Contributor
B: Arturo Anguiano, Quest Diagnostics (c29).

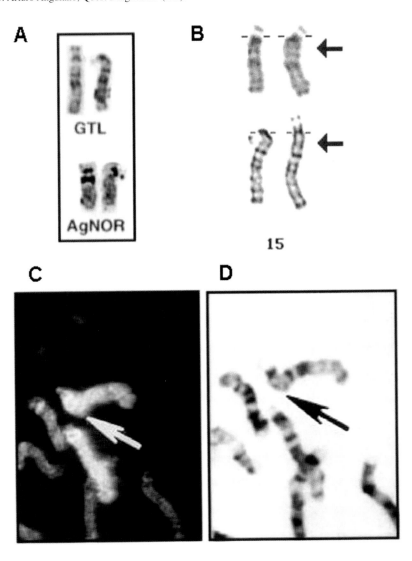

Chromosome 15: Summary

As with the other acrocentric chromosomes, the centromere, short arm and satellite regions of chromosome 15 are variable in size and staining properties. Variants by G-banding are represented (**Plate 41**) and by Q-banding (**Plate 42**). Some common variants and their staining properties by different banding techniques are shown (**Plate 43**).

Heteromorphisms of chromosome 15 are of interest because of the variability in staining of the short arm in common with other D and G group chromosomes, but especially because of banding with alkaline Giemsa [1] and DA/DAPI [2,3] that particularly stain components of 1qh, 9qh, D- and G-group short arms, 16qh and distal Yqh regions. Early in situ hybridization studies revealed different but overlaping distributions of satellite DNA fractions (isolated by their different buoyant densities) to the various heterochromatic regions in the human karyotype [4–6]. A loose correlation was reported between alkaline Giemsa staining and the "classical" satellite III [7]. Current FISH and molecular technologies define satellite DNAs somewhat differently but localize sequences in the satellite III family to similar chromosome regions [see Chapter 7].

Current, widely used FISH analyses distinguish at least two classes of repetitive DNA in the heterochromatin of chromosome 15: (1) a chromosome 15-specific alpha satellite DNA in the pericentromeric region of chromosome 15 [8] and (2) a chromosome 15-specific subcomponent of satellite III DNA that comprises a major component of the short arm of chromosome 15 [9,10]. Cross-hybridization of a chromosome 15-specific satellite III with other D-group chromosomes was reported in 5.5% of subjects in one study, and was correlated with additional DA/DAPI-positive signals on those chromosomes [11]. Cross-hybridization of the widely used chromosome 15-specific satellite III probe (D15Z1), as an extra signal specifically on the short arm of a chromosome 14, has been found in approximately 12% of individuals in two separate studies [12,13]. Examples are represented in the present volume (**Plate 69**).

Variations in the size of the classical satellite region of chromosome 15 are also evident by FISH. We know of at least one case (**Plate 44a–c**) with a diminutive short arm on a chromosome 15 by G-banding that shows loss of the classical satellite sequence D15Z1 but has a normal-size alpha satellite signal. In another case (**Plate 44 d–g**), a very large short arm on a chromosome 15 is shown by FISH to have a duplication of the classical satellite sequence. Homology between various satellite III DNA families among acrocentric chromosomes possibly accounts for the fact that almost all breakpoints in Robertsonian translocations occur in the satellite III DNAs [14,15] (see Chapters 8 and 9).

Homology between the short arm of chromosome 15 and distal Yq is suggested by the high frequency of Q-bright satellites on chromosome 15. Q-bright satellites in fact occur on all of the acrocentric chromosomes with the majority having nothing to do with the bright sequences on the end of the Y chromosome. Occasionally, however, translocations do occur between an acrocentric short arm and the distal long arm of the Y (**Plates 45,46**). When they occur they almost always involve chromosomes 15 or 22. Distinction between Y/15 and Y/22 translocations from other bright variants can be made by special treatments such as addition of distamycin A to cultures (see Part II, Chromosome 22), staining

220

with DA/DAPI and, more recently, by FISH or other molecular testing. Verma *et al.* [16] present one case in which origin from Yq could be eliminated by such techniques but the extra material on 15p still could not be identified.

Also of interest regarding heteromorphism of chromosome 15 is the close proximity of genes causing Angelman and Prader-Willi syndromes. Zackowski *et al.* [17] and Butler [18] have questioned whether larger, darker staining centromeric and short arm variants of chromosome 15 by GTG banding are more frequent in the deleted chromosomes than in the normal homologs in Angelman and Prader-Willi syndrome cases. However, Butler points out that in a FISH study of deleted chromosomes with D15Z1 (classical satellite probe), although there were variations in the size of the signal that could be determined to be heritable, such differences did not correlate with deletion [12]. Butler [18] concluded that some of the GTG size increases might be due to the deletion bringing non-heterochromatic GTG-positive regions into close proximity to the centromere. However, the large 15p variants Zackowski *et al.* [17] observed in AS patients were heritable from the mother.

Euchromatic variants

Proximal euchromatic variants in 15q (**Plate 47b–d**) have also been noted [19,20]. In these cases elongation of the 15q11.2 band has been noted in both phenotypically normal and abnormal patients. Riordan and Dawson [21] studied six clinically normal patients using probes for PWS/AS regions and found two groups: (1) those with duplication of PWS/AS probes and (2) those without, but who had a large D15Z variant (see Chapter 6). It should be noted that cases that do not include the Prader-Willi/Angelman (PWS/AS) region are usually familial and without phenotypic effect, whereas those that include the PWS/AS region can be *de novo* or familial and associated with developmental delay, minor malformations and/or autism [22–23]. Cumulative evidence indicates that cases with autism or autistic-like behavior are maternally derived whereas paternally derived cases usually have a normal phenotype [23–24]. The incidence of dup(15) is unknown, but the estimated prevalence among patients with mental retardation and/or developmental delay is 0.17–0.5% [25]. From these observations it is evident that any suspected case of dup(15)(q11q13) should be tested with FISH probes to determine whether or not the PWS/AS region is duplicated.

References

1. Bobrow M, Madan K, Pearson PL (1972). Staining of specific regions of human chromosomes, particularly the secondary constriction of No. 9. Nature New Biol. 238:122–4.
2. Schweizer D (1980). Simultaneous fluorescent staining of R-bands and specific heterochromatic regions (DA-DAPI bands) in human chromosomes. Cytogenet Cell Genet. 27:190–3.
3. Babu A, Macera MJ, Verma RS (1986). Intensity heteromorphisms of human chromosome 15p by DA/DAPI technique. Hum Genet. 73(4):298–300.
4. Jones KW, Prosser J (1973). The chromosomal localization of human satellite DNA III. Chromosoma (Berl.). 42:445–51.
5. Gosden JR, Mitchell AR, Buckland RA, Clayton RP, Evans HJ (1975). The location of four human satellite DNAs on human chromosomes. Exp Cell Res. 92:148–58.
6. Miklos GL, John B (1979). Heterochromatin and satellite DNA in man: Propeties and prospects. Am J Med Genet. 31:254–80.
7. Buhler EM, Tsuchimoto T, Jurik L, Stalder GR (1975). Satellite DNA III and alkaline Giemsa staining. Humangenetik. 26:329–33.

8. Choo KH, Earle E, Vissel B, Filby RG (1990). Identification of two distinct subfamilies of alpha satellite DNA that are highly specific for human chromosome 15. Genomics. 7:143–51.

9. Higgins MJ, Wang HS, Shtromas I, Haliotis T, Roder JC, Holden JJ, White BN (1985). Organization of a repetitive human 1.8 kb KpnI sequence localized in the heterochromatin of chromosome 15. Chromosoma. 93:77–86.

10. Fowler C, Drinkwater, R, Skinner J, Burgoyne L (1988). Human satellite–III DNA: an example of a macrosatellite polymorphism. Hum Genet. 79:265–72.

11. Smeets DF, Merkx GF, Hopman AH (1991). Frequent occurrence of translocations of the short arm of chromosome 15 to other D-group chromosomes. Hum Genet. 87:45–8.

12. Stergianou K, Gould CP, Waters JJ, Hulten MA (1993). A DA/DAPI positive 14p heteromorphism defined by in situ hybridization using chromosome 15-specific probes D15Z1 (satellite III) and p-TRA-25 (alphoid). Hereditas. 119:105–10.

13. Shim SH, Pan A, Huang XL, Tonk VS, Wyandt HE (2002). FISH variants with D15Z1 in clinical cases. Am J Hum Genet. 71:307A.

14. Gravholt CH, Friedrich U, Caprani M, Jorgensen AL (1992). Breakpoints in Robertsonian translocations are localized to satellite III DNA by fluorescence in situ hybridization. Genomics. 14:924–30.

15. Bandyopadhyay R, Berend SA, Page SL, Choo KH, Shaffer LG (2001). Satellite III sequences on 14p and their relevance to Robertsonian translocation formation. Chromosome Res. 9:235–42.

16. Verma RS, Kleyman SM, Conte RA (1996). Molecular characterization of an unusual variant of the short arm of chromosome 15 by FISH-technique. Jpn J Hum Genet. 41:307–11.

17. Zackowski JL, Nicholls RD, Gray BA et al. (1993). Cytogenetic and molecular analysis in Angelman syndrome. Am J Med Genet. 46:7–11.

18. Butler MG (1994). Are specific short arm variants or heteromorphisms over-represented in the chromosome 15 deletion in Angelman or Prader-Willi syndrome patients? Am J Med Genet. 50:42–5.

19. Butler MG, Greenstein MA (1991). Molecular cytogenetics of Prader-Willi and Angelman syndromes. Lancet. 338:1276.

20. Brookwell R, Veleba A (1994). Proximal 15q variant with normal phenotype in three unrelated individuals. Clin Genet. 31:311–14.

21. Riordan D, Dawson AJ (1998). The evaluation of proximal 15q duplications by FISH. Clin Genet. 54:517–21.

22. Browne CE, Dennis NR, Maher E, et al. (1997). Inherited interstitial duplications of proximal 15q: genotype-phenotype correlations. Am J Med Genet. 61:1342–52.

23. Bolton PF, Dennis NR, Browne CE, Thomas NS, Veltman MWM, Thompson RJ, Jacobs P (2001). The phenotypic manifestations of interstitial duplications of proximal 15q with special reference to the autistic spectrum disorders. Am J Med Genet (Neuro Genet). 105:675–85.

24. Yardin C, Esclaire F, Laroche C, Terro F, Barthe D, Bonnefont J-P, Gilbert B (2002). Should the chromosome region 15q11q13 be systematically tested by FISH in the case of an autistic-like syndrome? Clin Genet. 61:310–13.

25. Moeschler JB, Mohandas TK, Hawk AB, Knoll W (2002). Research Letter. Estimate of the prevalence of proximal 15q duplication syndrome. Am J Med Genet. 111:440-42.

CHROMOSOME 16

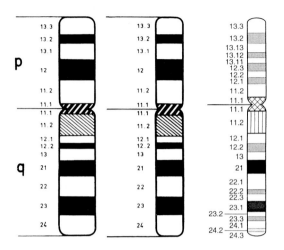

Plate 48. (**a**) Normal chromosomes 16 from five different subjects by G-banding showing increasing band resolution. (**b–e**) Pairs of chromosomes 16 from four different subjects showing 16qh+ (right hand chromosome in each pair). (**f**) Chromosome 16 by G-banding with extremely long qh region. (**g**) Pair of chromosome 16 homologs by G-banding showing striking discrepancy between a short qh region and a very long qh region in the same person. Pair of C-banded chromosomes from the same subject (extreme right).

Contributors
(a–e) Center for Human Genetics, Boston University (c1).
(f) Jacqueline Schoumans, Haukeland University Hospital (c21).
(g) Peter Benn, University of Connecticut Health Center (c11).

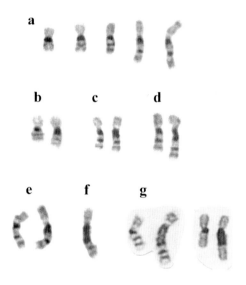

Plate 49. Euchromatic variants in chromosome 16. (**a**) Chromosome 16 ideogram and the homologous pairs from the fetus, mother, and a male sibling. (**A**) Ideogram at 400 band stage (arrow indicates the 16q21 band). Pair 16 from the fetus (**B**), the mother (**C**) and a male sibling (**D**) with the deleted 16q21 band in each pair (chromosomes at left) (see Chapter 6). (**b**) Increase of 16p arm by about one-third as a duplication variant [From Jalal SM, Schneider NR, Kukolioh MK, Wilson CN (1990). Euchromatic 16p heteromorphism: first report in North America. Am J Med Genet. 37:548–50, in two infants with unrelated abnormalities and three normal family members. This has been reported in a number of other cases (see Chapter 6)].

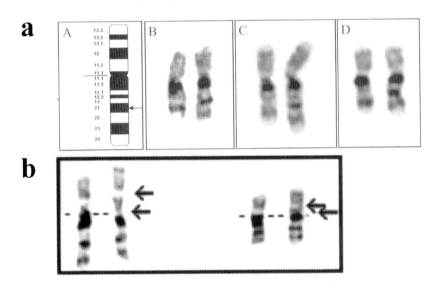

Chromosome 16: Summary

Approximately 38% of individuals, in a subsample of 400 7- and 8-year olds [1], showed a level-1size 16qh region (about the size of the non-heterochromatic portion of the short arm of chromosome 16) [2]. About 2–4% showed level-5-size variants (twice the size of 16p). No significant differences were reported between Black and White children. No cases of 16qh inversion were reported. In a separate study of 35 unrelated subjects (14 males and 25 females) studied by C-banding, 11 variants of chromosome 16 were recorded, nine of which were level 1. None involved inversion 16 [3]. Hsu *et al.* [4] also found no cases of inversion 16 in 6250 prenatal specimens representing four major population groups, and Potluri *et al.* [5] found no inversion 16 in 200 New Delhi infants. As with chromosomes 1qh and 9qh, variants of 16h are mainly visible by C-banding (**Plate 48**). One rare case of an inverted duplication involving alpha satellite DNA resulted in a C-negative band in a large 16qh region [6]. A very small 16qh C-negative region studied by molecular techniques showed a normal centromeric signal [7].

As with the other major heteromorphic regions, numerous studies have attempted to associate striking heteromorphisms of chromosome 16qh with various deleterious effects. Soudek and Sroka [8] found a higher frequency of 16qh in retarded individuals than in a control group. Buretic-Tomljanovich *et al.* [9] studied couples with two or more miscarriages, couples with a stillborn child, and couples with no history of miscarriages and at least two normal children. Their results suggested an increase in heterochromatin of chromosome 16 in couples with a stillborn or a malformed child.

Variations in size and location of the major heterochromatic regions have particularly been implicated in various cancers and leukemias (Chapter 5). Berger *et al.* [10] reported an excess in the amount of C-band heterochromatin on chromosomes 1, 9 and 16 and a higher incidence of inversions of 1qh and 9qh in breast cancer patients. They also noted a significant difference in C-band size of chromosome 16 between familial and sporadic breast cancer patients. Such differences, however, were *not* noted in other breast cancer series [11,12]. Differences in C-band heteromorphisms were also not seen in prostate cancer, relating to disease stage [13]. However, younger patients (less than 70 years old) had significantly higher frequencies of large C-bands on chromosome 1 and 16 compared to patients older than 70 years. Petkovic *et al.* [14] observed longer C-band segments on chromosomes 1, 9 and 16 in children with ALL than in controls.

Euchromatic variants

A number of studies have described an apparently innocuous euchromatic variant on the short arm of chromosome 16 (**Plate 49b**, see Chapter 6), first described by Thompson and Roberts [15] and appearing as an additional C-band-negative segment in the proximal short arm, which they later showed to be late replicating [16]. Additional cases (see Chapter 6) were reported by Pinel *et al.* [17], Bryke *et al.* [18], Jalal *et al.* [19], and Verma *et al.* [20].

Deletion of euchromatic band 16q21 (**Plate 49a**) has also been reported as a variant without apparent phenotypic effect in several reports (see Chapter 6).

References

1. Lubs HA, Patil SR, Kimberling WJ, *et al.* (1977). Q and C-banding polymorphisms in 7 and 8 year old children: racial differences and clinical significance: In: Hook EB Porter IH, editors. Population Cytogenetic Studies in Humans. New York: Academic Press, 1977, pp. 133–59.
2. Patil SR, Lubs HA (1977). Classification of qh regions in human chromosomes 1, 9 and 16 by C-banding. Hum Genet. 19: 377–80.
3. Craig-Holmes AP (1977). C-band polymorphisms in human populations. In: Hook EB, Porter IH, editors. Population Cytogenetics. Studies in Humans. New York: Academic Press, pp. 161–77.
4. Hsu LYF, Benn PA, Tannenbaum HL, Perlis TE, Carlson AD (1987). Chromosomal polymorphisms of 1, 9, 16 and Y in 4 major ethnic groups: a large prenatal study. Am J Med Genet. 26:95–101.
5. Potluri VR, Singh IP, Bhasin MK (1985). Chromosomal heteromorphisms in Delhi infants. III. Qualitative analysis of C-band inversion heteromorphisms of chromosomes 1, 9 and 16. J Heredity. 76:55–8.
6. Jalal SM, Law ME, DeWald GW (1993). Inverted duplication involving alpha satellite DNA resulting in a C-negative band in the qh region of chromosome 16. Am J Med Genet. 46:351–2.
7. Verma RS, Luke S, Mathews T, Conte RA (1992). Molecular characterization of the smallest secondary constriction region (qh) of human chromosome 16. Genet Anal Tech Appl. 9:140–2.
8. Soudek D, Sroka H (1979). Chromosomal variants in mentally retarded and normal men. Clin Genet. 16:109–16.
9. Buretic-Tomljanovic A, Rodojcic Badovinac A, Vlastelic I, Randic LJ (1997). Quantiative analysis of constitutive heterochromatin in couples with fetal wastage. Am J Reprod Immun. 38:201–4.
10. Berger R, Bernheim A, Kristoffersson U, Mitelman F, Olsson H (1985). C-band heteromorphism in breast cancer patients. Cancer Genet Cytogenet. 18:37–42.
11. Atkin NB, Brito-Babapulle V (1983). Chromosome 1 C-band heteromorphism in patients with carcinoma in situ and invasive carcinoma of the cervix uteri. Austral NZ J Obstet Gynecol. 23:73–6.
12. Kivi S, Mikelsaar AV (1987). C-band polymorphisms in lymphocytes of patients with ovarian or breast cancer. Cancer Genet Cytogenet. 28(1):77–85.
13. Lundgren R, Berger R, Kristoffersson U (1991). Constitutive heterochromatin C-band polymorphism in prostatic cancer. Cancer Genet Cytogenet. 51:57–62.
14. Petkovic I, Nakic M, Konja J (1991). Heterochromatic variability in children with acute lymphoblastic leukemia. Cancer Genet Cytogenet. 54:67–9.
15. Thompson PW, Roberts SH (1987). A new variant of chromosome 16. Hum Genet. 76:100–1.
16. Thompson PW, Roberts SH, Rees SM (1990). Replication studies in the 16p+ variant. Hum Genet. 84:371–2.
17. Pinel I, de Bustamante AD, Urioste M, Felix V, Ureta A, Martinez-Frias ML (1988). An unusual variant of chromosome 16. Two new cases. Hum Genet. 80:194.
18. Bryke CR, Breg WR, Potluri VR, Yang-Feng TL (1990). Duplication of euchromatin without phenotypic effects: a variant of chromosome 16. Am J Med Genet. 36:43–4.
19. Jalal SM, Schneider NR, Kukolich MK, Wilson GN (1990). Euchromatic 16p+ heteromorphism: first report in North America. Am J Med Genet. 37:548–50.
20. Verma RS, Kleyman SM, Conte RA (1997). Variant euchromatic band within 16q12.1. Clin Genet. 52:446–7.

CHROMOSOME 17

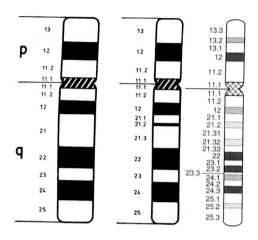

Plate 50. (**a**) Normal chromosomes 17 from five different subjects by G-banding showing increasing band resolution. (**b**) Large 17ph region (arrows) by G-banding. (**c**) Satellited 17p by G-banding (left) and by silver staining (middle and right). Arrows point to NOR region, visible as a constriction by G-banding and as dark staining by silver staining.

Contributors
(a) Center for Human Genetics, Boston University (c1).
(b) Patriciam Miron Brigham and Women's Hospital (c38).
(c) James M. Fink, Hennepin County Medical Center (c37).

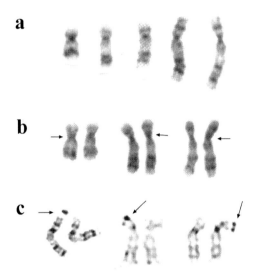

Chromosome 17: Summary

Both large and small variants of the centromeric region on chromosome 17 were reported by Lubs *et al.* [1] with a combined frequency of about 6%. The small centromeric region was more frequent in Caucasians and the larger region more frequent in Blacks. No significant differences were noted relating to IQ. In an Estonian population of normal adults, Mikelsaar *et al.* [2] reported 17ph+ to be more frequent in adult men than women. Among retarded children in their studies, multiple G-band variants were found in one patient that included 9q+, 13p−, 17ph− and Yq−.

Satellited 17

Several investigators, including Schmid and Bauchinger [3], Ferguson-Smith *et al.* [4], and Moores *et al.* [5] found cases with an apparent secondary constriction in the short arm of chromosome 17. Kuleshov and Kulieva [6], in a study of 6000 newborns, also mention a case with satellites on the short arms of 17 or 18. The constriction in these studies was not in every cell and often was present in low frequency. The variant was initially ascertained in subjects with various phenotypic abnormalities including trisomy 21, congenital heart disease, and cri-du-chat syndrome. In several instances normal carriers were reported as having aneuploid offspring [5,7,8], and the variant was observed in couples having multiple abortions [9]. Despite these observations the marker was also found in normal individuals [10] or was often familial and carried by normal relatives [11,12]. In at least one family it could be traced back several generations.

Schmid and Bauchinger [3] described the marker in five subjects with frequencies ranging from 10% to 100%. Of 350 metaphases examined from the five individuals, only seven were in satellite association. Whereas some reports described the variant 17 in satellite association, others, observing constrictions in 17p and finding no evidence of rearrangement with D or G group chromosomes, considered the variant to be a secondary constriction [11]. Oliver *et al.* [13] studied the 17p variant in four patients by silver staining. The absence of silver grain precipitate on chromosome 17 in all four patients supported the hypothesis that the 17p variant was a structural heteromorphism rather than translocated satellite material. Similarly, Patil and Bent [9] studied cells with satellited 17. The frequencies of silver staining and satellite association were compared for the 17ps variant with D and G group chromosomes. No cells with satellite association or silver staining of 17ps were observed.

Fragile site at 17p12

Some cases of reported satellited 17 may in fact represent a rare heritable fragile site on chromosome 17, fra(17)(p12) [14–16]. At least one case of homozygosity for this site has been reported in a healthy man [17]. Other studies [18] have shown a higher than expected incidence of fra(17)(p12) in patients with hematological disorders.

Identification of satellited 17

Differentiation of a satellited 17 from a fragile site is definitive when results are positive with Ag-NOR staining or other special staining techniques for acrocentric variants (**Plate 50**). Negative results may require chromosome painting to identify the material distal to the constriction as being from chromosome 17. In cases with a fragile site, however, all cells do not usually show the site. If heritable, the frequency of the site may be increased by special induction [19].

References

1. Lubs HA, Patil SR, Kimberling WJ *et al.* (1977). Q and C-banding polymorphisms in 7 and 8 year old children: Racial differences and clinical significance: In: Hook EB, Porter IH, editors. Population Cytogenetic Studies in Humans. New York: Academic Press, 1977, pp. 133–59.
2. Mikelsaar A-V, Tuur SJ, Kaosaar ME (1973). Human karyotype polymorphism. I. Routine and fluorescence microscopic investigation of chromosomes in a normal adult population. Humangenetik. 20:89–101.
3. Schmid E, Bauchinger (1969). Structural polymorphism in chromosome 17. Nature. 221:387–8.
4. Ferguson-Smith MA, Ferguson-Smith ME, Ellis PM, Dickson M (1962). The sites and relative frequencies of secondary constrictions in human somatic chromosomes. Cytogenetics 1:325–43.
5. Moores EC, Anders JM, Emanuel R (1966). Inheritance of marker chromosomes from a cytogenetic survey of congenital heart disease. Ann Hum Genet. 30:77–84.
6. Kuleshov NP, Kulieva LM (1979). [Frequency of chromosome variants in human populations] Chastota khromosmnykh variantov v populiatsiiakh cheloveka [Russian]. Genetika. 15:745–51.
7. Berg JM, Fauch JA, Pendrey MJ, Penrose LS, Ridler MA, Shapiro A (1969). A homozygous chromosomal variant. Lancet. 1:531.
8. Gustaavson KH, Kjessler B (1978). A variant chromosome 17 in a mother with repeated abortions and 46,XY/47,XXY Klinefelter son. Uppsala J Med Sci. 83:119–22.
9. Patil SR, Bent FC (1980). Silver staining and the 17ps chromosome. Clin Genet. 17:281–4.
10. Verma RS, Ved BS, Warman J, Dosik H (1979). Clinical significance of the satellited short arm of human chromosome 17 (17ps+): a rare heteromorphism? Ann Genet. 22:133–6.
11. Priest JH, Peakman DC, Patil SR, Robinson A (1970). Significance of 17ps+ in three generations of a family. J Med Genet. 7:142–7.
12. Sandstrom M, Jenkins EC (1973). A 17p marker chromosome familial study. Ann Genet. 16:267–9.
13. Oliver N, Francke U, Taylor KM (1978). Silver staining studies on the short arm variant of human chromosome 17. Hum Genet. 42:79–82.
14. Sutherland GR (1979). Heritable fragile sites on human chromosomes. I. Factors affecting expression in lymphocyte culture. Am J Hum Genet. 31:125–35.
15. Sutherland GR (1979). Heritable fragile sites on human chromosomes. II. Distribution, phenotypic effects and cytogenetics. Am J Hum Genet. 32:136–48.
16. Shabtai F, Klar D, Halbrecht I (1982). Chromosome 17 has a real fragile site at p12. Hum Genet. 61:177–9.
17. Izakovic V (1984). Homozygosity for fragile site at 17p12 in a 28-year old healthy man. Hum Genet. 68:340–1.
18. Murata M, Takahashi E, Minamihisamatsu M, *et al.* (1988). Heritable rare fragile sites in patients with leukemia and other hematologic disorders. Cancer Genet Cytogenet. 31:95–103.
19. Schmid M, Feichtinger W, Deubelbeiss C, Weller E. (1987). The fragile site (17)(p12): induction by AT-specific DNA ligands and population cytogenetics. Hum Genet. 77:118–21.

CHROMOSOME 18

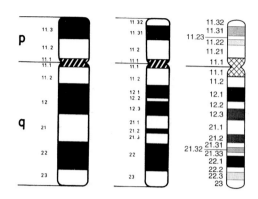

Plate 51. (a) Normal chromosomes 18 from five different subjects by G-banding showing increasing band resolution. (b) Two chromosome pairs from fetus (left) and one pair of chromosomes 18 from the father (right). Top: GTG-banding: bottom: CBG-banding [Figure 1, reprinted from Beverstock GC, Klumper F, Helderman V, Enden AT (1997). Yet another variation on the theme of chromosome 18 heteromorphisms? Prenat Diagn. 17(6):585–6.] Pair of 18's with discrepant size centromeric regions by GTG banding (c) and partial metaphase showing obvious discrepancy in size of alpha satellite signals (CEP 18, Vysis, Downers Grove, IL) by FISH in the 18-homologs (arrows, d). Both (c) and (d) are from a prenatal sample that showed a low percentage of non-cultured amniocyte cells with two alpha satellite signals by FISH with the same probe.

Contributors
(a) Center for Human Genetics, Boston University (c1).
(c, d) Texas Tech University Health Sciences Center (c43).

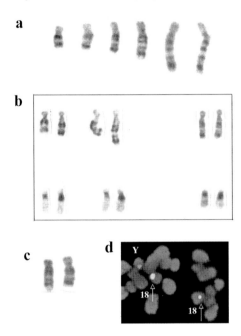

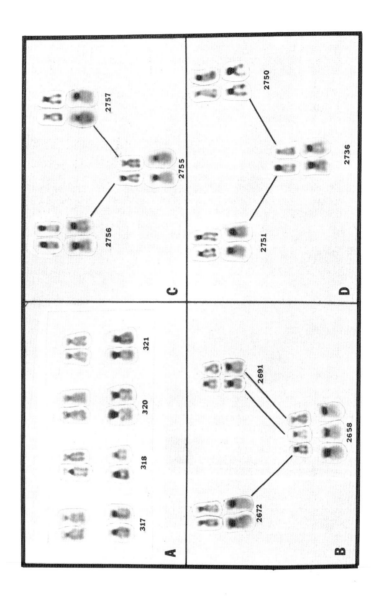

Plate 52. (**A**) The chromosome 18s from four different individuals treated with *Alu*I and stained by Giemsa (top row). The corresponding C-bands are shown below from the same individuals. The *Alu*I-resistant bands represent a small fraction of the C-bands and are usually located distally in the short arm (317, 320 and 321). Its location in the long arm (left homolog of 318) and the total absence (right homolog of 318) are normal variants. (**B**) Chromosome 18s from a family with Edward syndrome stained with *Alu*I (top) and CBG (bottom) techniques. The chromosomes from the mother (2672) are shown at the left while the father's (2691) are presented at the right. One of the chromosomes *18* (far left) in the proband (2658) is similar to the pattern seen in the mother while the remaining two (middle and right) closely resemble those of the father's, demonstrating the paternal origin. (**C, D**) The chromosome 18s from two normal families stained with *Alu*I (top) and CBG (bottom) techniques are also included to demonstrate their parental origin. The maternal chromosomes are shown to the left (2756 and 2751), while the paternal ones are presented to the right (2757 and 2750). The parental identification is also marked by lines [Figure 1, reprinted from Babu A, Verma RS (1986). The heteromorphic marker on chromosome 18 using restriction endonuclease AluI. Am J Hum Genet. 38(4):549–54.]

Plate 53. Partial karyotype depicting (**a**) diagrammatic representation of the normal 18 (left) and the duplicated 18p. (**b**) Prometaphase GTG-banded normal 18s (left in both pairs) and the duplication 18p chromosomes. Arrows denote the duplicated segment. (**c**) Partial C-banded karyotype revealing normal C-bands on E-group chromosomes including the normal number 18 and the duplicated 18. [Figure 1, reprinted from Wolff DJ, Raffel LJ, Ferre MM, Schwatz S (1991). Prenatal ascertainment of an inherited dup(18p) associated with an apparently normal phenotype. Am J Med Genet. 41:319–21.]

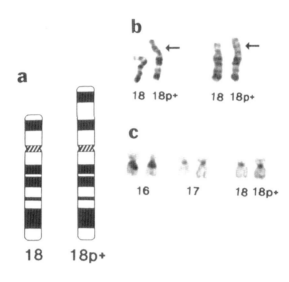

Chromosome 18: Summary

In an early study of 20 unrelated individuals, Craig-Holmes and Shaw [1] found one E-group chromosome with a small centromeric region (cen−) by C-banding. No cases with cen+ were described. McKenzie and Lubs [2], in their study of Q and C band variants, found variations in the centromeric regions of all of the chromosomes, with the exception of the Y, including chromosome 18. These were often more visible by C-banding than by Q-banding. Muller *et al.* [3], in a study of 375 newborns, found chromosome 18 with a double size C-band in about 1.1% of cases. In Q- and C-band studies of 7- and 8-year-olds, Lubs *et al.* [4] found a large 18cen in about 8% of White children and in about 15% of Black children. Heterochromatin in 18p was rarer, being found in 1–2% of both races. Differences in frequency between normal and mentally retarded groups were not significant.

Since these early studies, numerous reports have described heteromorphisms of chromosome 18, usually due to heterochromatin in the short arm (18ph+) and usually without phenotypic effect [5–8]. Bonfatti and colleagues [7, 8] describe heteromorphisms of pericentric regions of 18 that were detectable with alpha satellite probes by FISH but were almost undetectable by C-banding. Beverstock *et al.* [9] report an unusual variant of chromosome 18 with heterochromatin that extended from the centromere into the long arm. The region was lightly stained by GTG-banding, similar to 9qh or 16qh, and was C-band positive (**Plate 51**). Initially detected prenatally in both uncultured trophoblasts and in cultured villi, the variant was determined to be paternal in origin. Parents were both Spanish.

Babu and Verma [10] were the first to study the variability and heritability of AluI-resistant heteromorphisms of pericentric heterochromatin in chromosome 18 in normal individuals, and to determine the parental origin of the extra chromosome 18 in a case of Edward syndrome (**Plate 52**). In a subsequent study of 50 normal Caucasians and five cases of trisomy 18, Babu *et al.* [11] describe at least five size-classes, based on comparison with length of 18p, ranging from negative (class 1) to very large (class 5). The relative incidences for each of these classes were: (1) 11.3%, (2) 19.1%, (3) 29.57%, (4) 29.57% and (5) 10.4%. Location of heterochromatin was also classified into four types: I, absent (11.3%); II, on p-arm only (62.6%); III, on q-arm only (0.87%); and IV, on centromere, extending into both p and q (25.22%). Classes 1 and 5 were predominantly found in the trisomy 18 cases.

Euchromatic variants

One case reportedly has duplication of the entire short arm of chromosome 18 (**Plate 53**), without abnormalities [12]. Moog *et al.* [13] reported two patients with duplication/deletion and with tandem duplication, respectively, with developmental delay, mild/moderate mental rerardation and dysmorphic features. Abeliovich *et al.* [14] report a familial i(18p) that is mosaic in a mother who is mildly affected. The non-mosaic child has full tetrasomy 18p syndrome. Tetrasomy 18p has been associated with mild [15] to severe clinical anomalies [16,17]. The mechanism(s) contributing to the apparent range in phenotypes associated with 18p duplications at present remains unexplained.

References

1. Craig-Holmes AP, Shaw MW (1973). Polymorphism of human C-band heterochromatin. Science. 174:702–4.
2. McKenzie WH, Lubs HA (1975). Human Q and C chromosomal variations: Distribution and incidence. Cytogenet Cell Genet. 14:97–115.
3. Muller HJ, Klinger HP, Glasser M (1975). Chromosome polymorphism in a human newborn population. II. Potentials of polymorphic chromosome variants for characterizing the ideogram of an individual. Cytogenet Cell Genet. 15(4):239–55.
4. Lubs HA, Patil SR, Kimberling WJ et al. (1977). Q and C-banding polymorphisms in 7 and 8 year old children: racial differences and clinical significance. In: Hook EB, Porter IH, editors. Population Cytogenetic Studies in Humans. New York: Academic Press, pp. 133–59.
5. Pittalis MC, Santarini L, Bovicelli L (1994). Prenatal diagnosis of a heterochromatic 18p+ heteromorphism [letter]. Prenat Diagn. 14:72–3.
6. Zelante L, Notarangelo A, Dallapiccola B (1994). The 18ph+ heteromorphism. Prenat Diagn. 14:1096–7.
7. Sensi A, Giunta C, Bonfatti A, Gruppioni R, Rubini M, Fontana F (1994). Heteromorphic variant 18ph+ analyzed by sequential CBG and fluorescence in situ hybridization. Hum Hered. 44:295–7.
8. Bonfatti A, Giunta C, Sensi A, Gruppioni R, Rubini M, Fontana F (1993). Heteromorphism of human chromosome 18 detected by fluorescent in situ hybridization. Eur J Histochem. 37:149–54.
9. Beverstock GC, Klumper F, Helderman V, Enden AT (1997). Yet another variation on the theme of chromosome 18 heteromorphisms? Prenat Diagn. 17:585–6.
10. Babu A, Verma RS (1986). The heteromorphic marker on chromosome 18 using restriction endonuclease AluI. Am J Hum Genet. 38: 549–54.
11. Babu A, Verma RS, Patil SR (1987). AluI-resistant chromatin of chromosome 18: Classification, frequencies and implications. Chromosoma. 95:163–6.
12. Wolff DJ, Raffel LJ, Ferre MM, Schwartz S (1991). Prenatal ascertainment of an inherited dup(18p) associated with an apparently normal phenotype. Am J Med Genet. 41:319–21.
13. Moog U, Engelen JJ, de Die-Smulders CE et al. (1994). Partial trisomy of the short arm of chromosome 18 due to inversion duplication and direct duplication. Clin Genet. 46:423–9.
14. Abeliovich D, Dagan J, Levy A, Steinberg A, Zlotogora J (1993). Isochromosome 18p in a mother and her child. Am J Med Genet. 46:392–3.
15. Johnasson B, Mertens F, Palm L, Englesson I, Kristofferson U (1988). Duplication 18p with mild influence on phenotype. Am J Med Genet. 29:871–4.
16. Singer TS, Kohn G, Yatziv S (1990). Tetrasomy 18p in a child with trisomy 18 phenotype. Am J Med Genet. 36:144–7.
17. Pinto MR, Silva ML, Ribeiro MC, Pina R (1998). Prenatal diagnosis of mosaicism for tetrasomy 18p: Cytogenetic, FISH and morphological findings. Prenat Diagn. 18:1095–7.

CHROMOSOME 19

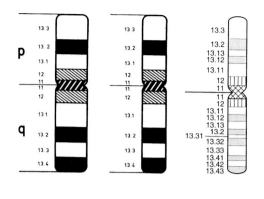

Plate 54. (**a**) Normal chromosomes 19 from five different subjects by G-banding showing increasing band resolution. (**b–d**). Variant 19's from three different subjects showing partial inversions and duplications in centromeric heterochromatin. (**e, f**) C-banding of 19's from subjects c and d, respectively.

Contributors
(a–b) Center for Human Genetics, Boston University (c1).
(c–f) Jacqueline Schoumans, Haakland University Hospital (c24).

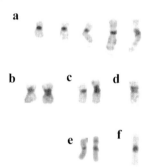

Chromosome 19: Summary

As with most other centromeric regions, variants of the centromeric heterochromatin of chromosome 19 were noted early [1–4]. Most of these reports described these variations as "rare", pericentric inversions, often ascertained through an abnormal proband, but considered in almost all cases to be unrelated to the abnormal phenotype [5–7]. Also, almost all cases of pericentric inversions were not associated with increased abortion rate or decreased reproductive fitness. However, in a review by Alessandro *et al.* [7], they describe three new families that all showed a "high frequency of abortions" as well as one "unclarified perinatal death". Such anecdotal studies, however, inherently have considerable bias. Almost no attention has been paid to subtle structural differences in these cases, although structural differences in C-banding are also occasionally evident (**Plate 54**). Verma and Luke [8] demonstrated four different classes of variants in pericentromeric heterochromatin of chromosome 19 from 50 normal individuals using Alu digestion followed by Giemsa staining.

References

1. Jacobs PA, Buckton KE, Cunningham C, Newton M (1974). An analysis of breakpoints in structural rearrangements in man. J Med Genet. 11:50–64.
2. Crossen PE (1975). Variation in the centromeric banding of chromosome 19. Clin Genet. 8:218–22.
3. Sutherland GR, Gardiner AJ, Carter RF (1976). Familial pericentric inversion of chromosome 19, inv(19)(p13q13) with a note on genetic counseling of pericentric inversion carriers. Clin Genet. 10:54–9.
4. Gardner HA, Wood M (1979). Variation in chromosome 19. J Med Genet. 16:79–80.
5. Jordan DK, Taysi K, Blackwell NL (1980). Familial pericentric inversion 19. J Med Genet. 17:222–5.
6. Tharapel AT, Ward JC, Wiggins L, Wilroy RS Jr (1986). Pericentric inversion of chromosome 19: Prenatal diagnosis and genetic counseling. Prenat Diagn. 6:75–8.
7. D'Alessandro E, DeMatteis Vaccaraella C, Lo Re ML *et al.* (1988). Pericentric inversion in chromosome 19 in three families. Hum Genet. 80:203–4.
8. Verma RS, Luke S (1991). Heteromorphisms of pericentromeric heterochromatin of chromosome 19. Genet Anal Tech Appl. 8:179–80.

CHROMOSOME 20

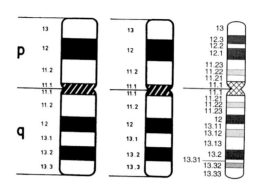

Plate 55. (**a**) Normal chromosomes 20 from five different subjects by G-banding showing increasing band resolution. (**b**) Chromosomes 20 from two different cells from one individual showing 20ph+ by GTG-banding. Chromosome is maternal in origin. (**c–f**) Pairs of chromosomes 20 by GTG-banding (**c**), by CBG-banding (**d**), by DAPI staining (**e**) and by FISH (**f**) with alpha satellite probe D20Z1 (CEP20, Vysis, Downers Grove, IL). The chromosome at right of each pair has 20ph+.

Contributors
(a, c–f) Center for Human Genetics, Boston University (c1).
(b) K Yelevarthi and J Zunich, Indiana University, NW Medical Center (c14).

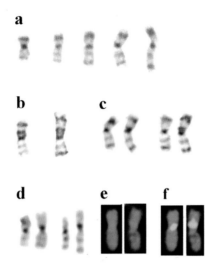

Chromosome 20: Summary

Variants of the centromeric region of chromosome 20 are rare. Only two cases of 20ph+ are reported [1,2]. A third case was submitted to this volume as a normal variant (Yelevarthi and Zunich, **Plate 55b**). A fourth case was detected in a patient with infertility (Center for Human Genetics, unpublished). The 20ph+ in one of the published cases was also detected in a couple with recurrent miscarriages [2]. In both of these cases the 20ph+ was positive by G and C banding and showed a larger signal by FISH with alpha satellite probe D20Z1 (**Plate 55, c–f**). In addition to 20ph+. Pericentric inversions in 20h also appear to be rare, there being only one reported prenatal case [1] that is known to us. In conclusion, it appears that variants of the centromeric region of chromosome 20 are both rare and of uncertain significance with regard to pregnancy loss.

References

1. Petersen MB (1990). Rare chromosome 20 variants encountered during prenatal diagnosis. Prenal Diagn. 6:363–7.
2. Romain DR, Whyte S, Callen DF, Eyre HJ (1991). A rare heteromorphism of chromosome 20 and reproductive loss. J Med Genet. 28:477–8.

CHROMOSOME 21

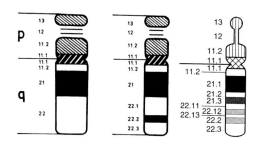

Plate 56. (**a**) Chromosomes 21 from six different subjects showing variations by GTG-banding in the size and staining of the short arm without satellite (far left) and with satellite (far right). (**b**) Large (right) vs. typical (left) short arms of pair of chromosome 21's by GTG-banding. Pair of chromosomes by silver staining at right is from the same subject. (**c**) Chromosomes 21 by G-banding (left) from three different subjects showing variations in size and intensity of staining of satellites. (**d**) Pair of chromosomes (left) by G-banding and from the same subject by Q-banding (right). (**e**) Pair of 21's stained by G-banding (left) showing large dark satellites and by silver staining (right) showing large NOR region (far right). (**f**) Pair of 21's by G-banding showing large dark short arm (right). (**g**) Pair of 21's by G-banding showing large dark satellite (right).

Contributor
Center for Human Genetics, Boston University (c1).

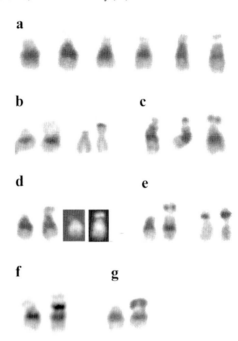

Plate 57. (**a**) Three pairs of chromosomes 21 from the same subject showing large dark satellite by G-banding. (**b**) Pair of chromosomes 21 from the same subject showing intense staining by Q-banding. (**c**) Chromosome 21 from same subject showing large satellite to hybridize with alpha satellite probe, DYZ1 (Vysis, Downers Grove, IL), indicating its origin from the distal end of the Y long arm.

Contributor
Center for Human Genetics, Boston University (c1).

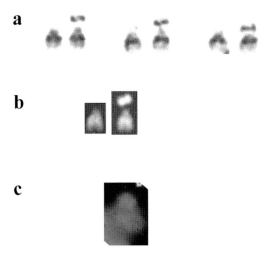

Plate 58. Fifteen different variants of chromosome 21 from a population of 39 unrelated people. Each chromosome is serially printed to reveal heteromorphisms not visible at an exposure generally chosen to define the overall banding pattern. [Figure 6, reprinted from Olson SB, Magenis RE, Lovrien EW (1986). Human chromosome variation: the discriminatory power of Q-band heteromorphism (variant) analysis in distinguishing between individuals, with specific application to cases of questionable paternity. Am J Hum Genet. 38(2):235–52.]

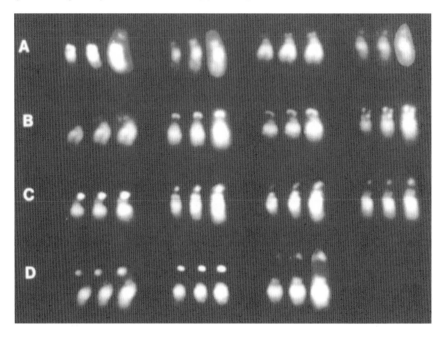

Chromosome 21: Summary

Numerous studies have attempted to show a relationship between striking variants (**Plate 56**) such as large bright satellites, double satellites, large or double NOR's and an increased risk for non-disjunction, leading to trisomy 21 in Down syndrome (see Chapter 5). Similarly, numerous early studies attempted to show a higher frequency of satellite association in parents of Down syndrome children. However, with the advent of banding techniques, it was shown that there was no difference in the frequency of satellite association in parents of trisomy 21 children and controls [1–4].

Occasionally, large bright satellites have been shown to be due to a translocation between the acrocentric chromosome and the distal end of a Y chromosome. The majority of translocations between the Y and an acrocentric involve chromosomes 15 or 22. These often have a distinctive morphology from typical satellites and can be distinguished by special techniques such as adding distamycin to cultures [5] or staining with distamycin A and DAPI (see Part II, Chromosome 22) or can be identified by FISH. A few cases involve chromosome 21 (**Plate 57**).

Because of their stability, Q-band variants of chromosome 21 (**Plate 58**) and other acrocentric chromosomes, have been particularly useful in paternity studies and in determining parental origin of the extra chromosome 21 in trisomy 21 (see Chapter 5). However, satellites that move around have occasionally been reported. Gimelli *et al.* [6] described a prominent, brightly fluorescent "jumping satellite" that was first observed on a normal 22 in a male carrier of the balanced translocation, t(10;22). A daughter and a son, who both inherited the balanced translocation, however, had the prominent satellite on the der(22)t(10;22). In the fetus of a chromosomally normal pregnancy of the daughter, the satellite was again on a normal chromosome 22. Farrell *et al.* [7] report two families: one family had an unusually large paternal 21 short arm that prenatally was found on the short arm of a chromosome 13 in the fetus. In a second family a paternal prominent short arm on a chromosome 15 moved to a chromosome 14 in some cells from a fetus. An interesting case of an extreme variant of an unstable satellite was also reported by Livingston *et al.* [8] in a woman who had symptoms related to occupational exposure to organophosphate pesticides. Chromosome studies, which revealed a slightly increased frequency of sister chromatid exhange (SCE), also revealed a Q-bright giant satellite that was present on a chromosome 21 in 15% of cells, on a chromosome 22 in 83% of cells, and on both 21 and 22 in 2% of cells. The woman's mother had the same giant satellite on a chromosome 22 in all of her cells. A study of the affected woman's chromosomes, 3 years post-exposure, revealed a similar distribution to chromosomes 21 and 22, even though her SCE rate was significantly less than at the time of her symptoms.

One case of a very large C-band positive short arm on a 21 in the mother of a child with 21/21 translocation Down syndrome was reported [9]. This extreme variant of 21 was not necessarily attributed to be a cause of the translocation trisomy in the child. No comparable examples of such extreme heteromorphism of 21ph have subsequently been reported.

Other notable variants of acrocentric chromosomes are those that show an apparent absence of heterochromatin or a short arm. Mayer *et al.* [9], in a study of C-band variants in 516 patients with mental retardation, report 16 patients with unusual heteromorphisms, including one with 21p− and trisomy 21. In a previous study of 1300 patients they had found only one other case of 21p− also in a family with Down syndrome due to a t(21q21q). Other instances of 21p− associated with Down syndrome were reported by Shaw [11], de Grouche [12] and Ballantyne et al. [13]. Although no causal relationship has been shown, it is conceivable that centromeric function could be affected in some of these cases, leading to non-disjunction, especially if such a chromosome arose from a broken dicentric chromosome [14]. The incidence of cases with 21p− is also of interest in assessing trisomy prenatally in non-cultured amniocytes by FISH using alpha satellite probes. Several cases of chromosome 21p− or 21 aneuploidy escaping detection because of low fluorescence have been reported [15–17]. Verma et al. [18] also looked at intensity of FISH signals in pericentromeric regions of chromosome 21 in 15 normal individuals and 12 individuals with trisomy 21, and classified them into five size categories ranging from negative (1) to very large (5). According to them, at least 3% of chromosomes 21 did not show a hybridization signal. A similar study by Lo et al. [19] in 17,000 morphologically normal chromosomes revealed 3.7% of chromosomes 21 failed to show a signal, compared to 0.12 % for chromosome 13 and 17 and 0% for all other chromosomes.

References

1. Cooke P, Curtis DJ (1974). General and specific patterns of acrocentric association in parents of mongol children. Humangenetik. 23:279–87.
2. Taysi K (1975). Satellite association: Giemsa banding studies in parents of Down's syndrome patients. Clin Genet. 8:319–323.
3. Yip MY, Fox DP (1981). Variation in pattern and frequency of acrocentric association in normal and trisomy 21 individuals. Hum Genet. 59:14–22.
4. Jacobs PA, Mayer M (1981). The origin of human trisomy: a study of heteromorphisms and satellite associations. Ann Hum Genet. 45:357–65.
5. Spowart G (1979). Reassessment of presumed Y/22 and Y/15 translocations in man using a new technique. Cytogenet Cell Genet. 23:90–94.
6. Gimelli G, Porro E, Santi F, Scappaticci S, Zuffardi O (1976). "Jumping" satellites in three generations: a warning for paternity tests and prenatal diagnosis. Hum Genet. 34:315–18.
7. Farrell SA, Winsor EJ, Markovik VD (1993). Moving satellites and unstable chromosome translocations: clinical and cytogenetic implications. Am J Med Genet. 46:715–20.
8. Livingston GK, Lockey JE, Witt KS, Rogers SW (1985). An unstable giant satellite associated with chromosomes 21 and 22 in the same individual. Am J Hum Genet. 37:553–60.
9. Mayer M, Matsuura J, Jacobs, P (1978). Inversions and other unusual heteromorphisms detected by C-banding. Hum Genet. 45:43–50.
10. Tuncbilek E, Bobrow M, Clarke G, Taysi K (1976). A giant short arm of no. 21 chromosome in mother of 21/21 translocation mongol. J Med Genet. 13:411–12.
11. Shaw M (1962). Familial mongolism. Cytogenetics. 1:141–79.
12. De Grouche J (1970). 21p− maternal en double exemplaire chez un trisomique 21 [French]. Ann Genet (Paris). 13:52–5.
13. Ballantyne GH, ParslowMI, Veale AM, Pullon DH (1977). Down's syndrome and the deletion of short arms of a G chromosome. J Med Genet. 14:147–50.
14. Lebo RV, Wyandt HE, Warburton PE, Li S, Milunsky J (2002). An unstable dicentric Robertsonian translocation in a markedly discordant twin. Clin Genet. 62:383–9.
15. Lebo RV, Flandermeyer RR, Diukman R, Lynch ED, Lepercq JA, Golbus MS (1992). Prenatal diagnosis with repetitive in situ hybridization probes. Am J Med Genet. 43:848–54.

16. Bossuyt PJ, Van Tienen MN, De Gruyter L, Smets V, Dumon J, Wauters JG (1995). Incidence of low-fluorescence alpha satellite region on chromosome 21 escaping detection of aneuploidy at interphase by FISH. Cytogenet Cell Genet. 68:203–6.
17. Conte RA, Mathews T, Kleyman SM, Verma RS (1996). Molecular characterization of 21p- variant chromosome. Clin Genet. 50:103–5.
18. Verma RS, Batish SD, Gogineni SK, Kleyman SM, Statda DG (1997). Centromeric alphoid DNA heteromorphisms of chromosome 21 revealed by FISH-technique. Clin Genet. 51:91–3.
19. Lo AWI, Liao GCC, Rocchi M, Choo KHA (1999). Extreme reduction of chromosome-specific α-satellite array is unusually common in human chromosome 21. Genome Res. 9:895–908.

CHROMOSOME 22

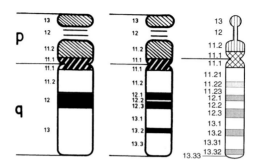

Plate 59 (**a**) Chromosomes 22 by G-banding from eight different subjects showing variation in size of the short arm. (**b**) Chromosomes 22 from eight additional subjects showing variation in size of and staining of the satellites and short arms. (**c–f**) Additional banding techniques on selected chromosomes: (**c**) chromosome with very long short arm, stalk and satellite by (left to right) G, Q-, C- and NOR-staining. Note lack of C-banding except at the centromere and on Q-bright satellite. A constriction just below the satellite corresponds to the NOR (far right). (**d**) Pairs of homologs from the same subject by G-banding (left) and by Q-banding (right). Note apparent lack of a dark satellite by G-banding and very bright terminal satellite by Q-banding (right-hand chromosome of each pair). (**e**) Pairs of homologs from the same subject by G-banding (left), Q-banding (middle) and NOR-staining (right). Note dark band in middle of short arm is Q-bright and is flanked by two NOR regions. (**f**) Chromosome 22 with long pale-staining short arm by G-banding (left) and two NORs (right).

Contributor
Center for Human Genetics, Boston University (c1).

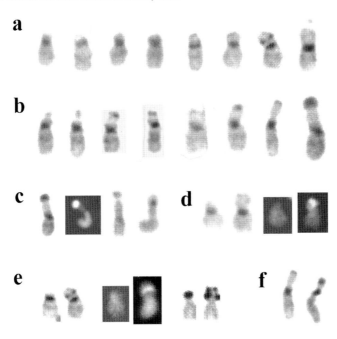

Plate 60   Twenty-four different variants of chromosome 22 from a population of 39 unrelated people. Each chromosome is serially printed to reveal heteromorphisms not visible at an exposure generally chosen to define the overall banding pattern. The large bright satellites in D-6 are relatively uncommon and were present in only one person of the population selected. [Figure 7, reproduced from Olson SB, Magenis RE, Lovrien EW (1986). Human chromosome variation: the discriminatory power of Q-band heteromorphism (variant) analysis in distinguishing between individuals, with specific application to cases of questionable paternity. Am J Hum Genet. 38(2):235–52.]

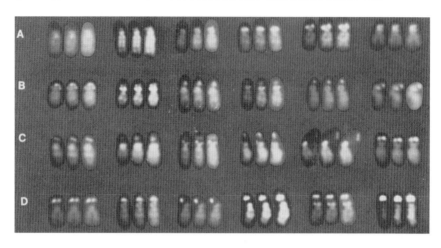

Chromosome 22: Summary

As with the other acrocentric chromosomes, the centromere, stalk, short arm and satellite regions are highly heteromorphic with, perhaps, some of the most striking variants observed in this group of chromosomes (**Plate 59**). While Q-bright variants (**Plate 60**) are not observed more frequently on chromosome 22 than on chromosome 13, bright variants of the short arm are more frequent. The frequency of bright satellites is similar to the other acrocentrics but is less than in chromosome 14. Very large bright satellites on chromosome 22 are rare, but have involved an exchange with distal Yq sequences more frequently than chromosomes 13, 14 or 21 and less frequently than chromosome 15. Special techniques such as staining with distamycin A and DAPI [1,2] have also been used to distinguish Q-bright Y chromatin from other Q-bright heterochromatin. In other cases distamycin A has been added to cultures to cause under-condensation of heterochromatin originating from Yqh [3–6]. Currently, FISH using a probe specific for the satellite sequences in Yqh provides a more definitive test. In most cases these translocations are familial, involving only the repetitive sequences of the Yqh region and acrocentric chromosome, and are of little or no clinical consequence [7]. A few cases of males with translocations between a Y and an acrocentric are oligospermic and presumably have a dicentric chromosome. Alves *et al.* [7] showed that such a dicentric chromosome resulted in malsegregation at meiosis, explaining the observed oligospermia.

The rare occurrence of an unstable satellite that moved from chromosome 22 to other acrocentric chromosomes was discussed in the summary for chromosome 21 [8,9]. A case of a prominent satellite moving from a t(10;22) to a normal 22 was also discussed [10].

The pericentromeric region and short arm of chromosome 22 consist of several types of repetitive DNA including contiguous arrays of 1, 3 and β satellites [11–14]. Two cases of extreme variants consisting of very large short arms on 22 were characterized by Conte *et al.* [15] who showed they were quite different in their organization. The first variant had a tandem duplication of p11.2–p11.3. The second variant had lost the β-satellite and ribosomal DNA regions and showed amplification of satellite III. Such detailed analysis of striking variants of heteromorphisms of the acrocentric chromosomes has not been done on a large scale. At least one group of investigators has shown the presence of expressed sequences within the heterochromatin of chromosome 22 [16].

Chromosomes 14 and 22 share alpha satellite sequences, so that the centromeres of these two chromosomes cannot be distinguished by FISH. Of interest, however, is the observation of several investigators of cross-hybridization of the chromosome 13/21 alpha satellite DNA to chromosome 22, detected in the prenatal screening of common chromosomal aneuploidies by FISH, emphasizing the need for caution in using repetitive probes for screening for the common aneuploidies by interphase FISH [17–19] (see Chapters 8 and 9 for a more detailed discussion of satellite sequences).

References

1. Spowart G (1979). Reassessment of presumed Y/22 and Y/15 translocations in man using a new technique. Cytogenet Cell Genet. 23:90–4.

2. Funderburk SJ, Klisak I, Sparks RS, Carrel RE (1982). Familial Y-autosome translocation in two unrelated girls. Ann Genet. 25:119–22.
3. Schmid M (1979). Demonstration of Y/autosomal translocations using distamycin A. Hum Genet. 53:107–9.
4. Cohen MM, Frederick RW, Balkin NE, Simpson SJ (1981). Identification of Y chromosome translocations following distamycin A treatment. Clin Genet. 19:335–42.
5. Schmid M, Schmidtke J, Kruse K, Tolsdorf M (1983). Characterization of a Y/15 translocation by banding methods, distamycin A treatment of lymphocytes and DNA restriction endonuclease analysis. Clin Genet. 24:234–9.
6. Schimd M, Hungerford DA, Poppen A, Engel W (1984). The use of distamycin A in human lymphocyte cultures. Hum Genet. 65:377–84.
7. Alves C, Carvalho F, Cremades N, Sousa M, Barros A (2002). Unique Y/13 translocation in a male with oligozoospermia: cytogenetic and molecular studies. Eur J Hum Genet. 10:467–74.
8. Livingston GK, Lockey JE, Witt KS, Rogers SW (1985). An unstable giant satellite associated with chromosomes 21 and 22 in the same individual. Am J Hum Genet. 37:553–60.
9. Gimelli G, Porro E, Santi F, Scappaticci S, Zuffardi O (1976). "Jumping satellites" in three generations: a warning for paternity testing and prenatal diagnosis. Hum Genet. 34:315–18.
10. Farrell SA, Winsor EJ, Markovik VD (1993). Moving satellites and unstable chromosome translocations: clinical and cytogenetic implications. Am J Med Genet. 46:715–20.
11. Rocchi M, Archidiacono N, Antonacci R et al. (1994). Cloning and comparative mapping of recently evolved human chromosome 22-specific alpha satellite DNA. Somatic Cell Mol Genet. 20:443–8.
12. Antonacci R, Rocchi M, Archidiacono N, Baldini A (1995). Ordered mapping of three alpha satellite DNA subsets on human chromosome 22. Chromosome Res. 3:124–7.
13. Mullenbach R, Pusch C, Holzmann K, Suijkerbuijk R, Blin N (1996). Distribution and linkage of repetitive clusters from the heterochromatic region of human chromosome 22. Chromosome Res. 4:282–7.
14. Shields C, Coutellle C, Huxley C (1997). Contiguous arrays of satellites 1, 3, and beta form a 1.5 Mb domain on chromosome 22p. Genomics. 44:35–44.
15. Conte RA, Kleyman SM, Laundon C, Verma RS (1997). Characterization of two extreme variants involving the short arm of chromosome 22: are they identical? Ann Genet. 40:145–9.
16. Blin N, Scholz M, Wissinger B, Mullenbach R, Pusch C (1997). Expressed sequences within pericentromeric heterochromatin of human chromosome 22. Mamm Geneome. 8:859–62.
17. Verlinsky Y, Ginsberg N, Chmura M, et al. (1995). Cross-hybridization of the chromosome 13/21 alpha satellite DNA probe to chromosome 22 in the prenatal screening of common chromosomal aneuploidies by FISH. Prenat Diagn. 15:831–4.
18. Biancato JK (1996). Re: Cross-hybridization of the chromosome 13/21 alpha satellite DNA probe to chromosome 22 in the prenatal screening of common aneuploidies by FISH [letter]. Prenat Diagn. 16:769–70.
19. Tardy EP, Toth A (1997). Cross-hybridization of the chromosome alpha satellite DNA to chromosome 22 or a rare polymorphism? Prenat Diagn. 17:487–8.

CHROMOSOME X

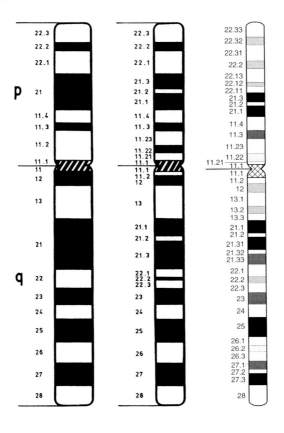

Plate 61.   X chromosomes of increasing G-band resolution from five different subjects.

Contributor
Center for Human Genetics, Boston University (c1).

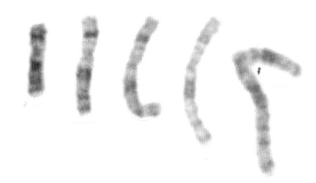

Plate 62. Representative FISH images from the proband and mother. (**a**) Interphase FISH of uncultured amniocytes hybridized with chromosome 18 (aqua), X (green) and Y alpha satellite probes demonstrating two 18 (aqua) signals (arrowheads), but only one X signal (arrow). Metaphase from cultured amniocytes hybridized with a BAC probe located within an X alpha satellite probe, showing a typical X chromosome signal (arrowhead), and a markedly reduced X signal (arrow). (**c**) Metaphase FISH from cultured amniocytes with a BAC probe located within a few hundred kilobases of DXZ1 on the long arm. [Figure 1, reprinted from Tsuchiya K, Schueler MG, Dev VG (2001). Familial X centromere variant resulting in a false-positive prenatal diagnosis of monosomy X by interphase FISH. Prenat Diagn. 21:852–5.]

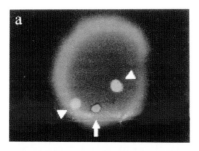

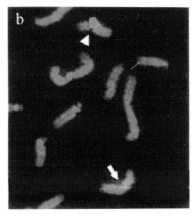

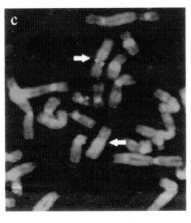

Chromosome X: Summary

McKenzie and Lubs [1] reported C-band heteromorphisms for the centromere of every human chromosome except the Y, but including the X chromosome. One Xcen+ variant was found in 77 newborns from Grand Junction, CO, in a child whose parents were Mexican-American. In a study of 400 7- and 8-year olds (Lubs *et al.* [2]), six cases with Xcen+ were found by C-banding; five were Caucasian; one was Black. Friedrich *et al.* [3] studied the reliability of a blind assessment of X centromere origin by C-band variations (by size and whether heterochromatin was in the centromere, in Xp or in Xq) in 22 girls with Turner syndrome, compared with assignment of parental origin by RFLP analysis. In 19 cases they were able to trace the X centromere to the mother in total agreement with RFLP analysis. More recently, one case of false-positive diagnosis of monosomy X by FISH was reported [4], due to a discrepancy in size of the alpha satellite DXZ1 signal, observed in metaphase, and resulting in only one scorable signal in interphase (**Plate 62**).

References

1. McKenzie WH, Lubs HA (1975). Human Q and C chromosomal variations: Distribution and incidence. Cytogenet Cell Genet. 14:97–115.
2. Lubs HA, Patil SR, Kimberling WJ et al. (1977). Q and C-banding polymorphisms in 7 and 8 year old children: racial differences and clinical significance. In: Hook EB, Porter IH, editors. Population Cytogenetic Studies in Humans. New York: Academic Press, pp. 133–59.
3. Friedrich U, Larsen TB, Nielsen J (1991). Diagnostic reliability of the cytogenetic centromere heteromorphism in the human X chromosome. Clin Genet. 40:465–6.
4. Tsuchiya K, Schueler MG, Dev VG (2001). Familial X centromere variant resulting in a false-positive prenatal diagnosis of monosomy X by interphase FISH. Prenat Diagn. 21:852–5.

CHROMOSOME Y

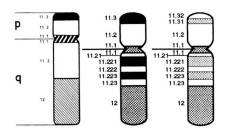

Plate 63. (**a**) Y chromosomes from five different individuals showing increasing length of the qh region by G-banding. (**b–d**) Y chromosomes of different length from three different individuals showing comparison of qh regions by G-banding (left) and Q-banding (right). (**e**) Y chromosomes from a population of 39 unrelated individuals showing variations in fluorescent portion of the Y long arm with scores (for qh size) ranging from 1 (left) to 5 (right). [Part of Figure 2, Olson SB, Magenis RE, Lovrien EW (1986). Human chromosome variation: the discriminatory power of Q-band heteromorphism (variant) analysis in distinguishing between individuals, with specific application to cases of questionable paternity. Am J Hum Genet. 38(2):235–52.]

Contributor
(a–d) Center for Human Genetics, Boston University (c1).

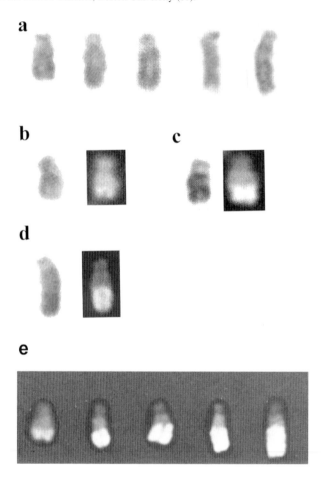

Plate 64. Comparison of Yqh fluorescence of three different size Y chromosomes from three different individuals in metaphases (A, C, E) and in interphase cells (B, D, F) (H.E. Wyandt, unpublished).

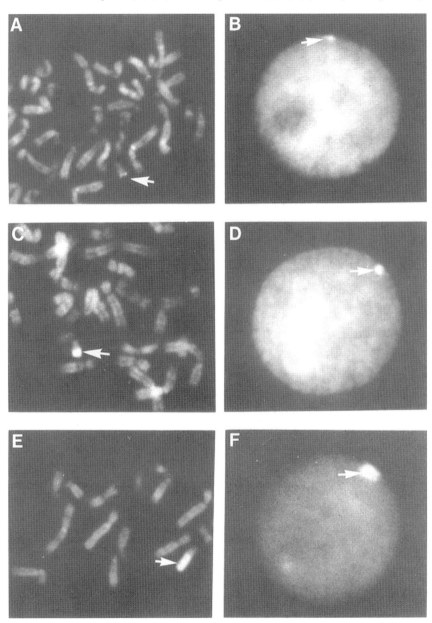

Plate 65. (**a–c**) Y chromosomes with pericentric inversions from three different individuals with pair at far right (**c**) showing the same Y chromosome by G and Q-banding. (**d**) Intrachromosomal insertion, ins(Y)(p11.2q10q11.23) by G-banding (left) and by Q-banding (2nd from left). FISH analysis with DYZ1/DYZ3 (Vysis) is shown (middle), with D15Z3 alone (2nd from right) and SRY (far right) (Xin Li Huang and H.E Wyandt, unpublished). (**e**) Diagram of mechanism of formation of (d) with rearranged chromosome at far right showing results of FISH and banding analysis [Xin Li Huang and H.E Wyandt, unpublished]. Chromosome, present in a fetus and in the father, was unstable in the father (see Y summary). Intact SRY region was also confirmed by molecular analysis. (**f**) Satellited, non-fluorescent Y chromosome studied by different FISH analyses using D15Z1, green (a,b), DYZ1, red and DYZ3, green (c), Y WCP, spectrum orange (d), and Xq/Yq telomeric associated sequence, red (e) probes on (A) the proband and (B) the father. The chromosome 15 specific classical satellite DNA probe (D15Z1) indicates chromosome 15 as the origin of the satellites. In (a) and (b) chromosomes 15 and Y of the proband and father come from the same metaphase. The negative signal for the Yq telomeric probe (e) suggests loss of Yqter on the Y[nfqs] [Figure 2, reprinted from Verma *et al.* (1997). Characterization of a satellited non-fluorescent Y chromosome (Y[nfqs]) by FISH. Med Genet. 34:817–18.]

Contributor
(a–e) Center for Human Genetics, Boston University (c1).

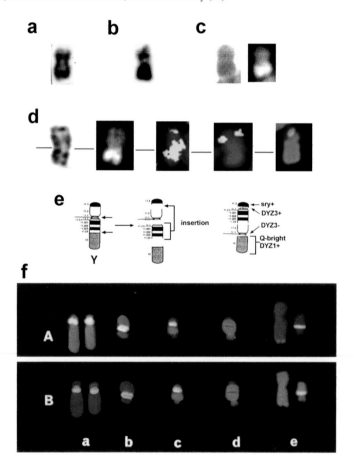

Plate 66. (**a–d**) Familial satellited Y chromosome (B. Haddad and H.E. Wyandt, unpublished) by G-banding (arrow, **a**), Q-banding (**b**), C-banding (**c**) and silver staining (**d**). (**e, f**) Satellited Y from a different family (father and son) by G and Q banding (**e, f**) and silver staining also shown (**f**, far right). (**g–l**) Satellited Y in a third family (father and son) by G-banding (**g**), Q-banding (**h**), silver staining (**i**) and by FISH (**j, k**). Probes include alpha satellite DYZ1 for Yqh alone (j), DYZ1 and DYZ3 (alpha satellite specific for the centromeric region), and D15Z1 (satellite III specific to the short arm of chromosome 15) with probe for SNRPN in 15q11.2 (**l**). Probe for D15Z1 (green) present on the satellited Y chromosome is indicated by the large arrow. The small arrows indicate two chromosomes 15. Orange signals represent SNRPN.

Contributor
(e–k) Center for Human Genetics, Boston University (c1).

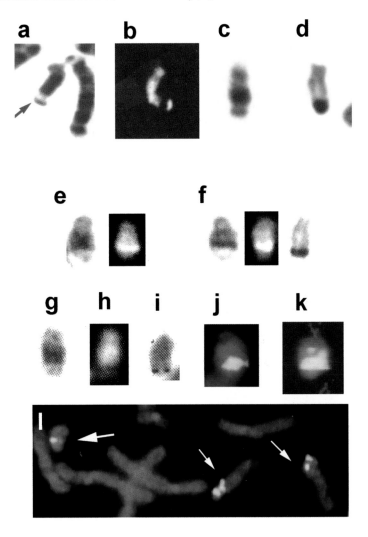

Chromosome Y: Summary

The distal end long arm of the Y chromosome, along with 1q, 9q and 16q, is one of the most variable in length in the human genome. Early reports recognized that variability in the length of the Y long arm was not associated with any consistent clinical pattern [1–4]. The size of the Y can vary from smaller than a G-group chromosome to as large as a D-group chromosome in apparently normal and fertile men (**Plates 63, 64**). The distal Q-bright end of the Y is dark by G-banding and C-banding. With quinacrine banding it was determined that the length of the brightly fluorescent distal end of the Y accounted for most of the size differences [5–7]. The distal Q-bright region in large Ys is often composed of two fluorescent bands that are especially visible in prophase [8, 9]. Other variant forms of the Y in normal males include pericentric inversions and satellited Ys (**Plates 65, 66**).

Nielsen and Friedrich [10] studied the length of the Y chromosome in 140 newborn boys (a 10% random sample of 1400 newborns) compared with Y length in 407 criminal males. They suggested a correlation between the size of the Y and risk of criminality. Nielsen [11] found 58 boys in 11,148 consecutive newborns had a large Y. Mothers of these boys had 22% spontaneous abortions compared to 13% among 4895 mothers of boys without Yq+.

In small Y's the Q-bright region may be greatly diminished in size or even absent [12, 13]. It was early noted that Y chromosomes lacking a Q-bright region are more likely to be associated with minor anomalies and infertility [14, 15].

Variations in length

Gosh and Singh [16] studied the Y chromosome in 100 individuals in each of two Indian populations and noted that 5% of Rajputs and 3% of Punjabis had a long Y. Verma and colleagues [17–19] studied the variation in the size of the Y chromosome in White, American Black and various Indian populations. They calculated indices of Y length compared to chromosomes 19 and 20 (F) in 60 White normal males and classified them into five groups: I, Y/F < 0.8 (0%); II, 0.81–0.94 (15%); III, 0.95–1.09 (66.7%); IV, 1.1–1.23 (13.3%); V, > 1.23 (5%). In comparison, the Y/F indices for the American Blacks were: 0% in group I, 3.3% in group II, 56.7% in group III, 30% in group IV and 10% in group V. In East Indians, results for the Y/F indices were: 0% in group I, 1.42% in group II, 15.7% in group III, 58.7% in group IV and 24.3% in group V. Variation in total length was also compared for f/F and nf/F indices. In general the greatest correlation was between total length (F) and length of the fluorescent segment (f), a lesser correlation was found between total length (F) and length of the non-fluorescent segment (nf), and no correlation was found between length of the f and nf. Nevertheless, the mean non-fluorescent segment (f/F) indices, which ranged from 0.42 to 0.47, was largest for the East Indian group and smallest for the American Blacks. The mean nf/F indices ranged from 0.57 to 0.73 and were clearly largest for the East Indian group. Hence, the frequency of longer Y's was highest for East Indians and American Blacks. However, in East Indians, the longer Y's also reflected an increase in size of the non-fluorescent (nf) segment compared to Black and Caucasian populations. Other studies of Asian populations have shown more variation in the size of the Y than in the White population [20,21]), and have shown that the non-fluorescent portion of the Y chromosome long arm also varies in length [7,22].

Inversion Y

Pericentric inversion is a rare Y-variant (**Plate 65**) reported in approximately 1–2 per 1000 cases in various populations [23]. Such high frequency may depend on the population being studied. A study of 14,835 consecutive newborns in a Japanese population found one case with a pericentric inversion in the Y [24]. On the other hand, inversion Y was found in 5.7% of a Gujarati Muslim Indian population of South Africa [25], shown by molecular polymorphism studies [26] to have a common origin. In a study of a large Taiwanese population of 6286 unrelated males, the frequency was 0.27%. Pericentric inversions in the Y are generally considered to be normal variants with no apparent effect on fertility [17,23]. However, a handful of recent cases have been reported in infertility studies [27–30]. Two cases have been associated with asthenonecrozoospermia and oligospermia, respectively. Although the inversion, inv(Y) (p11q11), appeared to be the standard type, DNA analysis revealed interstitial microdeletions [27]. One case with oligospermia and inv(Y)(p11q11) [29] was revealed by FISH to have a break in Yq11, through the DAZ gene. A few reports of multiple anomalies [30], association with other chromosome aneuploidies [31] or increased fetal wastage [32] appear to be spurious and most likely coincidental. Two cases of atypical Y rearrangements are noteworthy. Rivera *et al.* [33] report a three generation family with an unstable familial Y chromosome with a single Cd-positive constriction that occasionally assumed an acrocentric appearance, presumably due to an inversion. FISH with DYZ3 revealed a signal outside the primary constriction. Another case showing a similar aspect, but interpreted to be a possible insertion (**Plate 65d, e**) was detected prenatally and was also present in the father [Huang and Wyandt, unpublished]. Mosaicism was present in the father who had cells showing loss of a Y and cells with two Ys. The two cases [33] appear to be similar in that both showed alpha satellite signals away from the primary constriction supporting the idea that either alpha satellite is not necessary for centromere function or a new class of latent heteromorphism called a "neocentromere" was induced by the rearrangement (see Chapter 8).

Satellited Y

A familial satellited Y (Yqs) chromosome first reported by Genest *et al.* [34] was ascertained in a patient with trisomy 21. A second case reported by Schmid *et al.* [35] had congenital heart defects, hexadachtyly and a fragile 17p. Two sisters died with congenital heart defects and the father was shown to have Yqs and a fragile 17p. In a third family reported by Genest et al [34,36,37], also ascertained through a child with Down syndrome, the Yqs could be traced back, patrilinearly, 10 generations (over 300 years). Additional cases were reported in the post-banding era by Howard-Peebles and Stoddard [39] and others [40–42]. In all, 14 families were reported and reviewed in detail by Schmid *et al.* [35]. Observations of the frequent association of the Y constriction with the satellites of D- and G-group chromosomes indicated probable origin from an acrocentric chromosome. Silver staining detected NOR regions in all but one of the mentioned families. Chromosomal variants by Q, G, C and other special stains revealed different breakpoints and independent origins for all 14 families. Most cases of Yqs do not themselves cause phenotypic abnormalities. All of the cases described except one [41] were familial and transmitted patrilinearly through several generations. Despite the fact that several of these families were ascertained through a child with congenital abnormalities or other chromosome abnormality, most progeny of Yqs carriers were phenotypically normal with no specific malformations. Verma *et al.* [42] describe a familial non-fluorescent satellited Y chromosome in a prenatal sample. Subsequent studies by FISH (**Plate 65d**) revealed the satellited material to be from chromosome 15. Additional examples of satellited Y chromosomes characterized by different banding techniques and FISH are shown to also have satellites derived from chromosome 15 [43] with breakpoints in or close to satellite III sequences (**Plate 66**).

References

1. El-Alfi O (1970). A family with a large Y chromosome. J Med Genet. 7:37–40.
2. Makino S, Muramoto T (1964). Some observations on the variability of the human Y chromosome. Proc Jpn Acad. 40:757–61.
3. Bishop A, Blank CE, Hunter H (1962). Heritable variation in the length of the Y chromosome. Cytogenetics. 5:34–52.
4. Cohen MM, Shaw MW, MacCluer JW (1966). Racial differences in the length of the human Y chromosome. Cytogenetics. 5:34–52.
5. Bobrow M, Pearson PL, Pike MC, El-Alfi OS (1971). Length variations in the quinacrine-binding segment of human Y chromosomes of different sizes. Cytogenetics. 10:190–8.
6. Laberge C, Gagne R (1971). Quinacrine mustard staining solve the length variations of the human Y chromosome. Johns Hopkins Med. 128:79–83.
7. Schnedl W (1971). Fluoreszenzuntersuchugen uber die Langenvariabiliatat des Y-Chromosoms beim Menschen [German]. Humangenetik. 12:188–94.
8. Sperling K, Lackman I (1971). Large human Y chromosome with two fluorescent bands. Clin Genet. 2:352–5.
9. Kim MA, Bier L, Pawlowitzki IH, Pfeiffer RA (1971). Human Y chromosome with two fluorescing bands after staining with quinacrine derivates. Humangenetik. 13:238–40.
10. Nielsen J, Friedrich U (1972). Length of the Y chromosome in criminal males. Clin Genet. 3:281–5.
11. Nielsen J (1978). Large Y chromosome (Yq+) and increased risk of abortion. Clin Genet. 13:415–16.
12. Borgoankar DS (1971). Non-fluorescent Y chromosome. Lancet. 15:1017.
13. Wahlstrom J (1971). Are variations in length of Y chromosome due to structural changes? Hereditas. 69:125–8.
14. Tishler PV, Lamborot-Manzur M, Atkins L (1972). Polymorphism of the human Y chromosome: fluorescence microscopic studies on the sites of morphologic variation. Clin Genet. 3:116–22.
15. Robinson JA, Buckton KE (1971). Quinacrine fluorescence of variant and abnormal human Y chromosomes. Chromosoma (Berl). 35:342–52.
16. Ghosh PK, Singh IP (1975). Morphological variability of the human chromosomes in two Indian populations – Rajputs and Punjabs. Humangenetik. 29(1):67–78.
17. Verma RS, Evans-McCalla M, Dosik H (1982). Human chromosomal heteromorphism in American Blacks. VI. Higher incidence of longer Y owing to non-fluorescent (nf) segment. J Med Genet. 19:297–301.
18. Verma RS, Huq A, Dosik H (1983). Racial variation of a non-fluorescent segment of the Y chromosome in East Indians. J Med Genet. 20:102–6.
19. Verma RS, Dosik H, Scharf T, Lubs HA (1978). Length heteromorphisms of fluorescent (f) and non-fluorescent (nf) segments of human Y chromosome: classification, frequencies and incidence in normal Caucasians. J Med Genet. 15:277–81.
20. Hsu LYF, Benn PA, Tannenbaum HL, Perlis TE, Carlson AD (1987). Chromosomal polymorphisms of 1, 9, 16 and Y in 4 major ethnic groups: a large prenatal study. Am J Med Genet. 26:95–101.
21. Hou JW, Wang TR (1999). Study of human Y chromosome polymorphism in Taiwan. Acta Paediatr Twaiwan. 40:302–4.

22. Soudek D, Laraya P (1974). Longer Y chromosome in criminals. Clin Genet. 6:225–9.
23. Shapiro LR, Pettersen RO, Wilmot PL, Warburton D, Benn PA, Hsu LYF (1984). Pericentric inversion of the Y chromosome and prenatal diagnosis. Prenat Diagn. 4:463–5.
24. Maeda T, Ohno M, Matsunobu A, Yoshihara K, Yabe N (1991). Cytogenetic survey of 14,835 consecutive liveborns. Jinrui Idengaku Zasshi. 36:117–29.
25. Bernstein R, Wadee A, Rosendorff J, Wessels A, Jenkins T (1986). Inverted Y chromosome polymorphism in the Gujerati Muslim Indian population of South Africa. Hum Genet. 74:223–9.
26. Spurdle A, Jenkins T (1992). The inverted Y chromosome polymorphism in the Gujarati Muslim Indian population of South Africa has a single origin. Hum Hered. 42:330–2.
27. Tomomasa H, Adachi Y, Iwabuchi M et al. (2000). Pericentric inversion of the Y chromosome of an infertile male. Arch Androl. 45:181–5.
28. Giltay JC, van Golde RJ, Kastrop PM (2000). Analysis of spermatozoa from seven ICSI males with constitutional sex chromosomal abnormalities by fluorescence in situ hybridization. J Assist Reprod Genet. 17:151–5.
29. Causio F, Canale D, Schonauer LM, Fischetto R, Leonetti T, Archidiacono N (2000). Breakpoint of a Y chromosome pericentric inversion in the DAZ gene area. A case report. J Reprod Med. 45:591–4.
30. Acar H, Cora T, Erkul I (1999). Coexistence of inverted Y, chromosome 15p+ and abnormal phenotype. Genet Couns. 10:163–70.
31. Motos GMA (1989). Pericentric inversion of the human Y chromosome. An Esp Pediatr. 31:583–7.
32. Toth A, Gaal M, Laszlo J (1984). Familial pericentric inversion of the Y chromosome. Ann Genet. 27:60–1.
33. Rivera H, Vassquez AI, Ayala-Madrigal ML, Ramirez-Duenas ML, Davalos IP (1996). Alphoidless centromere of a familial unstable inverted Y chromosome. Ann Genet. 39:236–9.
34. Genest P, Bouchard M, Bouchard J (1967). A satellited human Y chromosome: An evidence of autosome gonosome translocation. Canad J Genet Cytol. 9:589–95.
35. Schmid M, Haaf T, Solleder E et al. (1984). Satellited Y chromosomes: structure, origin, and clinical significance. Hum Genet. 67:72–85.
36. Genest P (1978). [A satellited Y chromosome]. [French]. Ann Genet. 21:237–8.
37. Genest P (1979). [Remarks on a satellited Y chromosome]. [French]. Sem Hop. 55:799–80.
38. Genest P, Laberge C, Poty J, Gagne R, Bouchard M (1970). Transmission d'un petit "Y" durant onze generation dans une lignee familiale [French]. Ann Genet (Paris). 13:233–8.
39. Howard-Peebles PN, Stoddard GR (1976). A satellited Yq chromosome associated with trisomy 21 and an inversion of chromosome 9. Hum Genet. 34:223–5.
40. Bayless-Underwood L, Cho S, Ward B, Robinson A (1983). Two cases of prenatal diagnosis of a satellited Yq chromosome. Clin Genet. 24:359–64.
41. Turleau C, Chavin-Colin F, Seger J, Sorin M, Salet D, de Grouche J (1978). Satellited Y chromosome (Yqs) and nucleolar organizer occuring de novo. Ann Genet. 21:239–42.
42. Verma RS, Gogineni SK, Kleyman SM, Conte RA (1997). Characterization of a satellited non-fluorescent Y chromosome (Y[nfqs]) by FISH. J Med Genet. 34:817–18.
43. Shim SH, Pan A, Huang XL, Tonk VS, Wyandt HE (2002). FISH variants with D15Z1 in clinical cases. Am J Hum Genet. 71:307A.

Plate 67. Deletion variant at 2q telomeric region involving the locus D2S2986 was reported in a mentally retarded child and a normal father. The Vysis subtelomere probe (**A**) that was normal did not include D2S2986, but the Cytocell probe set that did include D2S2986 (**B**) was deleted in the child and father. The 2pter is green and 2qter is orange. This deletion variant occurs in about 8% of the population (Jalal *et al.*, 2000; see Chapter 6).

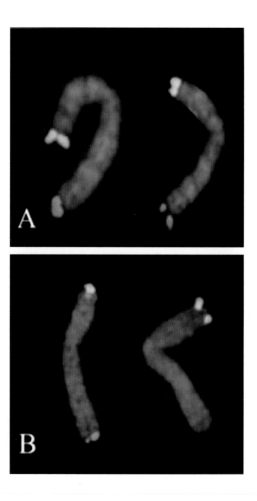

Plate 68. Four cases showing what may or may not be normal variants at the telomeric ends of four different chromosomes (four different cases) showing loss of subtelomeric sequences (arrows) from 2q (**a**); from 8p (**b**); from 10q (**c**) and from 22q (**d**). In each case there appears to be no detectable loss of material by G-banding (pairs of chromosomes at left). Note that the loss from 8p (**b**) is not total, and in fact an intermediate loss of sequences was seen in the father (Huang *et al.*, unpublished). All of these cases were submitted for FISH analysis because of idiopathic mental and developmental retardation. In all such cases it is imperative that chromosomes of both parents also be studied by FISH, preferably using probes from the same source (see Chapter 7), and confirmed, if possible, by additional molecular studies to demonstrate actual loss of genes.

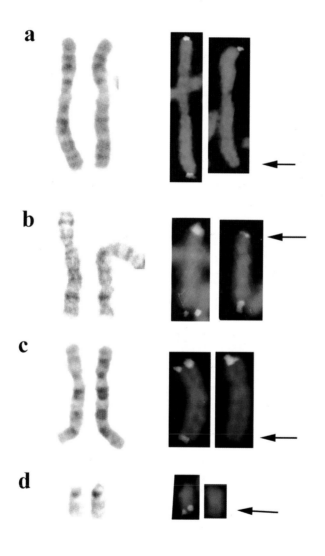

Plate 69. (a) Apparently common variant of chromosome 14 seen with the chromosome 15-specific probe for satellite III sequences (D15Z1). Partial karyotypes of 14s and 15s from three different cases showing extra signal (green) with D15Z1 on the short arm of a chromosome 14 (left hand pair of chromosomes in each row). Chromosomes 15 (right-hand pair in each row) shows green signal with D15Z1 and orange signal with probe for SNRPN in 15q11.2. Last row shows two normal-appearing 14s by G-banding from one of the cases. (**b**) Metaphase showing two chromosomes 14 with a signal with D15Z1 (arrows). Two normal 15s have signals for D15Z1 (green), for SNRPN (orange) in proximal 15q and for PML (orange) in distal 15q.

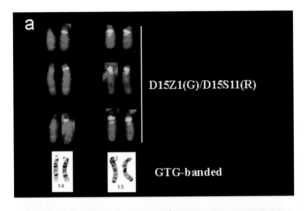

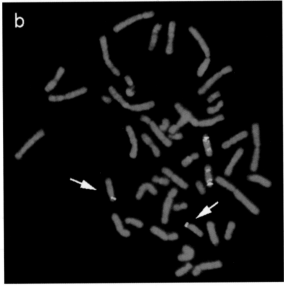

FISH VARIANTS: SUMMARY

A new class of variants is emerging that may sometimes be below the limits of resolution by standard chromosome banding. These variants become visible by fluorescent *in situ* hybridization (FISH). In some cases they may not be totally innocuous (see Chapter 7). In other cases they appear to be normal variants. The most common of these is deletion of a subtelomeric region on chromosome 2 (Plate 67, see Chapter 6). Other subtelomeric deletions are shown in Plate 68, any one of which may or may not be a normal variant. Although parental chromosome studies using the same probes are recommended to confirm whether or not such deletions are familial, not all cases are so easily resolved. For example, an apparent loss of signal was from 8p was consistently seen in a child with developmental delay (Plate 68b). However, a similar but less dramatic discrepancy in signal size was seen in the father's 8's. This case was not resolved by FISH analysis and, in fact, some other form of molecular analysis is required to determine if such a finding is real or artifact.

Plate 69 shows another aspect of heteromorphism by FISH analysis. Namely, cross-hybridization occurs for repetitive DNA sequences that are present on more than one chromosome. In fact, the challenge has been to find sequences among these repeated sequences that are specific for particular chromosomes (see Chapters 7–9). D15Z1 is a commercially available probe (Vysis, Downers Grove, IL) that is usually specific for a variable number of sequences on the short arm of chromosome 15. However product literature indicates cross-hybridization with sequences in the short arm of a chromosome 14 (Plate 69a) which occurs about 12% of the time [1,2]. Occasionally, both 14's may have this variant signal (Plate 69b). The likelihood of such an occurrence is approximately 1 per 300 individuals. If seen in an individual with anomalies, the possibility of uniparental disomy needs to be ruled out [2].

References

1. Stergianou K, Gould CP, Waters JJ, Hulten MA (1993). A DA/DAPI positive human 14p hetero-morphism defined by fluorescent in-situ hybridization using chromosome 15-specific probes D15Z1 (satellite III) and p-TRA-25 (alphoid). Hereditas 119:105–110.
2. Shim SH, Pan A, Huang XL, Tonk VS, Varma SK, Milunsky JM. FISH variants with D15Z1 (2003). Am J Gen Tech (in press).

Index

275

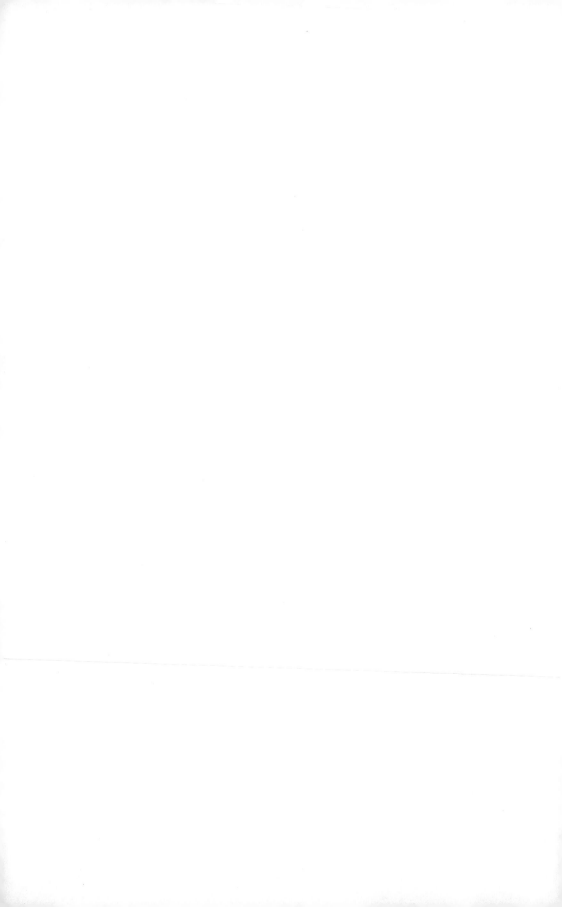